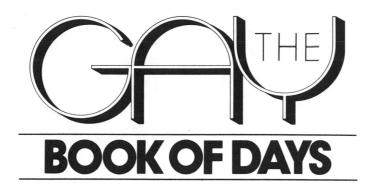

# THE GAY

## BOOK OF DAYS

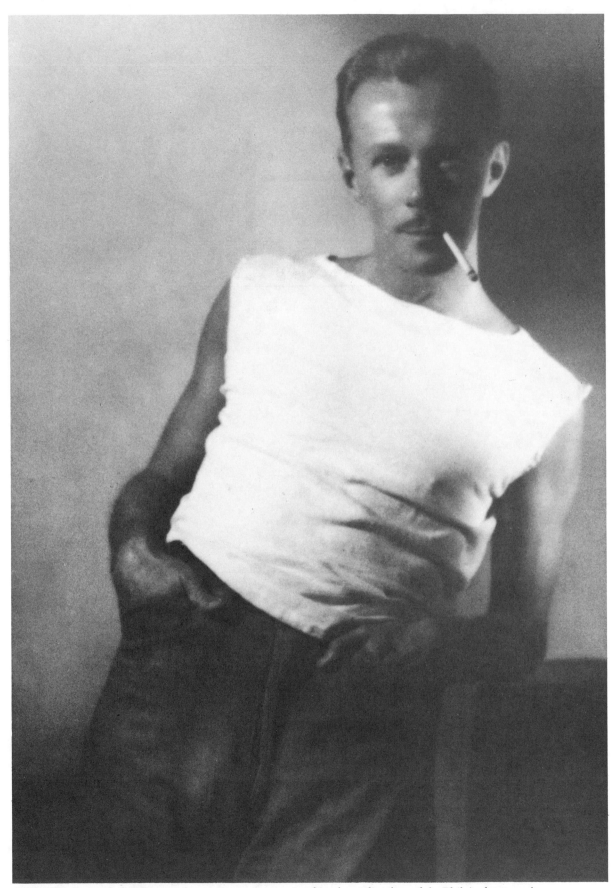

**Samuel M. Steward:** Scholar, teacher, writer, tattoo artist, friend — and author of the Phil Andros novels.

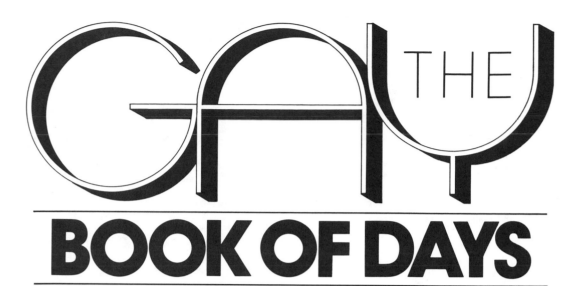

# THE GAY BOOK OF DAYS

An Evocatively Illustrated Who's Who of Who Is, Was, May Have Been, Probably Was, and Almost Certainly Seems to Have Been Gay During the Past 5,000 Years

## BY MARTIN GREIF

A MAIN STREET PRESS BOOK

LYLE STUART, INC. · SECAUCUS, NEW JERSEY

Published by Lyle Stuart Inc.
120 Enterprise Avenue
Secaucus, New Jersey 07094

Published simultaneously in Canada by Musson Book Company
A division of General Publishing Co. Limited
Don Mills, Ontario

Designed by Frank Mahood
Produced by The Main Street Press
Manufactured in the United States of America

This book includes the names of both homosexual and heterosexual people. The inclusion of
any person's name in this book is in no way to be construed as an implication that he or she
is homosexual unless explicitly stated.

Library of Congress Cataloging in Publication Data

Greif, Martin
   The gay book of days.

   "A Main Street Press book."
   Bibliography: p. 219
   Includes index.
   1. Homosexuals—Biography.   2. Birthday books.
I. Title
HQ75.2.G73 1982      306.7'66'0922      82-10714
ISBN-0-8184-0384-5

## FOR MOLLY

*Vale canis nobilis et fidelis.*
*Sit tibi terra levis.*

# Contents

Foreword by Samuel M. Steward   9

Introduction                    11

**1.** JANUARY                  14

**2.** FEBRUARY                 34

**3.** MARCH                    48

**4.** APRIL                    62

**5.** MAY                      78

**6.** JUNE                     96

**7.** JULY                     114

**8.** AUGUST                   134

**9.** SEPTEMBER                154

**10.** OCTOBER                 170

**11.** NOVEMBER                186

**12.** DECEMBER                200

Bibliography                    219

Index                           220

# Foreword

There's never been a book quite like this one.

There are lots of Books of This and Books of That: Books of Hours, of Kells, of Martyrs, but *The Gay Book of Days* is not like any of them. It is rowdy, rambunctious, and racy. It is sprightly and gay — both in the modern usage of that second word, and in the "merrie" sense of jollity and wit.

Gays are sometimes thought of as lonely and melancholy creatures, but that has never been entirely true. This book proves what fun they've had, against all odds, for at least fifty centuries past — and will undoubtedly continue to have until Armageddon arrives. Even then they'll probably be squabbling with the ushers for the best seats in the house. Gays will always be around; they always have been. Everyone might as well relax and get used to them. So long as they pay their rent, they have no intention of being evicted from the human boarding house.

This is a book of gossip, but it must be remembered that in the wildest gossip there is always a nugget of truth. In its original meaning the word *gossip* had the form *God-sib,* referring to "God-relative" and applied to godparents at christenings. Then it shifted to mean a woman's best friend; Chaucer's Wife of Bath was always consulting with her good friend, her "gossip." And finally the word was altered to mean the talk itself of intimate friends — the pastime of old women chattering over the back fence, and old men talking in taverns about sex and stuff. The young discovered its attractions, for the love of gossip is universal and flows around the world in all latitudes. And one of the best examples and collections of gossip is right here in your hands, in *The Gay Book of Days.*

Who would ever imagine that the Danish tenor Lauritz Melchior was actually the personal Great Dane of writer Hugh Walpole? Or that Melchior and poet Hart Crane owned common stock in a well-proportioned sailor? That Cole Porter and Jackie O's daddy were once an item? That both Winston Churchill and Marilyn Monroe strayed occasionally from the straight and narrow? Or that the saintly inventor of the American Dream, Horatio Alger, wore his wickedness like a sulfurous halo?

You'll find them all here, their peccadilloes and fetishes and hangups and pleasures.

This book is unusual in that the compiler, Martin Greif, uses humor to make some very serious points that might otherwise seem shrill or somber. There is, of course, a method to his madness. He has a world view that is mischievous and witty and sometimes downright ornery. His humor is like that of Swift and Firbank combined; it can bite and tickle both at the same time. With tongue in cheek, he can destroy with a stroke, puff up with a metaphor, inflate or deflate according to what he had for lunch — and leave the reader helpless with laughter, shock, or outrage.

Samplings of this book, which was long in gestation, have delighted ever-enlarging audiences of the annual *Gay Engagement Calendar,* as riotous and informative a thing as was ever put on any market. But here in this volume, the snippets from the calendar are wonderfully and excitingly expanded, given their proper or improper treatment, and preserved in a permanent form for posterity's pleasure. The gossip in the book gives you an earful, and there's also an eyeful waiting in the exotic and amusing illustrations. Read it any way you want. If you are strong-willed, you may be able to restrict yourself to one entry a day, but chances are that you will sit down and get hooked—and read it all from cover to cover. And then you will probably suffer from over-reading, foundered on brilliance, surfeited with sophistication.

Come join the jolly crew in these pages. You may never be the same again.

SAMUEL M. STEWARD

# Introduction

Why a *Gay Book of Days?* Well, why not? Everybody likes to celebrate birthdays, or almost everybody. In fact, if we think about it for a moment, we're almost inundated by a wave of birthdays every day of every week. Is there a classical music station on the air that doesn't feature a daily "anniversary concert," honoring a composer or performer born that day? And how many morning wake-up shows broadcast a list of famous personalities, sandwiched between the orange juice commercial and the weather report? And what about the horoscopes in supermarket tabloids, the ones that read like the offspring of a Chinese fortune cookie and Rona Barrett? Don't they usually provide a list of celebrity birthdays to gull the great American hausfrau into thinking that her wagon is somehow hitched to Robert Redford's star or that she shares something in common, say a garbage pickup on Wednesdays, with Nancy Reagan? Come to think of it, is there anyone on earth who isn't ready at the slightest provocation to recite the names of famous people born on his or her own special day? Aside from the singular impossibility of remembering the words to "The Star-Spangled Banner," this is probably the only universal human trait shared by everyone from Katmandu to Cooch Behar.

Birthdays. There's no escaping them. For every interest, for every specialty, someone has compiled a list of daily birthday celebrants: Movie stars and show-biz personalities, classical and popular composers, writers, rock stars, liberated women, athletes, blacks, well-known southpaws from around the globe, and, for all one knows, even Serbo-Croatian dentists from Illinois. Why not, then, a book of days devoted to the most interesting homosexuals in history, a gay calendar of saints and sinners, famous, not so famous, and infamous?

The book you are about to read is an entertainment. It is neither a reference book nor a political tract. It was written for my own enjoyment and with the intention of giving pleasure to others. If that pleasure is derived from the basic information contained within its pages, very well and good. If it comes from sharing my peculiar vision of human history, so much the better. And if it stems from an appreciation of the extraordinary breadth and variety of the homosexual experience throughout the centuries, the book's central theme, then that is best of all. If, on the other hand, the book offends or angers—or, even worse, leaves the reader totally cold—then let's be candid with each other: What on earth can I do about it now?

At its core, this is a book about the comedy of sex. In the frenzied pursuit of the object of one's affection, human beings are almost always at their antic worst. Two squirts of adrenalin and we're off and running, all reason and good sense thrown as caution to the wind. The lengths to which we will go in making fools of ourselves for just a simple roll in the hay are known intimately to each of us. How willingly we submit to tiny irrationalities: walking around the block three times to avoid being too early for a date, for example, or buying six dollars worth of magazines at the corner newsstand in stupefying embarrassment just because the guy you've been following has stopped to buy a pack of cigarettes before deciding whether you're worth talking to or not. Momentary flights of sanity, these, and no real harm done. But when Cupid suddenly whacks you over the head with a twenty-pound sledge, watch out. The bouts of irrationality are then more violent, longer lived, downright dangerous—attacks of weeping, for example, jealousy, and even homicidal rage. One of the wonders of God's democracy is that none of us, great or small, rich or poor, is immune to such behavior once Cupid's quiver hits us in the quim. The cosmic joke, of course, is that whatever our other accomplishments—art, music, literature, architecture, science—we're all of us most human when scratching our privates. Leonardo, Beethoven, and Marie Antoinette scratched theirs, just as you and I scratch ours. In satisfying the universal itch, the great are no different from the humble. For this reason, many of the famous personalities treated in these pages are seen at their most human—when in love or in hot pursuit of love—hence, at their silliest. If this be considered irreverent, a trivialization of the great, so be it.

*The Gay Book of Days* is certain to cause mild outrage in several quarters. I am not particularly concerned about the Anitas, Jerrys, and Nancys of this world since, given its subject, they won't read the book anyway. And if they should choose to burn it, which is perfectly OK with me, they'll at least have to pay for each copy first before tossing it in the fire. If I offer no apologies to the right, I have none for the left as well. But I do propose the following explanations for what will undoubtedly appear to radicals as grievous crimes committed against their holy writ. My sins are obvious and predictable:

(1) *Given the serious nature of the subject and the less than Christian charity shown gay people during the past 2,000 years or so, I have treated homosexuality lightly, even humorously.* To this charge I plead guilty—but by reason of self-defense. I have already read far too many books so shrill in their special pleading that my gritted teeth had to be pried apart by chapter 2—and books so deadly somber, so tediously self-righteous and high-minded that lifting my hand to turn a page was a monumental effort. I will not apologize for laughter. What's more, I urge us all to contemplate the satirist's highly sensible answer to the ancient question, "What makes life worth living?" The answer, of course, is "to be born with the gift of laughter and a sense that the world is mad."

(2) *By failing to distinguish between gays and lesbians—"gays" being homosexual males and "lesbians" homosexual females—the book is not politically "correct." It should have been called* The Gay and Lesbian Book of Days, *since both male and female homosexuals are included within its pages.* To this charge I say, oh nuts. Since I do not use such antiquated words as "poetess," "Negress," and "aviatrix" when I mean poet, black, or aviator who happens to be female, why should I be pushed into antediluvian sexism at this late date? By "gay" I simply mean "homosexual," male or female.

(3) *I am "elitist" because only well-known people appear in this book, and not Tom, Dick, Harry, Bruce, Mary, Jean, and Joan, the "real" gay people.* Awww, come off it. Who is interested in ordinary people? Do Rex Reed, Johnny Carson, or Merv Griffin interview ordinary people? Does Ronald Reagan? Of course not. People want the lowdown on the high life, all the poop they can get on the big guys, the rich, the famous, the celebrated. Or, to put it another way, if as an average Joe I'm willing to exclude my own birthday from this book, why in hell should I include yours?

(4) *I am a vulgarian, skewing both history and its superstars with sophomoric wit and naughty*

*words*. There's nothing that I can do about the wit, but I can and will defend the language. Since some gays have been known on more than one occasion to do more than just hold hands, I have therefore had to find an appropriate way of saying so. I cannot believe that when Lord Byron prepared to mount his young friend Nicolò Giraud, he said: "I'd like to sexual intercourse you, Nicky." If a great poet wouldn't say anything so antiseptic, why should I?

(5) *I do not prove that everyone mentioned in this book was gay.* Of course I don't. There's no way to dig up someone dead for several centuries and ask, is there? In dealing with the past, all one can reasonably do is weigh the available evidence and come up with an educated guess. While I'd not presume that George Washington was in fact the mother of his country, it's interesting nonetheless to note that a number of his contemporaries thought he was. And though there's no questioning the heterosexuality of Winston Churchill, he may very well have messed around with other chaps when he was a young man, as his mother said he did. He attended English public schools, didn't he?

(6) *I have exploited a sensitive subject for personal gain and, moreover, haven't a serious bone in my body.* It remains to be seen whether or not this book will make me rich, although it's doubtful that anyone will attempt to turn it into a movie or a musical. As to my bones, this book is no less "serious" than any other book. Its seriousness is cumulative, as is its meaning. In the end it does not say that gay is good or that gay is bad. It merely says that gay is, has been, and always will be a vital part of the human experience. That homosexuality has been a natural condition of kings, composers, engineers, poets, housewives, and bus drivers, and that it has contributed more than its share of beauty and laughter to an ugly and ungrateful world should be obvious to anyone who is willing to peer beneath the surface.

There are, no doubt, other objections to the controversial content of *The Gay Book of Days*, and even possible praise, but why ruin a perfectly fine day? Besides, you've already paid for this book, so why not peruse its pages and get on with it?

*11 July 1982*
*Pittstown, New Jersey*

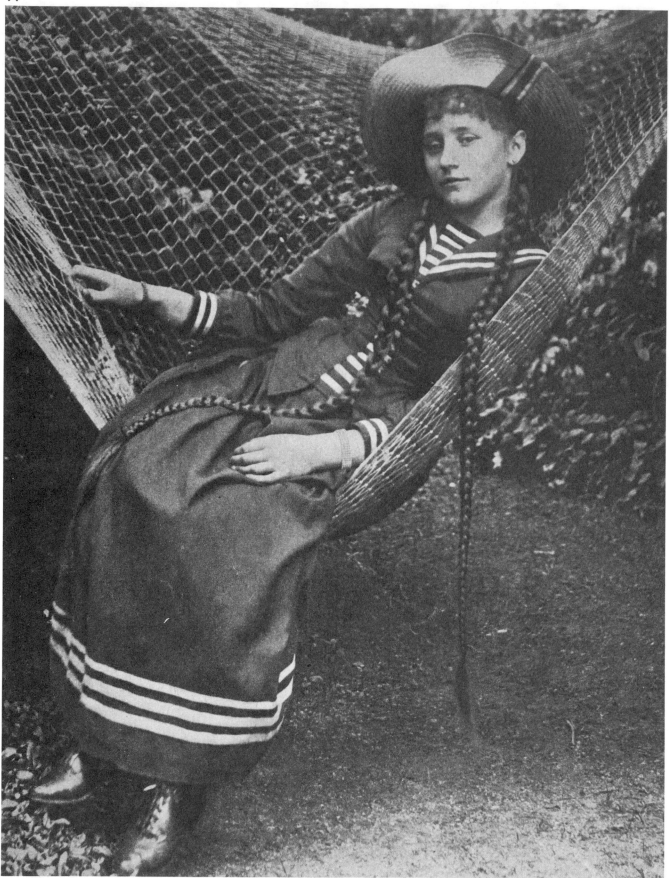

**Sidonie Colette:** "I find pleasure in looking at women in each other's arms, waltzing well."

# JANUARY

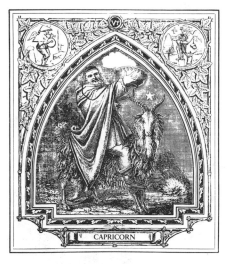

CAPRICORN

**Capricorn** (December 21st to January 19th), a cardinal earthly sign ruled by the dour old man, Saturn, is unemotional, solemn, and lacking in humor. The adjective "saturnine" aptly sums up the qualities of the sign. At the same time, the Capricornian is tough, determined, and practical. Although he moves slowly, he is very difficult to stop once he has set his mind on a goal. He is a good organizer and has the ability to withstand and overcome hardships. The typical Capricornian takes life earnestly and is generally an enthusiastic upholder of tradition and authority. When fully developed he has a fine historic sense and a strong interest in the past. At his worst, he has an intense desire to influence others—to manage them, mother them, direct, protect, persuade, convert, pervert, wheedle, attract, or meddle with them in one way or another.

# 1.

**E. M. FORSTER, b. London, 1879.** It has become fashionable, in the years since Edward Morgan Forster's death at 91 in 1970, and especially since the posthumous publication of his 1914 gay novel, *Maurice,* a year later, to scoff at this master craftsman's brilliant fiction. But it was not always so. From 1924, when Forster published his masterpiece, *A Passage to India,* until his death almost a half-century later, no new novel appeared, and yet by one of the great paradoxes of 20th-century literature, his reputation continued to grow. The so-called lean years, however, saw Forster active as critic, essayist, and public figure, especially in the debate of political and moral issues. But it was the publication of *Maurice,* suppressed during its author's lifetime and badly dated by

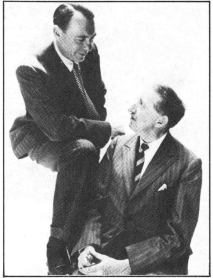

**Bob Buckingham and E. M. Forster:** Lower-class top, upper-class bottom.

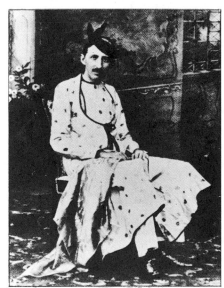

**E. M. Forster in India:** Love the dress, but hate the hat.

the time of its release, that provided modern critics with the chisel to chip away at Forster's pedestal. "*Maurice,*" writes one, "shows why his imagination failed him: he was crippled by his sexual condition." In

short, since fags don't know how to write about love between the sexes, and since in his day Forster couldn't exactly write about pansy love, he stopped writing novels, period. Yes, it *is* true that Forster was not particularly good at delineating any kind of sexual relationship between a man and a woman (Katherine Mansfield complained, "I can never be perfectly certain whether Helen [in *Howards End*] was got with child by Leonard Bast or by his fatal forgotten umbrella. All things considered, I think it must have been the umbrella.") Yet the unique power of any Forster novel stems not from the depiction of heterosexual love, but from an acute observation of English hypocrisy. Forster came of age during the trials of Oscar Wilde. The viciousness of English hypocrisy was not lost on him. It resulted in both his public silence about his homosexuality, and in the savage indictment of English morality that runs through all his exquisitely written novels, from *Where Angels Fear to Tread* (1905) to *A Passage to India*. Forster's detractors are fond of painting him as an over-refined, mousy introvert, a mama's boy who was uninitiated in the rites of sex until a grown man. Yet he had as his lover for half a century a virile, handsome, married London policeman named Bob Buckingham, who granted Forster his most elemental wish: "to love a strong young man of the lower classes and be loved by him and even hurt by him." How many of you, even in the meat racks and slings of our modern backroom sinks, could fulfill *that* fantasy today?

**J. EDGAR HOOVER, b. Washington, D.C., 1895.** In some future time, when the late director of the Federal Bureau of Investigation is no longer a figure of considerable controversy, perhaps in two or three thousand years, an unbiased biographer may possibly solve the riddle of the forty-four-year friendship between bachelor buddies J. Edgar Hoover and Clyde Tolson. Now, anyone who has ever seen the simple-minded G-man flicks of Depression Hollywood knows that it was A-OK for even the most stolid law-and-order man to have a close buddy, usually forgotten by the final fade-out in favor of a marcelled cutie with a Peter Pan hat. But there was simply no Warner Bros. precedent for the flatfoot walking into the sunset with the gumshoe buddy himself, living with him in domestic bliss for more than four decades, and finally leaving him his entire worldly goods and possessions after departing for right-wing heaven. Were they gay? Were they womanizing lechers? Or were they merely two ageing turnips? The very presence in these pages of J. Edgar Hoover, whom Truman Capote once called a "killer fruit," will anger almost everyone. Gays most certainly don't want to claim him. But then, neither do most straights. Poor J. Edgar. Only Clyde Tolson could have loved that bulldog face.

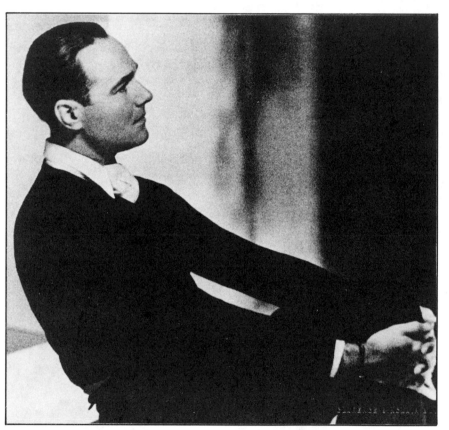

William Haines: The marine came; he went.

**WILLIAM HAINES, b. Staunton, Virginia, 1900.** Bill Haines was a remarkably popular star of silent movies whose good looks and baby face enabled him to play the same role over and over. More often than not, he played the wisecracking, penniless young man who won the millionaire's daughter in the final reel. In real life, as *New York Times* obituaries always put it when a famous corpse is homosexual, "he never married." Blessed with a very pleasant speaking voice, Haines made the transition from silents to talkies with ease and continued to play the boyish roles that endeared him to the ladies. Although he was later to become Hollywood's most successful interior decorator, a second career that made him as rich as any of the stars whose homes he designed, he was unprepared for the disaster that befell him in 1935. Caught in a downtown YMCA with a U.S. serviceman, Haines was immediately fired by Louis B. Mayer who shrewdly realized that the public would soon tire of a middle-aged boy anyway. His last film was entitled, with ironic appropriateness, *The Marines Are Coming.*

**JOE ORTON** (né **John Kingsley Orton**), b. Leicester, England, 1933. "I have high hopes of dying in my prime," Joe Orton confided to his diary in July, 1967, when he was only thirty-four years old. Less than one month later, Britain's most promising comic playwright was murdered by his lover, Kenneth Halliwell, in the London flat they had shared for fifteen years. By then Orton had already attracted a coterie with his outrageous black farces, notably *Entertaining Mr. Sloane* (1964) and *Loot* (1966), both of them savagely comic expressions of his contempt for social institutions as well as his delight in shocking people.

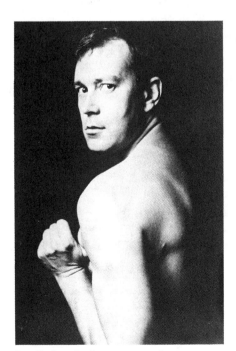

**Joe Orton:** An irreverent genius.

His twitting of authority first came into public view when he and Halliwell were arrested for having mutilated and then pasted pornographic pictures in over 200 library books. His ensuing six-months prison sentence confirmed his conviction that a mere facade covers the hypocrisy and viciousness of the police, as well as those of the Church and most other social institutions, including sex—in and out of the marriage bed. Orton's life with Halliwell was very much a gay version of *A Star Is Born,* with Halliwell the struggling, unpublished writer fading into obscurity as his wildly promiscuous lover became famous. A few months before Halliwell bashed in Orton's skull with a hammer and then killed himself, Orton had reflected in his diary on having allowed a one-night stand to mount and enter him: "It was a most unappetising position for an internationally-known playwright to be in." When, two months later, his body was found, it was lying ass-up in a pool of blood.

# 2.

**CAREY THOMAS, b. Baltimore, Maryland, 1857.** There's no getting around the fact that Carey Thomas was a remarkable woman, even though she came out of Baltimore at a moment in history when that city was home to many remarkable women, Etta and Claribel Cone and Gertrude Stein among them. (The fate of that progressive city in the 20th century can be summed up by naming the most extraordinary "woman" to have emerged from Baltimore in our time—Divine.) Carey Thomas, older than the others, served as pioneer for them all, Divine probably but not necessarily excepted. A brilliant and headstrong young woman who refused to accept

the conventional subordinance of women in 19th-century America, she fought a series of battles in order to live a life of her own—first with her father to attend Sage College, the women's division of Cornell University; then with John Hopkins University, and the universities at Leipzig and Zurich for the right to pursue graduate studies; finally with the trustees of Bryn Mawr College to become dean and later president of that distinguished school. Not the least of this extraordinary woman's accomplishments was her role in creating the medical college at Johns Hopkins (on condition that women be admitted) and her prescience in hiring as one of her teachers at Bryn Mawr a young history instructor named Woodrow Wilson. There were a number of women in Carey Thomas's life, all but one of whom provided her with a loving domestic life marred only by their unfortunate tendency to die young, leaving Carey widowed no fewer than five times. The one exception was Mamie Gwinn, a teacher at Bryn Mawr who made Thomas's life a living hell for almost thirty years. The unequal triangle of Carey, Gwinn, and Gwinn's married boyfriend, a Bryn Mawr professor, is the basis of Gertrude Stein's early novel, *Fernhurst.* It remains a living testament to a passionate and painful episode in the life of one of the greatest women of the 19th century, who in matters of love was as ordinary as the rest of us.

# 3.

**JOHANNES VON MÜLLER, b. Neunkirch, Switzerland, 1752.** That the name of this once famous Swiss historian is hardly a household word is not exactly surprising. It would probably be easier to climb the Matterhorn in a blizzard than to tackle Müller's monumental *Geschichten der Schweizer* (Swiss History), a project that occupied most of his life and took him more than forty years to complete. And it would probably be more practical to climb the Matterhorn as well, since Müller's tome (18 volumes in French translation) is now considered hopelessly unreliable, even though in its day it greatly stirred Swiss nationalism and had a profound influence. Müller rates a place in this book because of his favorite extracurricular activity—writing love letters to Charles Victor de Bonstetten, a young, devastatingly handsome Swiss writer whose greatest talent was apparently turning on academic types who had passed through menopause at twenty-two. (We'll meet Charlie again when he causes that grayest of English poets, Thomas Gray, to do nip-ups at fifty-three.) Müller's love letters, among the loveliest ever penned, were published in 1835, a quarter of a century after his death. Long before then, however, Goethe had gone on record declaring Müller's homosexuality. It was another classic case of it taking one to know one.

# 4.

**MARSDEN HARTLEY, b. Lewiston, Maine, 1877.** One of America's earliest modern painters, Hartley was in Paris "at the creation" to be influenced by the Cubists and in Germany to be influenced by the Expressionists before developing an abstract style uniquely his own. Although he flits almost inconspicuously through the pages of the biographies devoted to his famous contemporaries, he has yet to be the subject of a major biography of his own. Strange, considering the company he kept. Among Hartley's acquaintances were

a telephone directory of contemporary homosexuals, including William Sloan Kennedy, the biographer of Longfellow, Whittier, and Holmes; Thomas Bird Mosher, the publisher of Whitman and one of the earliest American publishers of Oscar Wilde; Horace Traubel, socialist editor of the *Conservator* and Whitman's secretary; Peter Doyle, Whitman's trolley conductor lover; Gertrude Stein; the American painter Charles Demuth; writer and publisher Robert McAlmon, whose "notorious" Greenwich Village wedding to the lesbian writer "Bryher" Hartley attended in 1921; Wallace Gould, fellow Lewiston poet who dedicated his *Children of the Sun* to Hartley in 1917; actor George de Winter; writer Djuna Barnes; and poet Hart Crane—to name just a few. Although few seem to know it, Hartley was also a fine poet. His *Selected Poems,* out of print for almost forty years, is worth rediscovery. The love of Hartley's life was Karl von Freyburg, a young German soldier killed in battle in 1914. This was Hartley's greatest tragedy, an event mirrored in a series of contemporary abstractions that are teeming with boldly outlined forms, violent in color, and aggressively painted. The dead soldier was twenty-two; the painter, fifteen years his senior, grieved for the rest of his life.

# 5.

**RICHARD HEBER, b. London, 1773.** Anyone who has been privileged to attend a meeting of a certain famous American bibliophilic club on the East Coast realizes in a flash that a majority of the tuxedo-clad gentlemen gathered to discuss their common passion—book collecting—is rich, recondite, Republican, and

remarkably gay. Their ancestor of ancestors was English book collector Richard Heber, who made a habit of attending continental book sales, purchasing sometimes single volumes, sometimes whole libraries. He did not confine himself to the purchase of a single copy of a work. "No gentleman," he remarked, "can be without three copies of a book, one for show, one for use, and one for borrowers." He is known to have owned 150,000 volumes and probably many more. And why is Heber included in this book? Because he was forced to leave England in exile after public disclosure of his "unnatural acts," that's why. One wonders whether aristocratic Richard licked his index finger whenever he turned over a page!

# 6.

**SHERLOCK HOLMES, b. North Riding, Yorkshire, England, 1854.** What? Sherlock Holmes? Why list the famous hawk-nosed detective, a figment of Arthur Conan Doyle's imagination, when today is also the birthday of the very real King Richard II of England (b. 1367), whom even the staid *Encyclopaedia Britannica* calls "tall, handsome, and effeminate"? Why? Because Sherlock, whom his creator almost named "Sherrinford," is simply more interesting. And, besides, almost everyone who has read Shakespeare knows about Richard, whereas almost no one realizes that Sherlock was gay. Holmes, of course, was the world's first consulting detective, a vocation he followed for twenty-three years. In January, 1881, he was looking for someone to share his new digs at 221B Baker Street, and, there being no pink pages in *The Advocate* in those days, nor any "personals" in *The New York Review of Books,* a

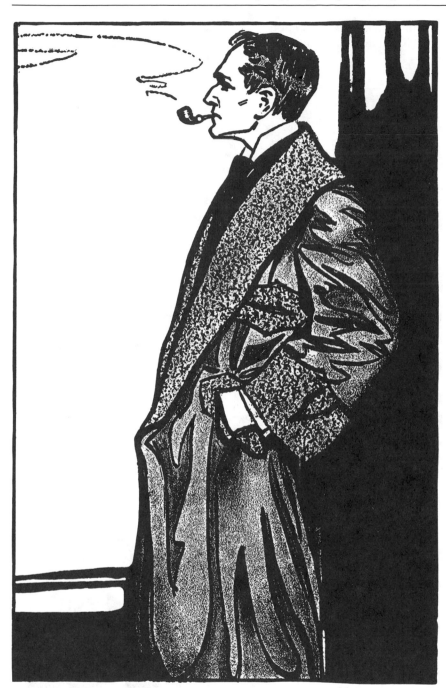

**Sherlock Holmes:** Was Irene Adler just a blind to protect his real true love?

Woman," in which the famous creator of Nero Wolfe (himself hardly a butch stud) reveals that Watson and Holmes were the most extraordinary gay team in sleuthing history.

# 7.

**FRANCIS POULENC, b. Paris, 1899.** Throughout his career, Poulenc probably composed more from instinct and aural experience than any major composer of this century. He was a musical natural and would doubtless have invented his own means of composing it if none had existed previously. Nonetheless, he studied music formally with gay pianist Ricardo Viñes, of whom he later said, "I owe him everything." In his *Paris Diaries,* Ned Rorem recalls Poulenc chasing pretty Arab boys through the back streets of French North Africa—much like Delacroix and Saint-Saëns before him. But his one great love was the great French baritone Pierre Bernac, for whom he wrote many of his most beautiful songs. For nearly twenty-five years they appeared more or less regularly as an art-song team, touring Europe,

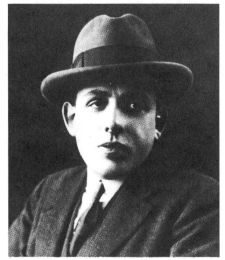

**Francis Poulenc:** Les Six and Le Sexe, Arab boys and Pierre Bernac.

friend introduced him to Dr. John H. Watson. Before agreeing to share the flat, the two men, immediately attracted to each other, listed their respective character deficiencies. Holmes admitted to smoking a smelly pipe, although he didn't mention that he was frequently turned on by cocaine. Watson owned up to a peculiar habit of leaving his bed at odd hours of the night. "I have another set of vices," he admitted, but, then, so did Sherlock. The two became friends and roommates for the rest of their lives. For the sordid details of the famous marriage of true minds that followed, read Rex Stout's astonishing "Watson Was a

North Africa, and North America repeatedly. Their many recordings together, like those of Benjamin Britten and Peter Pears, will enable future generations to understand and enjoy the creative offspring of one of the greatest marriages in music history.

**ROBERT DUNCAN and CHESTER KALLMAN, b. Oakland, California, and Brooklyn, New York, 1919 and 1921, respectively.** Duncan and Kallman are two poets born on the same day, two years, two coasts, and two worlds apart. A leading poet of the San Francisco Renaissance, Duncan is easily recognizable as a member of the international avant garde. The first poet to use the word *cocksucker* in print, and the first to strip to the buff during poetry readings, he is nonetheless in spirit, if not in fact, a modern romantic whose best work is instantly engaging by the standards of the purest lyrical traditions. Duncan has lived for over thirty years with the painter Jess Collins, even though their life together has not become the stuff of popular literary legend. The same cannot be said for Chester Kallman who, though a good poet in his own right, will be known forever as W. H. Auden's lover. When Isherwood and Auden came to America in the late '30s, Kallman and fellow Brooklyn College student Harold Norse—both young, blonde, and handsome—attended an Isherwood/Auden reading in order to flirt with the celebrated writers. Only Isherwood flirted back; Auden was near-sighted. When, two days later, eighteen-year-old Kallman showed up at the Englishmen's apartment, Auden, apprised of the young hunks by Isherwood, answered the doorbell and exclaimed, "But it's the wrong blonde!" Isherwood, it seems, had particularly hankered after Norse. Chester Kallman entered Auden's apartment and, in a manner of speaking, didn't leave until the great poet's death thirty-four years later.

# 8.

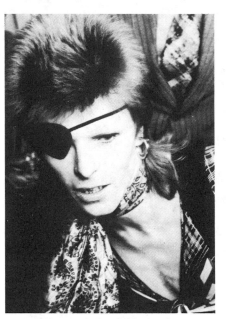

**David Bowie:** plink, plank, punk.

**DAVID BOWIE** (né David Jones), **b. London, 1947.** In recent years, the former *enfant terrible* of punk has acquitted himself as a competent actor on screen (*The Man Who Fell to Earth*) and on stage (*The Elephant Man*). But when he was at the top of the charts in the early '70s, the rock star's acting was of an entirely different stripe: he was fond of staging a mock blow job of his guitarist Mike Ronson before a delighted audience of shrieking fourteen-year-olds. And then, of course, there were his songs about lesbians in the army and the one about Queen Bitch, a young dude who "dresses like a queen but . . . can kick like a mule," not to mention the one about the stud who "came on so loaded, man, well-hung, and snow-white tan." In 1976, the same year that Jimmy Carter admitted to *Playboy* that he had lusted in his heart after women, thereby forever losing the support of the pinch-faced, thin-lipped, blue-rinse set of American patriots, David Bowie confided to his *Playboy* confessor that he was bisexual, as was his wife. "Angela and I knew each other," he said, "because we were both going out with the same man." 'Fessing up has injured his career not one whit.

# 9.

**RICHARD HALLIBURTON, b. Brownsville, Tennessee, 1900.** Richard Halliburton was the quintessential preppie. And in the Ivy League of yore, preppieness and gayness often went hand in hand. When Halliburton's Chinese junk, *Sea Dragon,* was lost in the Pacific in 1939, he still looked very much as he had at Lawrenceville and Princeton—trim, muscular, and innocently handsome. His athletic prowess and world-wide adventures had titillated a generation of vicarious thrill-seekers and had been happily ex-

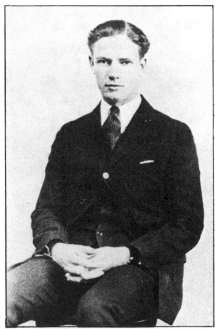

**Richard Halliburton:** He climbed mountains and other rocks as well.

ploited by both the media and Halliburton's many best-selling books. And it's easy to see why. He climbed the Matterhorn in 1921; swam the Hellespont in 1925 and the Panama Canal (from the Atlantic to the Pacific) in 1928; and flew over 50,000 miles around the world in his own airplane, *The Flying Carpet,* between 1928 and 1931, thereby milking the adoration of an aviation-mad public. He starred in his own documentary films and lectured, for stiff fees, to large audiences throughout the world. But between exploits he managed to find the time to exercise his gayness. As Roger Austen writes in *Playing the Game,* Halliburton "had a special fondness for YMCAs, spent the night with Rod La Rocque, went flying with Ramon Navarro, and settled down with another bachelor in Laguna Beach." And how was his adoring public to know? Hadn't his books been filled with his appreciation of "Kashmiri maidens, Parisian ballerinas, and Castillian countesses"? "Halliburton," writes John Paul Hudson with acute insight, "certainly did a lot of straight-approved things, though his exploits were self-stretching and not competitive—which is the gay way."

# 10.

**SAL MINEO, b. The Bronx, New York, 1939.** One of the articles of faith of the James Dean cult that grew out of the actor's early death in 1955 is that Sal Mineo "turned queer" after the auto wreck that took his co-star's life. As the story goes, young Mineo left a séance in which he had attempted in vain to contact his fallen friend, only to wreck his own car. His life was spared, but the words "James Dean" suddenly appeared indelibly on his smashed

windshield. Supposedly, he was gay from that moment on. One can take or leave that bizarre coming-out story, but it seemed perfectly obvious to gay audiences almost three decades ago that Mineo and Dean only had eyes for each other. The Hollywood Code and the mores of the '50s may have dictated that Dean win Natalie Wood and her pointed uplift bra at the end of *Rebel Without a Cause,* but anyone with half a brain knew that it should have been Mineo's Plato and Dean's Jim who embraced at the climax. Sal Mineo grew up to produce a revival of *Fortune and Men's Eyes* and to star in a West Coast production of James Kirkwood's *P.S. Your Cat Is Dead,* both of which enabled him to say without a word, "I'm gay; so what?" Rumors that he spent his off hours in the company of rough trade have led to lurid speculation about his grisly murder in 1976. Such is Hollywood fame and popular legend that no one wants to believe that, like so many innocent Americans these days, he was "merely" mugged, robbed, and left to die just a few short steps from the safety of his home.

**GILLES DE RAIS, b. Machecoul, Brittany, 1404.** If one is to believe his confession, and there is good reason not to, Gilles de Rais had run through his fortune and was convinced that sacrificing young boys to

Satan would restore his riches. Somewhere along the way, he decided that sodomizing his victims before killing them would satisfy both his needs and the Devil's, and so more and more boys disappeared in his castle, never to be seen again. When Gilles was arrested on charges of blasphemy, the grisly murders were uncovered. He confessed to having killed some 150 boys "for the pleasure and gratification of my senses." Gilles had been an ally of Joan of Arc, so there is reason to suspect that the murders were the invention of the Church.

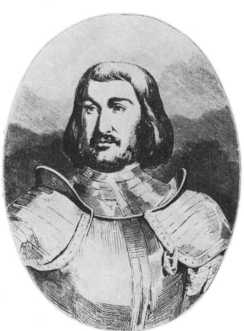

**Gilles de Rais:** Is the Bluebeard legend based on him?

# 11.

**ALEXANDER HAMILTON, b. Nevis, British West Indies, 1757.** One wonders what the present occupants of 1600 Pennsylvania Avenue would think if they knew of the ruckus caused a couple of centuries ago by Alexander Hamilton

and George Washington, the American patriots who became the first secretary of the treasury and the first president of the United States respectively. George, whom everyone knows had no children of his own, surrounded himself with a circle of

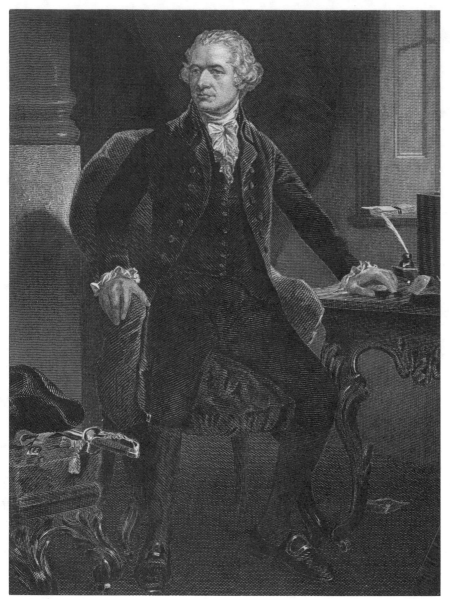

**Alexander Hamilton:** Those aren't love letters; they're classical exercises!

# 12.

**EDITH EMMA COOPER, b. Kenilworth, Warwickshire, England, 1862.** Together with her aunt (and lover), Katherine Harris Bradley, Edith Cooper wrote poetry and plays under the joint pseudonym "Michael Field." Edith called Katherine "Michael" and Katherine nicknamed Edith "Henry," and for the rest of their lives they were known to each other and to their friends by these male names. Where the surname "Field" came from is anybody's guess. Among Michael and Henry's closest friends were the famous Royal Academy painters, Charles Ricketts and Charles Shannon, who lived together near them in a relationship comparable to their own. (What Charles and Charles called each other needn't concern us here.) The poems of "Michael Field" are rich in love lyrics to women, and they were well received until it was discovered that the "male" poet was in fact two women. From that time on their work was treated with ever-increasing coldness by the literary world. Of course, several well-known people knew the identity of "Michael Field" from the beginning, including Robert Browning, who was a friend. But even Browning asked for an explanation when *Long Ago*, based on fragments from Sappho, appeared in 1889. The friendship of Michael and Henry with the Brownings is telling. The Brownings wrote their poetry separately. The two women, on the other hand, wrote theirs jointly, believing themselves to be "two bodies joined as one." The contrast was not lost on "Michael Field": "These two poets, man and wife, wrote alone; each wrote, but did not bless and quicken one another at their work; *we are closer married.*"

young male revolutionaries whom he called his "family." Among his favorites were John Laurens, who once fought a duel to defend George's honor sullied by some cad for reasons now lost to history; and Alexander Hamilton, who was known to be something of a prick-tease. George, whose hips were a bit shy of Elsa Maxwell's, was thought by his enemies to be a bit soft on the boys and was suspected of being overly fond of young Hamilton in particular. Between 1779 and 1782, Hamilton and Laurens exchanged a series of love letters, reprinted in Jonathan Katz's *Gay American History,* in which "Laurens addressed Hamilton as 'My Dear' and offered flowery protestations of undying affection, to which Hamilton responded with the touching declaration: 'I love you'." To this day the letters are explained away on the grounds that 18th-century men "were classical scholars whose thoughts and actions were colored by the grandeur of antiquity." Oh.

# 13.

**HORATIO ALGER, b. Revere, Massachusetts, 1834.** In 1866 Horatio Alger moved from Brewster, Massachusetts, where he had been a Unitarian minister, to New York City. The experiences gained in his efforts to improve the condition of street boys in that famous city of "lights and shadows" became the raw material of over 100 books that he eventually wrote for boys. By leading exemplary lives, struggling valiantly against poverty and adversity, Alger's heroes gain wealth and honor. His juvenile fiction, particularly the *Luck and Pluck* and *Tattered Tom* series, was amazingly popular and left a strong mark upon the character of a generation of American youth. What no one understood at the time, however, was the reason for Alger's arrival in New York, not to mention an interesting correlative to his atavistic concern for boys. Back in Brewster, a special parish investigating committee of the Unitarian church had charged their minister with "gross immorality and a most heinous crime, a crime of no less magnitude than the abominable and revolting crime of unnatural familiarity with boys." Considering what Alger had been accused of doing to two lads named John Clark and Thomas S. Crocker before he hightailed it out of Brewster, is it any wonder that his first boys' book was called *Ragged Dick*?

# 14.

**YUKIO MISHIMA, b. Tokio, Japan, 1925.** The reputation of this Japanese poet-dramatist-novelist-actor-essayist-body-builder has gone

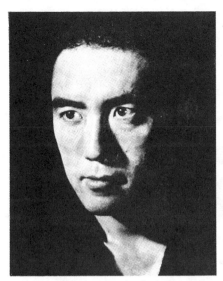

Yukio Mishima: When he died, his mother said, "My lover has returned to me."

steadily downhill since he committed ritual suicide, together with a youthful disciple named Masakatsu Morita, in a neo-fascist demonstration in 1970. Brilliantly written as they are, Mishima's many novels are morbid, sensational, and generally unpleasant, and his ugly and pointless death has underscored their essential meretriciousness. Oddly enough, Mishima seems destined to be remembered for those works, notably *Confessions of a Mask* and *Forbidden Colors,* that explore his homosexuality, and critics agree that these are both psychologically accurate and genuinely moving. Mishima equated the union of two men with the incarnation of Buddah and yearned for a return to "a time when the passive homosexual was given the seat of honor at the banquet and was the first to receive the Lord Buddha's saki cup . . . The organ of the male that was loved was called the 'Flower of the Law'; the organ of the man loving him was called the 'Fire of Darkness.'" And as the one would penetrate the other, he would chant: "Thy body is the deep seat of holiness, the ancient Tathagata of Buddha; thou art come into the world to save the multitude."

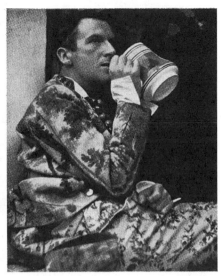

Cecil Beaton: Only he could get away with wearing brocades.

Poor Mishima. Modern Japan (and the rest of the world, for that matter) has a long way to go before it willingly passes that cup of saki.

**CECIL BEATON, b. London, 1904.** In these post-Stonewall days of macho gay males in matching *ensembles* of bulging muscles and hairy chests, it's hard to know what to make of Cecil Beaton. Photographer, costumier, writer, and raconteur, he was a snob, a man about town, a wit, and a bit of a shit. Beaton's many talents notwithstanding, Condé Nast was forced to let him go when a prank revealed his anti-Semitism to a hundred-thousand *Vogue* readers, many of them prominent Jews. Much of his wit, in fact, was tinged with bitchiness. Here he is on the close-cropped lesbians of the 1920s who cavorted around London in tailored suits, collars and cuffs, watchchains, and carnations: "Why, my dear, they look and talk like ventriloquist's dummies." In Truman Capote's still-unfinished *Answered Prayers,* he has Beaton say, "The most distressing fact of growing older is that I find my private parts are shrinking." To which his friend Greta Garbo replied, "Ah, if only I could say the same."

The capstone of Cecil Beaton's career was the knighthood bestowed on him by Queen Elizabeth in 1972. One wonders what he thought of the Queen Mum's hats.

**PIERRE LOTI (né Louis Marie Julien Viaud), b. Rochefort, France, 1850.** A French naval officer who was neither well-educated nor particularly interested in books, Loti began to write when a friend persuaded him to record some of his bizarre experiences in Constantinople. The result was *Aziyadë,* a book which, like so many of Loti's, is half a romance, half an autobiography. Thereafter he continued to write novels which were mainly reminiscent of his travels. Like the American writer Charles Warren Stoddard, whom he in so many ways resembles, Loti wrote of the South Seas and the Far East in a fruity, overripe style that would likely cause a modern reader to break out into hives. His pseudonym is said

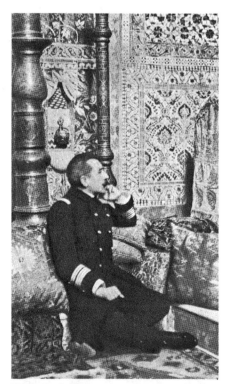

Pierre Loti: The perfumed poet within his very own mosque.

to have been due to his extreme shyness in early life, which made his comrades call him after *le Loti,* an Indian flower which grows in unfrequented spots. Suspended from the Navy for his part in some unspecified "scandal," Loti was described by a contemporary as "having made lavish use of scent and cosmetics, varnished his nails, glued a curl over his brow, and invariably circled his dreamy eyes with violet shadows." No wonder his playmates thought him a rare flower. No wonder sailors have more fun.

# 15.

**MOLIÈRE (né Jean Baptiste Poquelin), b. Paris, 1622.** What? The famous French playwright and actor gay? Impossible! Wasn't he as straight as Tartuffe was hypocritical or Le Bourgois Gentilhomme a parvenu? Well, not exactly. Molière was successful, which meant that he had enemies. He wrote with a sharp pen, which meant that his enemies were out for blood. Because of the many vicious stories that circulated about him, it's often difficult to separate truth from tongue-wagging. But this much seems sound: When he was in his late forties, Molière fell in love with fifteen-year-old Michel Baron, "the talented young actor whom he had taken into his own home after removing him from a company of child actors of which he was the star." Molière's wife, twenty-one years his junior, screamed bloody murder. The boy, not exactly dumb, moved out. Molière ordered him back. The wife said, "Choose! It's either him or me . . . er, he or I." Molière chose. Three years later, when the playwright died, Michel Baron was at his side. Curtain.

**IVOR NOVELLO (né David Davies), b. Cardiff, Wales, 1893.**

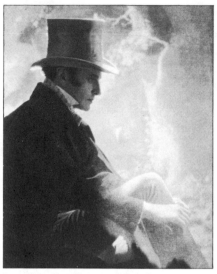

Ivor Novello: "Musical!" said Winnie.

Everyone knew that the dashing British matinee idol and operetta king was gay—except the ten million women who adored him, bought his Gramophone records, tore his clothes at the stage door, and believed the baloney about his romance with young Gladys Cooper cooked up by a press agent to mask the fact that the young man who had written the World War I marching song "Keep the Home Fires Burning" really preferred to take it up the bum. For the astonishing story of Ivor Novello's one-night stand with Winston Churchill—yes, Winston Churchill—see November 30.

# 16.

**GEORGE KELLY, b. Philadelphia, 1887.** George Kelly was a successful Broadway playwright, the uncle of Princess Grace of Monaco, a Philadelphia Kelly, and a confirmed homosexual, not necessarily in that order. Hardly poor to begin with, Kelly made a fortune from his popular plays, *The Torch Bearers, The Show-Off,* and *Craig's Wife.* The latter, because of its central character, Harriet Craig, who is apoplectic if there's so much as a single dog's hair on the living-room carpet, has become a camp symbol of overfastidiousness, thanks to the two film versions starring Rosalind Russell and Joan Crawford (at about the time that Christina was being whacked with the Bon-Ami can). Not long after George Kelly was caught in a hotel room with his pants down and had to pay off his young trick to buy his silence, he decided to settle down with someone more reliable and less expensive. He chose a mousy bookkeeper named William E. Weagley and thereafter declined any invitation that excluded his lover. Well, *almost* any invitation. The Philadelphia Kellys—a generation before Princess Grace's brother Jack and the transsexual Harlow were an item—would have none of it. Whenever "Uncle George" brought his companion around to call, Weagley was obliged to eat in the kitchen with the servants. So much for the City of Brotherly Love.

# 17.

**RONALD FIRBANK** (né Arthur Annesley Ronald Firbank), **b. London, 1886.** Firbank was an English novelist who wore two dressing gowns at once, stained his fingernails carmine, and lived in a black-walled London apartment surrounded by books bound only in blue leather. He was also gay, unhappy, chronically ill, neurotic, exceptionally wealthy, and a literary genius who combined the decadence and aesthetic exquisiteness of the 1890s with a secular love of Roman Catholic ritual. As a stylist and technical innovator, he is perhaps without peer. (Anthony Powell and Evelyn Waugh owe a great deal to him.) Firbank's best novels are *Caprice* (1917) and *Concerning the Eccentricities of Car-*

*dinal Pirelli* (1926), the story (one of the most hilarious ever written) of a mad cardinal who dies chasing a seductive choirboy around the altar. Firbank is reputed to have dined exclusively on champagne and flower petals. He died undernourished at an early age.

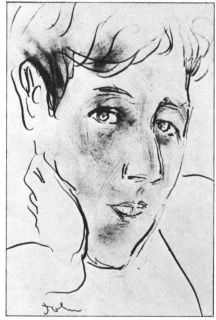

**Ronald Firbank:** Carmine nails, blue leather, champagne and flower petals.

# 18.

**PRINCE HEINRICH OF PRUSSIA, b. Berlin, 1726.** What do you do if you're king of Prussia and your kid brother is screwing all the pages, sleeping with the help, and graduating to love affairs with Italian tenors and visiting diplomats? You ship him off to the New World to become King of America, that's what. Prince Heinrich *was* the younger brother of Frederick the Great, and he *was* constantly in trouble for sleeping around, but his chance to become the American king didn't happen quite so simply. During the 1780s, Americans were as

politically fickle as they are now. Tired of the weak government under the Articles of Confederation, they thought that it was time for a change and hankered for a king. George Washington was their first choice, but he declined. Baron von Steuben, himself gay, thought that his old friend Heinrich would make a dandy king and let him know that the job was open, but Heinrich, wondering whether New World puritans ever put out, was slow in making up his mind. By this time, however, the American electorate had changed its stripes again and supported a Constitutional Convention rather than a monarchy. Thus the good old U.S.A. came within a whisker of genuflecting to a homosexual king and—if there's any historic truth to the entry for January 11—wound up with a constitutional queen instead.

# 19.

**NATACHA RAMBOVA, b. Salt Lake City, Utah, 1897.** In the Hollywood of the madcap Twenties, when stars had names like Nita Naldi and Pola Negri, a little glamor helped. Natacha Rambova, who in private life was Mrs. Rudolph Valen-

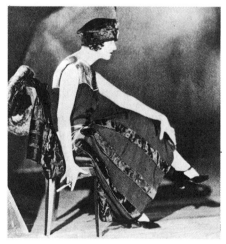

**Natacha Rambova:** The Russian emigrée from Salt Lake City.

tino, was a self-made exotic. Where else but in Hollywood could little Winifred Shaunnessy from Salt Lake City become a Russian aristocrat in Southern California exile? Rambova was reputed to be a prominent member of Alla Nazimova's lesbian sewing circle and was unkindly called, behind her back of course,

Valentino's husband. She made one movie, *When Love Grows Cold* (1925), that was really cold borscht. When her Hollywood days were over, she settled down and became (no kidding) a prominent Egyptologist, publishing learned tomes at the Princeton University Press under the name of, yes, Natacha Rambova.

somewhat exaggerated, there being "more men than women." Peggy Casertas, in *Going Down with Janis* —the title says it all—would have us believe otherwise; there were "more women than men," she says. This great dispute is likely never to be resolved, but we can all be grateful that Joplin didn't particularly care for German Shepherds.

# 20.

**ST. SEBASTIAN, b. Rome, 3rd Century A.D.** Sebastian is the patron saint of archers because he was bound to a stake and shot at with arrows. As the arrows stuck in his body, thick as pins in a pincushion, he was also made patron saint of pinmakers. And as he was a centurion, he is patron saint of soldiers. All very well and good, but Sebastian was also properly the patron saint of gays

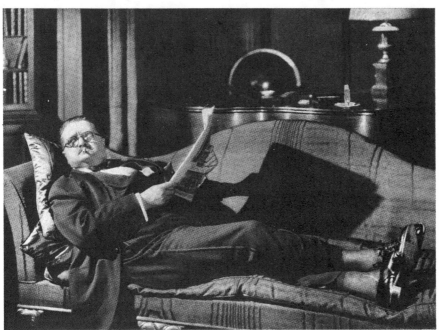

**Alexander Woollcott:** Too much estrogen, but not enough for motherhood.

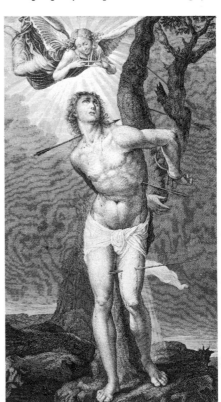

**St. Sebastian:** Stuck.

**ALEXANDER WOOLLCOTT, b. Phalanx, New Jersey, 1887.** Back in the days when American culture consisted of Mickey Rooney playing Shakespeare's Puck and Paul Muni impersonating Emile Zola, Alexander Woollcott was every Babbitt's idea of what a literary critic should be. One of the best-known journalists of his time, he exerted great influence on popular literary and theatrical tastes as the rotund drama critic for *The New York Times* and as a weekly radio reviewer called the "Town Crier." His gossipy essays, which only a doctoral candidate desperate for a dissertation subject would want to read today, were collected in several volumes. Woollcott was the model for Kaufman and

Hart's *The Man Who Came to Dinner* and even played the role on Broadway. Most of Woollcott's contemporaries considered the exceptionally effeminate critic gay. But his biographer contends that he was actually a turnip, rendered asexual because of a hormone imbalance. No wonder he once wept on Anita Loos's shoulder because he'd never become a mother.

**JANIS JOPLIN, b. Port Arthur, Texas, 1943.** Even schoolkids used to know that Janis did it with men and women both. Her two biographers differ only quantitatively. Janis's legendary sexual exploits with women, says Myra Friedman in *Buried Alive*, were true, although

because tradition made him a beautiful youth beloved by the emperor Diocletian, who turned against him for embracing Christianity. Sebastian lost his appropriateness as the official gay patron saint after the Stonewall Riots. Modern Sebastians, after all, shoot back.

# 21.

**DUNCAN GRANT, b. Rothiemurchus, Inverness-shire, Scotland, 1885.** When this famous English painter, decorator, and designer of textile, pottery, and theater decor died at ninety-three in 1978, the world press, in lengthy obituaries, mourned the passing of one of the last members of the Bloomsbury group, which had included, among others, Roger Fry, Clive and Vanessa Bell, and Virginia Woolf. Conspicuously missing from the obituaries was any mention that Grant had once been the lover of his cousin Lytton Strachey—that is, until he was stolen away from under Strachey's nose by someone even better known, the economist John Maynard Keynes. Since Strachey and Keynes had themselves been lovers, with Keynes possessing the extraordinary knack of expropriating anyone who shared Strachey's bed, Strachey's anguished cries when he lost Grant to his perpetual rival were heard from one end of Bloomsbury to the other. Today Grant's portraits of Strachey and Keynes are considered to be two of his three best works. The other is a portrait of the bisexual Virginia Woolf.

# 22.

**SIR FRANCIS BACON, b. London, 1561.** In addition to being a philosopher, essayist, and statesman,

Bacon was an innovative thinker whose greatest contribution was his application of the inductive method of modern science as opposed to the *a priori* method of medieval scholasticism. He urged full investigation in all cases, avoiding theories based on insufficient data. When the magnifying glass of Bacon's scientific method is applied to the known facts of his life, he emerges as one of the only personalities of his day accused of being gay whose homosexuality is easy to prove. Although Bacon's contemporaries Aubrey and D'Ewes mention in their writings his love of boys, particularly tow-haired red-cheeked lads from Wales—a letter from Bacon's

mother survives that leaves no doubt about sonny's escapades. In it Lady Anne rails against the steady stream of servants and envoys who were finding their way to Bacon's bed: "I will not have his cormorant seducers and instruments of Satan to him committing foul sin by his countenance to the displeasing of God and his godly true fear." She also denouced an effeminate Hispanic envoy with whom gay Francis was making it as "that bloody Perez and bed-companion of my son." One wonders what her other son, Roger Bacon, thought when he received this letter from mama. After all, he, too, was gay.

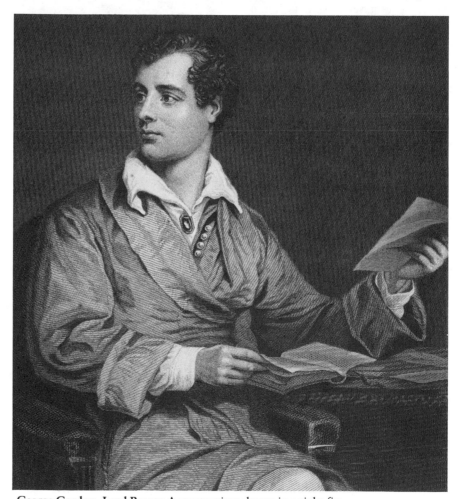

**George Gordon, Lord Byron:** A great writer always in a tight fix.

**GEORGE GORDON, LORD BYRON, b. London, 1788.** If only the improbably handsome poet's memoirs, *My Life and Adventures,* had not been burned because they were deemed too scandalous for publication, we would have today a document by one of the masters of English literature about the timelessness of sex. As it is, we are able to piece together aspects of the poet's private life that make him appear to us a uniquely sympathetic "modern" man. Byron was a champion of freedom, an enemy of cant and hypocrisy, an astonishingly erudite poet who was (we frequently forget) remarkably funny. He also had a ravenous sexual appetite, enjoyed the mysteries of love-making in all its varieties, and possessed a forceful masculine appeal, and the requisite physical equipment, to make him irresistible to women and men alike. That he once took his young French-Greek friend, Nicolò Giraud, to a physician to repair the boy's overworked anal sphincter, leaves little doubt about the poet's sexual proclivities. Among the many reasons for the breakup of his marriage, in addition to his wife's knowledge of his affair with his married half-sister, was his insistence that Lady Byron offer him what Nicolò had so diligently and dutifully provided. Lady Byron adamantly refused, apparently not caring to visit her husband's physician. At one point in his brief life, Byron considered leaving his entire fortune to Nicolò. Whether this was to have been done for love, for services rendered, or for an early version of workman's compensation is not entirely known.

**CONRAD VEIDT, b. Potsdam, Germany, 1893.** His face, it was said, should have been painted by the Renaissance masters. It was aristocratic, lean, sensuous, sinister, commanding, and most of all, enigmatic. Although he died at fifty, his career in films lasted from the period of German Expressionism to the Hollywood of World War II. Movie

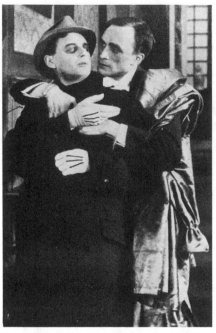

**Conrad Veidt** (right): A scene from *Anders als die Anderen.*

buffs know him as the star of *The Cabinet of Dr. Caligari,* as the cruel nobleman loved by Joan Crawford in *A Woman's Face,* and as Major Strasser in Bogart's *Casablanca.* But he was also a character right out of the pages of Christopher Isherwood's *Berlin Stories.* Isherwood, in fact, has recorded that the German actor was in regular attendance at the gay *lokals* of decadent Berlin. Significantly, he was the star of *Anders als die Anderen* (Different from the Others), a film sponsred by Magnus Hirschfeld's Institute for Sexual Science that pleaded tolerance for homosexuals. When Hitler came to power, the Institute and the film were burned. Among the first to flee Germany was the enigmatic gay actor.

# 23.

**FRANKLIN PANGBORN, b. Newark, New Jersey, 1893.** This unforgettable character actor built his

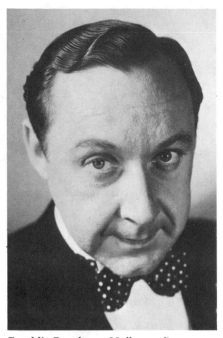

**Franklin Pangborn:** Hollywood's gay Stepin Fetchit?

entire thirty-year film career on playing prissy, fluttery clerks, bank tellers, assistant hotel managers, and department store floorwalkers. Was he in fact the gay Stepin Fetchit? Who cares. He was funny, had perfect comic timing, and brightened many an otherwise dreary picture by his amusing presence. And if Pangborn's public thought that sissies and sister-marys were one and the same, so what? They sure as hell don't think so now. Rest in peace, dear Franklin Pangborn.

# 24.

**THE EMPEROR HADRIAN, b. near modern Seville, Spain, 76 A.D.** "Hadrian," as John Paul Hudson writes, "was noted for his intelligent, circumspect rule of the vast Roman Empire, for building walls to stay the barbarian invasions, and for putting down the last serious revolt of the Jews, but it was his love for his flawless consort, Antinous, that posterity has chiefly remembered . . . When Antinous mysteriously drowned himself in the Nile, Hadrian plunged into an orgy of despair, then did all his vast power and wealth would allow to memorialize his lover, by building a city named for him. . . ." It is said that Antinous killed himself before the ravages of age could destroy his beauty. He was all of twenty-one. For a modern retelling of this tragic love story, and one of the few undisputed masterpieces of contemporary literature, read Marguerite Yourcenar's *Memoirs of Hadrian* if you've not already done so. And if you have, read it again.

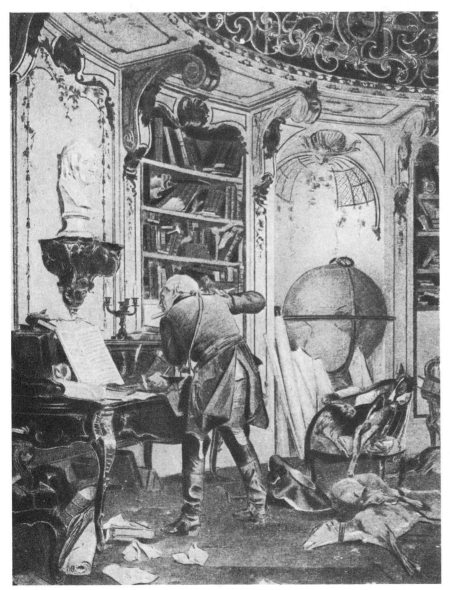

**Frederick the Great at Sans-Souci:** A life devoted to the arts.

## FREDERICK THE GREAT (Friedrich II), b. Berlin, 1712.
Frederick—or Frédéric as he came to call himself once intoxicated with the French language—was born to be a poet, a musician, an architect—anything but what his father wanted him to be, a ruthless warrior, a conquerer of nations. To escape the wrath of his tyrannical father, young Frederick enlisted the aid of his lover, the dashing Hans von Katte. Together they fled, but were soon captured. Forced to witness his lover's execution, which his father thought would toughen his sensitive son, the weeping prince blew his friend a kiss and begged forgiveness. The handsome lieutenant replied, "There's nothing to forgive, my lord," and went bravely to his death. Misery turned to joy when his father died not long after. At Sans-Souci, the magnificent palace he built at Potsdam, he came into his own. Women were totally excluded and all was literature, music, and gay love immortalized in bawdy verses written by the king himself. Frederick is viewed today as a dour misanthrope, but he was not without a touch of wit. On learning that a particularly well-endowed soldier had been arrested for "bestiality with his horse," he is reputed to have replied, "Fool—don't put him in irons; put him in the infantry."

# 25.

## W. SOMERSET MAUGHAM, b. Paris, 1874.
The famous playwright, novelist, and short-story writer was twenty-one years old when Oscar Wilde was brought to trial. Like many other Englishmen who saw first-hand the horrors of Victorian hypocrisy, he became publicly straight in England and discreetly gay on the Continent. That such behavior was in itself another form of hypocrisy, and that it eventually shattered the lives of Maugham's wife and daughter and ultimately himself, was the price he paid for respectability and for keeping out of jail. Maugham once said that his greatest mistake had been that "I tried to persuade myself that I was three-

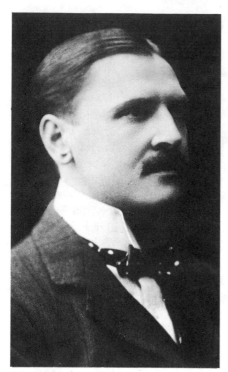

**W. Somerset Maugham:** He felt that loving men made his work second-rate.

fering character, *any* suffering character, to get on with it and simply grab her lady friend and kiss her squarely on the mouth. Of her several infatuations, the most important was probably Vita-Sackville West, since the fruit of this affair is the novel *Orlando*, considered by many to be the longest love poem in the English language. But whether any of Virginia Woolf's infatuations ever led directly to physical intimacy with another woman is not entirely certain. While writing *Mrs.*

*Dalloway,* she drops a hint in her diary: "Yesterday, I had tea in Mary's room and saw the red lighted tugs go past and heard the swish of the river. Mary: in black with lotus leaves round her neck. If one could be friendly with women, what a pleasure—the relationship so secret and private compared with relations with men." Had she acted on her instincts, the world had not been given *Orlando*. But then, she might not have walked into the sea and drowned herself.

quarters normal and that only a quarter of me was queer—whereas really it was the other way round." Despite his wealth, his fame, and his love for his secretary-companion Gerald Haxton, Maugham ended his days a bitter, unhappy man. But approaching senility had perhaps loosened up the old boy a bit. In his eighties, injected with cells from sheep fetuses (as had been Merle Oberon and Pope Pius XII), he delighted in demonstrating to uncomfortable guests his ability to achieve a rampant erection.

**VIRGINIA WOOLF, b. London, 1892.** Opinion about the experimental novels of this most celebrated member of the Bloomsbury group is divided. Some say that she is over-refined to the point of tedium, others that she created an original kind of novel. But on one point there seems to be universal agreement: the key to much of Virginia Woolf's writing is her lesbianism, so subtly, so cerebrally treated, that one longs for one suf-

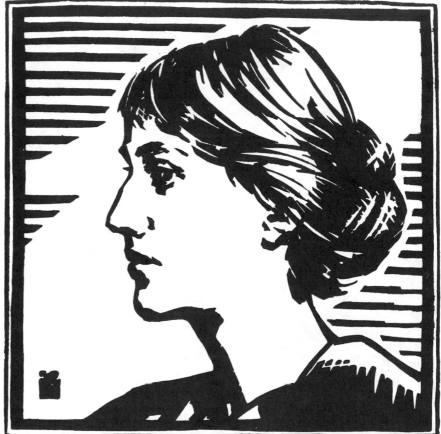

**Virginia Woolf:** Her love for Vita Sackville-West made her feel like "a real woman" for the first time.

**AARON FRICKE, b. Providence, Rhode Island, 1962.** "The simple, obvious thing would have been to go to the senior prom with a girl. But that would have been a lie—a lie to myself, to the girl, and to all the other students. What I wanted to do

was to take a male date. But as Paul Guilbert had shown the year before when he had attempted to take another man to the prom, such honesty is not always easy." So writes Aaron Fricke in *Reflections of a Rock Lobster: A Story About Grow-*

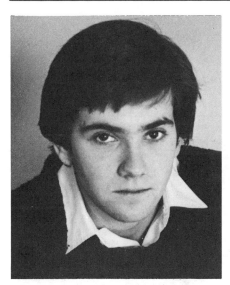

**Aaron Fricke:** Tomorrow's hope.

*ing Up Gay,* his engaging account of how he did, in fact, win the right to take a young man as his date to his high-school prom. That Aaron Fricke at seventeen risked everything—the scorn of his classmates, the disaffection of his parents, the anger of his community—is a tribute to his courage and sense of right. That he has written a book without a touch of self-pity or arrogance is a testimony of his humanity. In an age of cynicism, he offers us hope.

# 26.

**LORD GEORGE GERMAIN, b. London, 1716.** While you're cursing that smoky fireplace on a wintry January evening, think a thought or two of Lord George who, while in America as British Colonial Secretary, fell in love with handsome Benjamin Thompson of North Woburn, Massachusetts, who became his literal and figurative undersecretary. When it looked as if the Yankee rebels would win their battle for independence, Lord George and his American pal, now a Tory by marriage, fled to the mother country,

where Ben of North Woburn was elevated to the title of Count Rumford. What does this have to do with fireplaces on a wintry night? Count Rumford, who became one of the leading physicists of his day, was famous for having discovered the cause of smoky chimneys, although he was neither the first nor last to gain a title through a smoky hole.

# 27.

**LEWIS CARROLL (né Charles Lutwidge Dodgson), b. Daresbury, Cheshire, England, 1832.** What was the author of *Alice in Wonderland* anyway? Gay? A dirty old man? An Oxford suet pudding? Since the dead are notoriously silent, the psychiatrists and other necrophiliacs have run riot over Carroll's bones. The *Alice* books, writes one, reflect much "unassimilated phallic problems," a phrase composed, most likely, when all mimsy were the borogoves. "He had a horror of little boys," writes another, explaining Carroll's attraction to little girls. "This great aversion could hardly be anything else than an ambivalent sexual attraction to little boys, with the fear that he might yield to it . . . So little girls it had to be. . . ." Hmmm. "'Contrariwise,' said Tweedle-dee, 'if it was so, it might be; and if it were so, it would be; but as it ain't, it ain't. That's logic.'"

# 28.

**CHARLES GEORGE "CHINESE" GORDON, b. Woolwich, England, 1833.** A military hero of imperial Britain and a martyr at Khartoum, Gordon worried constantly about his inability to score with women, several times wishing himself either a

eunuch or a corpse. His wish to die in battle, which was eventually granted him, no doubt accounted for his almost legendary bravery. Although the record shows that he surrounded himself with beautiful young men, his sense of honor and his religious convictions make it doubtful that his soul was ever sullied, no less his pud. Still, he found a novel way to gratify his senses. He was fond of picking up street urchins, bathing them, feeding them, and mending their clothes with his very own needle and thread. Wasn't that sweet of him?

**GABRIELLE SIDONIE COLETTE, b. Saint-Sauveur-en-Puisaye, France, 1873.** The great French writer's affairs with women are well known, but equally so are her affairs with men. Colette's was a concept of androgyny in which everyone was predisposed to discover within himself, herself, and in other people, a subtle mixture of male and female components. "Once the precious tresses are cut," she wrote, "the breasts, hands, bellies, hidden, what is left of our female façades? In sleep, an incalculable number of women approach the form they would probably have chosen had their life awake not made them ignorant of themselves. And the same for men. I can still see the gracefulness of a sleeping man! From forehead to mouth, behind his closed eyelids, he smiled, nonchalant and sly as a sultana behind her grilled window. . . . And I, who would have in my stupidity 'really liked' to be completely a woman, I looked at him with a male regret." Ambivalence was Colette's middle name.

# 29.

**CHRISTIAN VII, b. Copenhagen, Denmark, 1749.** Sometimes, being king isn't any fun at all. Rejected by his father as effeminate and slightly feeble-minded, Christian was systematically debauched in his youth by nobles who schemed to control him once he gained the throne by supplying him with rough-trade bedmates who regularly beat the living daylights out of him. By the time he succeeded his father at sixteen, he was virtually insane. But his troubles were just beginning. Christian's personal physician, a German named Johann Struensee, took Christian's queen as his mistress, began to run the government, and assigned the king a lover of his own, a brute named Brandt who got his kicks by locking Christian in his room and pummelling him with his fists. Talk about pushy! But the villains eventually got theirs. The queen was summarily divorced, the physician and the brute each lost their right hand and head and were then drawn and quartered. Wouldn't this make a great musical?

# 30.

**HOWARD OVERING STURGIS, b. London, 1855.** Howard *who*, you say? Sturgis was a millionaire American expatriate who passed his life in England knitting, embroidering, and writing novels in the company of his live-in stud W. H. Smith, better known as "The Babe," who presumably slugged anyone who tittered at Howard's petit point. Not surprisingly, Sturgis failed as a novelist and would not be remembered were it not for his pallid—but for the time courageous—novel *Bedchamber*, about a young English nobleman who is both a homosexual and a utopian. George Santayana, who himself was gay, modeled the character of Mario in *The Last Puritan* on Sturgis. The famous Har-

vard philosopher, who like the rest of us could be a bitch at times, once called the knitting novelist "the perfect Victorian lady."

# 31.

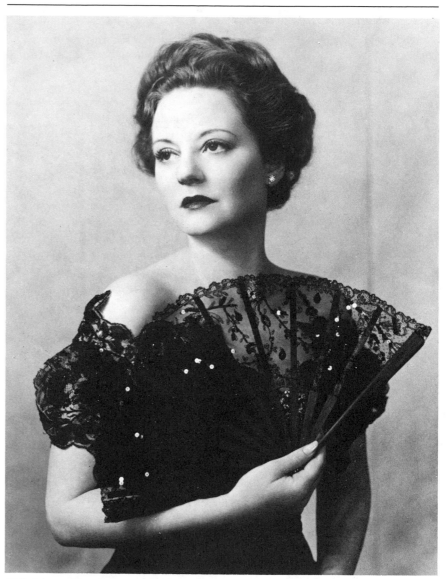

Tallulah Bankhead: "My family warned me about sex, daaahling, but they never never mentioned a word about women. . . ."

**TALLULAH BANKHEAD, b. Huntsdale, Alabama, 1902.** What can be said about this remarkable character that hasn't already been said? She liked men, she liked women, she especially liked herself. She could be a great actress on opening nights, and a parody of herself when she grew bored with a long run. She was the toast of London in the '20s and a flop in Hollywood in the '30s. She was a bit of a drunk, a bit of a junkie, a holy terror, and a saint. She could play the aristocratic Southern belle or out-curse a drunken sailor on shore leave. Of all her famous one-liners, this one perhaps sums her up the best: "I can say 'shit,' daaahling, I'm a lady."

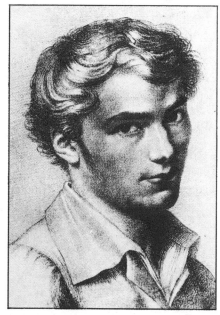

**Franz Schubert:** At 16 one of the beauties of his day.

**FRANZ SHUBERT, b. Vienna, 1797.** Far more is known about this great composer's music than about his life. Because his music became widely known only many years after his death at thirty-one, our knowledge of Schubert the man is based completely on the memoirs written by friends who lived long enough to see him famous. These are the recollections of the old, who, looking back at their youths, bathed the past in a glow of golden sentiment. No wonder Schubert has emerged a character out of Viennese operetta—a bohemian artist, poor but happy, who composed delightful melodies as the spirit moved him. But there is no knowing the real Schubert without knowing the friends with whom he lived from his early teens. Almost all never married, with the exception of one who married at the age of sixty. The others were suicides. That Schubert travelled in a circle that was predominantly gay seems fairly certain. That he suffered for years from syphilis that eventually killed him is also certain. That he himself was gay is more than likely. There is no evidence to prove otherwise.

## Other Personalities Born in January

1. **Rama VI,** King of Thailand, 1881
   **Charles "Badger" King,** Western poet, 1883

3. **Ethel F. L. R. Robertson,** English novelist, 1870

5. **Ian Young,** Canadian poet, 1945

6. **John Wieners,** American poet, 1934

8. **Francois,** Duke of Luxembourg, French general, 1628

9. **William Cory,** English poet, 1823
   **Henry Blake Fuller,** American novelist, 1857
   **Joan Baez,** American folk singer, 1941

10. **Johnnie Ray,** American popular singer, 1927
    **Craig Russell,** Canadian female impersonator, 1950

11. **Bayard Taylor,** American writer and diplomat, 1825

12. **Pierre Bernac,** French singer, 1899

13. **Adolf Hausrath ("George Taylor"),** German theologian and novelist, 1837
    **Oliver Messel,** English stage designer, 1904

15. **Franz Grillparzer,** Austrian dramatist, 1791
    **Mazo de la Roche,** Canadian novelist, 1879

   **Ernest Thesiger,** English-born American actor, 1879

17. **Oscar Browning,** English educator, 1837

19. **Edgar Allan Poe,** American writer, 1809
    **Edmund White,** American writer, 1950
    **Stan Persky,** American poet, 1941

21. **Christian Dior,** French couturier, 1905

22. **August Strindberg,** Swedish dramatist, 1849

23. **Thomas Sergeant Perry,** American writer, 1845
    **Sergei Eisenstein,** Russian filmmaker, 1898
    **James Spada,** American writer, 1950

24. **Farinelli,** Italian male soprano, 1703
    **Gustavus III,** King of Sweden, 1746
    **Mario Palmieri,** Italian activist, 1898

26. **Christopher Hampton,** English dramatist, 1946

27. **Leopold von Sacher-Masoch,** German novelist, 1836

29. **Frederick Delius,** English composer, 1863
    **Robin Morgan,** American feminist and poet, 1941

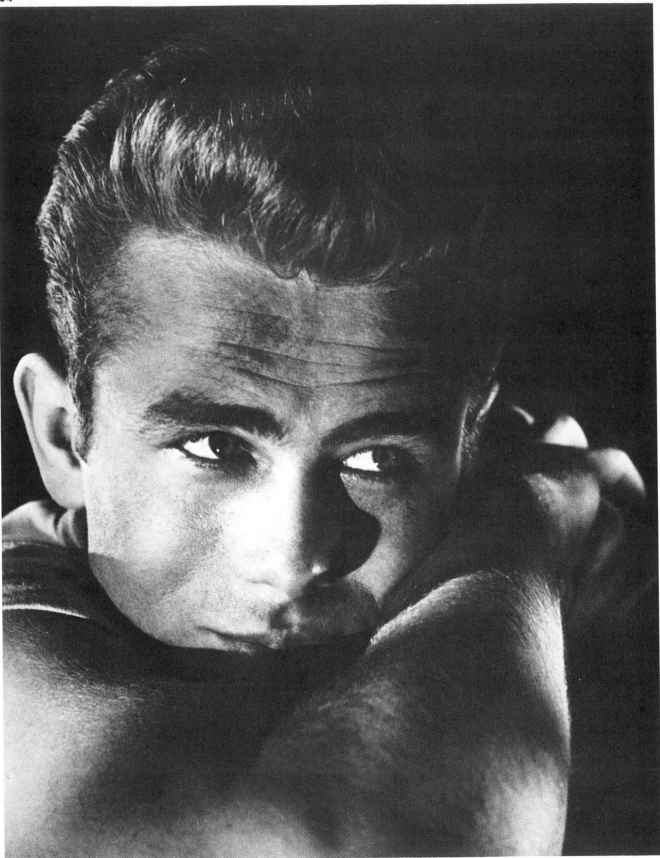

**James Dean:** When he died at twenty-four, an entire generation mourned.

# FEBRUARY

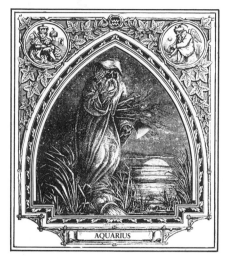

AQUARIUS

**Aquarius** (January 20th to February 18th), a fixed airy sign, shows some of the characteristics of Saturn, being serious and undemonstrative in emotion. But the sign also takes on some of the qualities of its ruler, Uranus. Whereas the Capricornian is a respecter of tradition, the Aquarian is the reverse—revolutionary, unconventional, and individual in his thought. He does not usually make close friendships, for his feeling is for humanity as a whole and often leads to altruism in the extreme. The Aquarian possesses an extraordinary breadth of vision; he is a truth seeker. His ways are neither militant nor aggressive. He can wait, and the longer he waits, the more clearly he knows the futility of seeking truth. He is willing to learn from anyone, for the only thing of which he is certain is that he knows very little.

## 1.

**LANGSTON HUGHES, b. Joplin, Missouri, 1902.** The great black poet was most widely known as the chronicler of Harlem, where he lived for many years. Unlike the generation of black writers that came after him, Hughes's approach to American racism was more wry than angry, sly than militant. But he helped set the mood for today's black movement. As a poet he was discovered, while working as a busboy in Washington, by Vachel Lindsay, himself gay. He was in no sense a traditional poet, but took his poetic form and material from folk sources, a great deal of his work expressing in words the spirit of the blues. With Countee Cullen, also gay, he was an outstanding figure in the Harlem literary renaissance of the 1920s. Hughes's greatest creation was perhaps Jessie

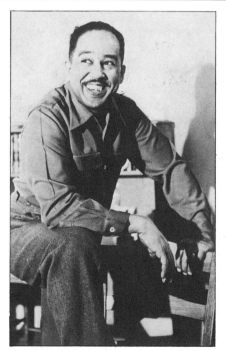

**Langston Hughes:** Rumor says yes.

B. Semple, or "Simple"—the humorous Harlem dweller who in several books "spoke his mind" sharply on matters of racial injustice. "White folks," said Simple with characteristic understatement, "is the cause of a lot of inconvenience in my life."

## 2.

**PRINCE WENZEL ANTON VON KAUNITZ, b. Vienna, 1711.** The great Austrian statesman, who single-handedly engineered an alliance between two traditional enemies, Austria and France, was also a bona-fide pluperfect eccentric. An arrogant and conceited fop who never tired of talking or of delivering interminable moral sermons (he once chewed Frederick the Great's ear for over two hours, having exacted from the Prussian King a promise that he'd not be interrupted), he was one of the greatest hypochondriacs of all time,

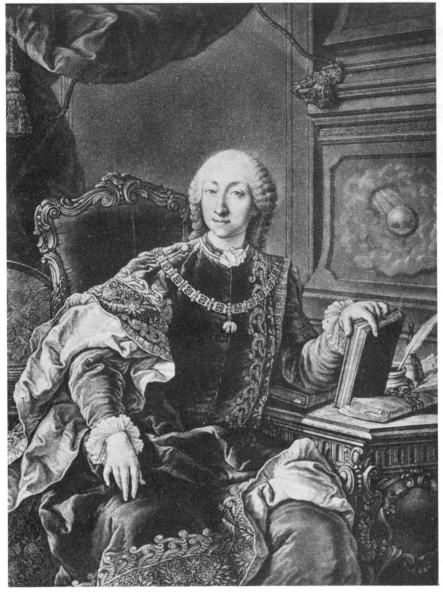

**Wenzel Anton von Kaunitz:** History records that he was a hero, a hypochondriac, and a homosexual. H-h-heavens!

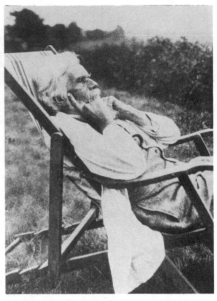

**Havelock Ellis:** When it rains, it pours.

refusing ever to allow fresh air within and placing a handkerchief over his mouth whenever venturing without. Given his extreme aversion to anything physical and his horror of natural bodily functions, it is hard to believe that he fathered four sons, no less that he was interested in shtupping boys, as contemporary rumor had it.

**HAVELOCK ELLIS, b. Croydon, Surrey, England, 1859.** Ellis's monumental seven-volume *Studies in the Psychology of Sex* (1897-1928) was not only of the greatest importance in changing the general Western attitude towards sex, but has influenced almost all writers on the subject since. Given the nature of his major interest, he was more than entitled to a full-fledged fetish all his own. A bisexual married to a lesbian, Ellis took particular enjoyment in peeing in his women after intercourse. Looking on the "golden water" as a symbol of love, he'd ask his "Naiad" or his "Water Nymph," as he called his lady friends, to urinate down her leg as they were walking the streets, hand in hand, in the rain. Dry cleaning, one should not forget, was infinitely cheaper in those days.

# 3.

**GERTRUDE STEIN, b. Allegheny, Pennsylvania, 1874.** Like the Cubist paintings she knew so well, Gertrude Stein was multifaceted, complicated, and occasionally impenetrable. So much has been written about her that it is difficult to know exactly what to make of this extraordinary woman, whose long and happy life with Alice B. Toklas she once summed up by writing, "I love my love with a b because she is peculiar." Was she a genius, a fraud, a bitch, a saint, over-rated, underrated, or a little of each? What she was more than anything else was honest, scrupulously so, perhaps the most honest writer of her

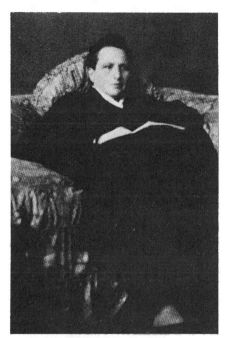

**Gertrude Stein:** Alice B. Toklas called her "Lovey."

time. Her early fiction, *Q.E.D.* and *Three Lives,* offers us the first realistic portrayal of lesbianism in the English language that is not veiled in misty metaphor or drowned in sickly sentiment. The very act of creating these books required an heroic courage that is inconceivable today. What she risked in breaking new ground, in writing about a subject scarcely known, no less understood, was the creation of works destined to cause shock and be called "ugly." As she later wrote in her inimitable style, ". . . When you make a thing, it is so complicated making it that it is bound to be ugly, but those that do it after you they don't have to worry about making it and they can make it pretty, and so everyone can like it when the others make it." Gertrude Stein was first. Keep her memory green.

# 4.

**THE AUTHOR OF THIS BOOK,**

b. New York City, 1938. Yes, I know it says in the Introduction that, as an average Joe, I'll exclude my birthday from the book. I was lying.

# 5.

**WILLIAM S. BURROUGHS, b. St. Louis, 1914.** The outline of his life is known to almost everyone: the flight from the riches of the Burroughs Adding Machine Company family to jobs as a newspaper reporter, private detective, exterminator; the tragic, but grimly comic, death of his wife when he tried to shoot a champagne glass off her head *à la* William Tell and missed; the escape into drugs and the fifteen-year addiction that led to his first novel, *Junkie,* and *The Naked Lunch,* which twenty years ago was thought to be required reading. But time seems to be working against the avant-garde writer. What once seemed new is now seen to be a pastiche of techniques borrowed from surrealism, science fiction, gothic. And yet . . . and yet . . . there's something in Burroughs that holds one, that resists too easy dismissal. Read the instructive pages given him in *Gay Sunshine Interviews,* in which he is questioned by a gay writer some twenty years his junior. It is the meeting of a giant and a pygmy that makes one want to re-read his books while simultaneously fearing for the future of the language.

# 6.

**RAMON NOVARRO (né José Ramon Samaniegos), b. Durango, Mexico, 1899.** *Ben-Hur*—bulging biceps lashing fleet steeds in the famous Colisseum chariot race; the whitest teeth that ever were; the

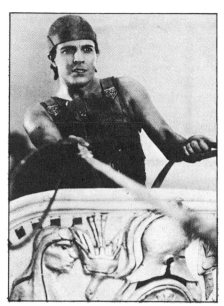

**Ramon Novarro:** Murdered with a lead dildo given him by Rudolph Valentino.

Roman tunic that one wishes were just a wee bit shorter: This is the picture of Ramon Novarro remembered by movie buffs. Many more films, however, made and kept him MGM's great Latin lover throughout the '20s and early '30s. He was one of Richard Halliburton's Hollywood bedmates and the actor forced to deliver one of the most memorable lines in movie history. (Says Novarro to Greta Garbo, who, as Mata Hari is registering worry, world-weariness, and pain: "What's the matter, Mata?") In the end, in 1968, this still-handsome actor was murdered by two hustlers, the lead dildo once given him by Rudolph Valentino reputedly the murder weapon.

# 7.

**JONATHAN, SON OF SAUL, b. Jerusalem, c. 1046 B.C.** No one knows exactly when the biblical Jonathan was born, of course. But since no one of any particular importance to gay history was born on

February 7, why not assign the day to this sweet young man, whose presence in Holy Writ has always been an embarrassment to fundamentalist preachers? The love of Jonathan for David, a love so deep that he foreswore his father out of loyalty to his beloved, has provided literature with both a powerful trope for male friendship and one of the most oft-quoted lines of Scripture, spoken by David at the death of his friend: "My brother Jonathan, thy love to me was wonderful, passing the love of women" (2 Samuel 1:26). The attempts to explain away this line are among the most dazzling examples of sophistry, ingeniousness, and wrong-headed mumbo-jumbo in 2,000 years of biblical exegesis. But *we* know what it means, don't we.

# 8.

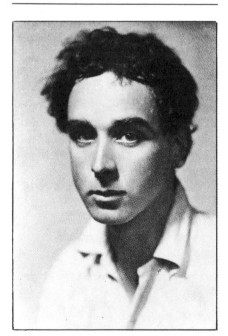

**Ralph Chubb:** Snips and snails, and puppy dogs' tails. . . .

**RALPH CHUBB, b. Harpenden, Hertsfordshire, England, 1892.** If you've ever wondered what an English eccentric is, as opposed to, say, an American eccentric or a German, then Ralph Chubb's your man. Cared for by a spinster sister even dottier than he, Chubb spent most of his life producing hand-printed books that reflected his obsession with pederasty (*The Heavenly Cupid, Water-Cherubs*). These elaborate fantasies about little boys, frequently poetic and beautifully illustrated with his own graphics, are fine examples of the bookmaker's art and make their author very much the William Blake of boy-love. It's often said that virgins make the best pornographers, a point not without relevance to Chubb, whose one and only sexual experience occurred when he was eighteen. Who knows what his books would have been like had he enjoyed it.

**JAMES DEAN (né James Byron), b. Marion, Ohio, 1931.** It's hard to explain to those who weren't there just what this brilliant, eccentric young actor meant to gay men (and young people of both sexes) during the McCarthy '50s. His brooding, unhappy, rebellious presence in the midst of adult corruption and hypocrisy made an entire generation identify strongly with him. When in *East of Eden* he walked fully clothed into a Turkish bath, where one towel-clad man said, "You make me hot, just looking at you," gay men laughed nervously in theaters around the world. His death at twenty-four resulted in the greatest wave of film-fan necrophilia since the passing of Rudolph Valentino. Almost thirty years later the rumors and the famous naked pictures continue to circulate, but a serious biography has yet to appear.

# 9.

**AMY LOWELL, b. Brookline, Massachusetts, 1874.** As her famous poem "Patterns" implies, Amy Lowell defied her era's stiff, brocaded mores regarding her sex and became a self-liberated woman. She was a militant literary leader in the development of modern American poetry and thumbed her patrician nose at the Boston Brahmins who raised eyebrows at her apparent lesbianism. One of the prominent Boston Lowells, she suffered the physical humiliation of extreme obesity, compensated for by the soul of a poet. Finding fulfillment from her relationship with the actress Ada Dwyer Russell, whom she called "Peter," she journeyed with Ada to London and organized a group of "Imagists," among them D. H. Lawrence, whose writings she championed. Returning to America she wrote ten volumes of verse in thirteen years and a monumental biography of John Keats, in addition to lecturing on modern poetry throughout America. One woman, a Wellesley graduate now eighty-five, remembers sitting with her classmates at Lowell's feet and worrying lest the immense poet fall and crush them. Amy Lowell, whose verse is fragile and ethereally

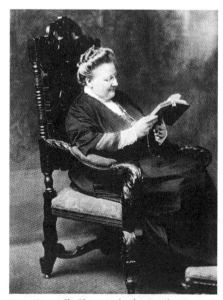

**Amy Lowell:** She smoked Manila cigars and called her actress lover "Peter."

beautiful, smoked Havana cigars and was said (by Mercedes de Acosta) to be able to spit a cigar tip into a spittoon fifteen feet away.

# 10.

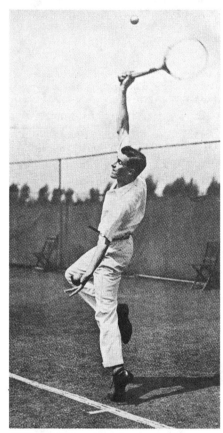

**William Tilden:** Tennis, anyone?

**WILLIAM "BIG BILL" TILDEN, b. Philadelphia, Pennsylvania, 1893.** Back in the dark ages, before one had to be a certified public boor in order to become a tennis star, Bill Tilden was tennis champion of the world and almost as popular a sportsman as Babe Ruth, his contemporary. A member of the Davis Cup team through the 1920s, he turned pro in 1931, when attempts were made to cash in on his immense popularity by turning him into a movie star, an attempt that failed. He came a cropper with the law

when caught in *flagrante delicto* with an adolescent boy, an event that shattered his career and life. Although Roman Polanski is still making films, albeit not in the home of the brave and land of the free, and Billie Jean King is still a reigning tennis queen, it was Bill Tilden's tragic luck to have been born fifty years too soon.

# 11.

**AHMED TEVFIK PASHA, Khedive of Egypt, b. Istanbul, 1845.** Aside from his wild, gay youth, from which he apparently "recovered" in order to please the English masters under whom he ruled, there's little here worth reporting. Once you've seen one wild, gay youth, you've seen them all.

# 12.

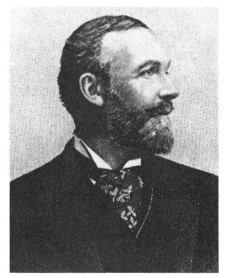

**Philipp zu Eulenburg-Hertefeld:** The German Oscar Wilde.

**PHILIPP, PRINCE ZU EULEN-BURG-HERTEFELD, b. Königsberg, Germany, 1847.** Those who

think that Oscar Wilde was the only popular figure crucified for the love that dare not speak its name, don't know their Geman history. The Eulenburg trial, if anything, was even smarmier than the Wilde case, since the reasons for "exposing" the well-liked and gentle Eulenburg were strictly political. The favorite of Kaiser Wilhelm II, Eulenburg had attempted to dissuade the emperor from a militaristic course and naturally had to be disposed of in the quickest way by the merchants of death. Smeared as a "degenerate" by his enemies, the oldest political dirty trick in the book, Eulenburg was swiftly ruined and conveniently out of the way. The indirect result of this ugly incident was World War I.

# 13.

**PINDAR, b. near Thebes, c. 518 B.C.** Why a Greek poet on February 13 when it's impossible to know the precise birth dates of the ancients? Because the one well-known modern gay born on this day is neither dead nor out of the closet, that's why. So this is as good a place as any to mention Pindar, the greatest lyric poet of ancient Greece, whose love for Theoxenus of Tenedos is celebrated in his verses.

# 14.

**ST. VALENTINE, martyred c. 270.** No, no, no, no, no. Don't jump to conclusions. St. Valentine was not gay, but neither did he have anything to do with the holiday for lovers that bears his name. That St. Valentine, one of the more boring Christian martyrs, is the patron saint of lovers is a mere fluke. You see, the Norman word *galatin,* meaning a lover, was often written and pronounced *valentin,* and through a natural confusion of names, St. Valentine became associated with love. Benjamin Franklin, that old straight lecher, hated this sentimental day. The periwigged cheapskate, you'll recall, preferred to have *old* lovers "because they were so much more grateful," by which he meant he could have his fun without spending any jack. Ben, I think, deserved to be straight. This deliberately goofy Valentine's message was brought to you through the courtesy of the celebrity whose name is discreetly hidden within this paragraph.

# 15.

**JOHN SCHLESINGER, b. London, 1926.** The great English film director is an unheralded pioneer. His *Midnight Cowboy* (1969) was kicked to pieces by the critics for being too gay, and by militant gays for not being gay enough. Even Vito Russo, in *The Celluloid Closet,* pummels the film for daring to present "homosexuals as losers and freaks." Didn't anyone bother to read James Leo Herlihy's book in which *everyone,* by virtue of living in the 20th century, is a loser and a freak? If Schlesinger got it between the eyes for *Midnight Cowboy,* his even better film, *Sunday, Bloody Sunday* (1971), was (in America, at least) a box-office bomb. Who was going to pay good money to see, yecch, anything as disgusting as two men kissing? A decade later Americans were queuing up around the block to see Michael Caine and Christopher Reeve kiss in *Death Trap* and actually applauding the big moment. Poor John Schlesinger. It never pays to be the first kid on the block.

# 16.

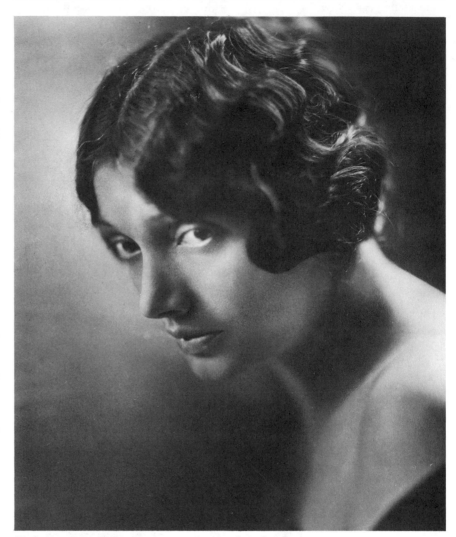

**Katharine Cornell:** Hers was a marriage made in heaven.

**KATHARINE CORNELL, b. Berlin, Germany, 1898.** *A Bill of Divorcement, Casanova, The Green Hat, The Age of Innocence, The Barretts of Wimpole Street, Romeo and Juliet, St. Joan, The Wingless Victory*—Katharine Cornell was one of the great actresses of the American stage, and starred in many of its greatest hits. For over forty years she and her husband, Guthrie McClintick, who produced most of her theatrical successes, were the envy of Broadway. Against all odds, considering their profession, theirs was a happy marriage, a successful business partnership, a close friendship. What they also shared in comon was their bisexuality, exercised to suit their needs, maturely, honestly. In many ways they were the American Vita Sackville-West and Harold Nicolson.

**SUSAN B. ANTHONY, b. Adams, Massachusetts, 1920.** If the federal government had deliberately set out to sabotage the first American coin to commemorate a woman, and per-

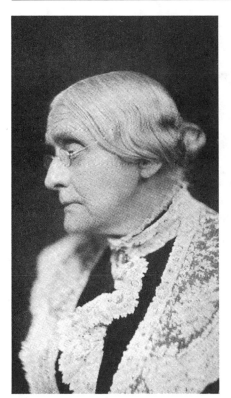

**Susan B. Anthony:** Love letters to "My Dear Chicky Dicky Darling."

haps it did, it could not have done better than to choose Susan B. Anthony as the honorand. Not merely the funny shape of the Anthony dollar killed it; the choice of Susan B. helped. It's not that the pioneering American feminist isn't a great figure worthy of respect and honor; she is. It's the confusion in the public mind as to who she was, most people thinking that she carried a hatchet and demolished saloons, the old bat. Carrie Nation she wasn't, but it's the clothes of her period that confuse and put off people. Every woman of a certain age looked like Whistler's mother then, or like doilies on an easy chair in mourning. What Susan B. needed was a modern image, the way the White Rock Girl and Betty Crocker have been periodically updated. Perhaps it would have helped to publicize her love letters to Anna Dickinson — the ones that began, "My Dear Chicky Dicky Darling."

**HORATIO FORBES BROWN, b. Nice, France, 1854.** Alas, poor Brown. When the English writer died in 1926, his executors burned almost all his unpublished works, attempting to hide what his acquaintances already knew. Like the tastes of so many of his upper-class colleagues, Brown's ran to sailors, footmen, tram conductors, and other strapping members of the lower orders. One of his surviving poems, a psychological gem, depicts a boring society musicale in which Brown can't keep his eyes off a broad-shouldered servant when he should be concentrating on the performing artiste. Each stanza ends with the line, "But I liked their footman John the best." And he did, too.

# 17.

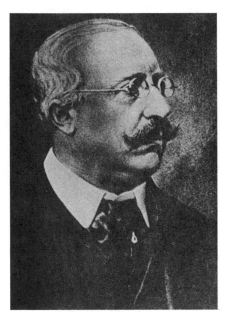

**Fritz Krupp:** At one of his parties, a general dropped dead in a pink tutu.

**FRIEDRICH ALFRED KRUPP, b. Essen, Germany, 1854.** Brought up, like Frederick the Great, to fulfill the ambitions of a father who hated him, the heir to the German munitions

empire spent much of his life waiting for his old man to die so that he could cut loose. And cut loose he did, particularly in Italy, where he consecrated a "holy" grotto — "the Hermitage of Fra Felice" — dedicated to entertaining Italian youths. Within the grotto, and dressed in the robes of a Franciscan monk, Fritz Krupp would frolic with his favorite boys as sex was accompanied by three violins and orgasms by fireworks. The crowning touch was a delightful bit of Teutonic kitsch: As in a Playboy Club with all the bunnies adolescent males, "members" were given keys, shaped like miniature golden bullets, and designed by Fritz himself. They would have been a laff-riot at Belsen-Bergen.

# 18.

**BILLY DE WOLFE, b. Wollaston, Massachusetts, 1907.** Billy De Wolfe was different from the other comedians who played harried, effeminate, prissy characters. He had a silly moustache that became his veritable trademark at a time when most men were smooth-faced. His favorite shtick was playing middle-class matrons taking tea, and in full drag, complete with hat and polka-dotted eye-veil. With the moustache a distinctive touch of incongruity, he was really very, very funny, looking as he did like Alice Toklas in late middle age, only better dressed.

# 19.

**CARSON McCULLERS, b. Columbus, Georgia, 1917.** When she was twenty-three, the gifted novelist and playwright wrote of "the hungry search of people for an escape from individual loneliness, for self-expression and for identification with what each most idealizes in human living." Her own hungry search led to marriage to the homosexual Reeves McCullers, who eventually killed himself; a love affair with composer David Diamond, who was simultaneously sleeping with her husband; to infatuations with Greta Garbo, Erica Mann, and other women; and to such works as *The Heart Is a Lonely Hunter, The Member of the Wedding,* and *Reflections in a Golden Eye.* Because of her sad life, or in spite of it, she remains compulsively readable.

# 20.

**ROBERT LYGON, SEVENTH EARL BEAUCHAMP, b. London, 1872.** In the years before the trial of Oscar Wilde, English aristocrats involved in homosexual scandals went into voluntary exile on the Continent until the heat died down at home. In the years immediately following the trial, public exposure was positively ruinous. The Seventh Earl Beauchamp is included here not because his situation was any better or worse than that of other "disgraced" men of his age, but because his case prompted one of the most famous lines in gay history. In hearing that the young man was homosexual, King George V remarked, "I thought they shot themselves." Unfortunately, so did far too many young people growing up gay.

# 21.

**HARRY STACK SULLIVAN, b. Norwich, New York, 1892.** In the

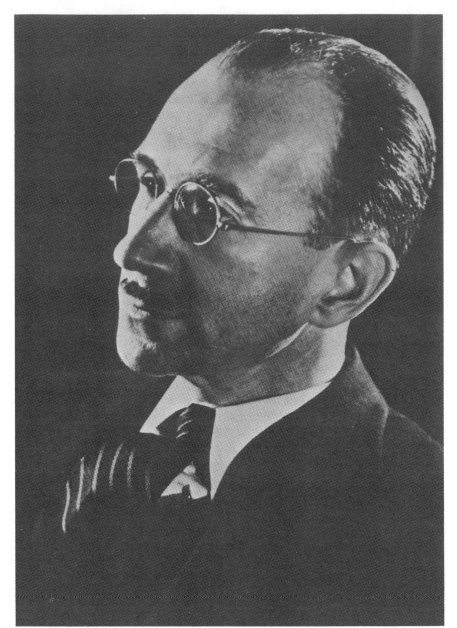

**Harry Stack Sullivan:** He adopted a fifteen-year-old male patient.

understanding of mental disorders, this influential psychiatrist believed that psychoanalysis, although essentially valid, needed to be supplemented by a thoroughgoing study of the impact of cultural forces upon the personality. In the years following his death in 1949, recognition of his accomplishments was intentionally overlooked because of his homosexuality. Sullivan, however, is now acknowledged as the prime developer of the interpersonal approach to psychiatry and as one of the greatest American psychiatrists of the century. Forgotten, finally, is his great "sin." In middle age he adopted a fifteen-year-old male patient, with whom he lived as "father" and "son" for more than fifteen years.

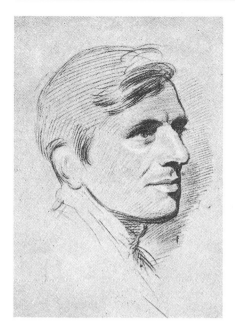

**Cardinal Newman:** A night in bed with the corpse of Brother Ambrose.

## JOHN HENRY, CARDINAL NEWMAN, b. London, 1801.

There's no denying that the great English churchman's most important work, the *Apologia pro Vita Sua,* contains many homoerotic passages of intense beauty, but there is little reason to suspect that his love for other men extended to the flesh itself. Newman was particularly devoted to his friend Brother Ambrose, fourteen years his junior. Grief-stricken by his death in 1875, the cardinal threw himself upon the deathbed and spent the night with the corpse. Newman joined his friend in death fifteen years later. By his own instructions, his body was buried in the same grave. By anyone's measure, theirs was a pretty close friendship.

## W. H. AUDEN, b. York, England, 1907.

Aside from graduate school courses in English literature, where life is taken very seriously, the question about the great English poet that most people want answered is: Did Auden write a poem about a blow job or didn't he? The answer is yes, he did. The poem, written in 1948 to

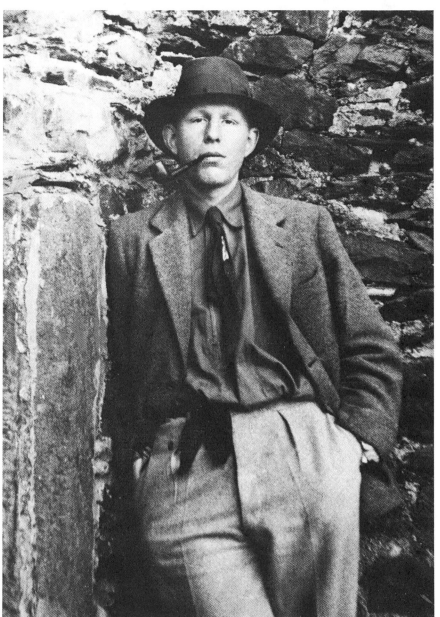

**W. H. Auden:** When his face developed its famous wrinkles, Igor Stravinsky remarked: "Soon we shall have to smooth him out to see who it is."

amuse hmself and his friends, is actually called "The Platonic Blow," although it sometimes appears in unauthorized form as "The Gobble Poem," hardly a title that a poet of Auden's quality would have chosen. After *Fuck You: A Magazine of the Arts* published the poem without the poet's permission in 1965, "A Platonic Blow" was issued in "a

Trade edition" of 300 copies and "a Rough Trade edition of 5 numbered copies, each with beautiful slurp drawings by the artist Joe Brainard." The poem's first two lines suggest its flavor: "It was a Spring day, a day for a lay, when the air/Smelled like a locker-room, a day to blow or get blown." Auden proudly admitted authorship in 1968.

# 22.

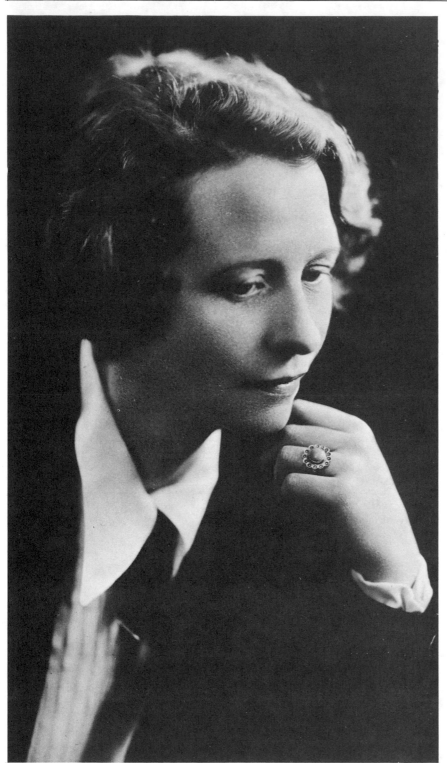

**Edna St. Vincent Millay:** In many of her most passionate poems, the sex of the beloved is uncertain, if not deliberately concealed.

**EDNA ST. VINCENT MILLAY, b. Rockland, Maine, 1892.** It's time for a new biography of this American poet, whose name sounds like the first line of a dirty limerick and whose life was most likely a bisexual romp, even though the early biographies make it difficult to know for sure. For the moment, the poems themselves will have to serve as biography, making it difficult to believe that the poet who dreamed of a lover with a "pink camellia-bud . . . beside a silver comb" was dreaming of anything other than another woman.

# 23.

**POPE PAUL II (né Pietro Barbo), b. Venice, 1417.** Exceptionally vain— and not without reason, since he was a very good-looking man—Paul wanted to take the name "Formosus I," the Well-Shaped, upon his election. Any name chosen would have been better than the one given him sarcastically by his successor, Pius II—"Maria Pietissima," Our Lady of Pity. All of this is rumor, of course, as is the story of his death of a heart attack while playing bottom to his favorite top. Popes have a lot of enemies, you know.

**GEORGE FREDERICK HANDEL, b. Halle, Lower Saxony, Germany, 1685.** Of the German composer who anglicized the spelling of his name upon removing to England, a contemporary wrote: "His social affectations were not very strong; and to this it may be imputed that he spent his whole life in a state of celibacy; that he had no female attachments of another kind may be ascribed to a better reason." What was the "better reason" that made Handel eschew not only marriage, but "female attachments of another kind," presumably mistresses or whores?

Was it the fear of syphilis or the possibility that the composer was homosexual? The evidence thus far is inconclusive, but the latter is more than probable.

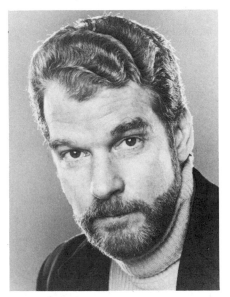

**Doric Wilson:** Funny, free-wheeling, irreverent . . . and razor-sharp.

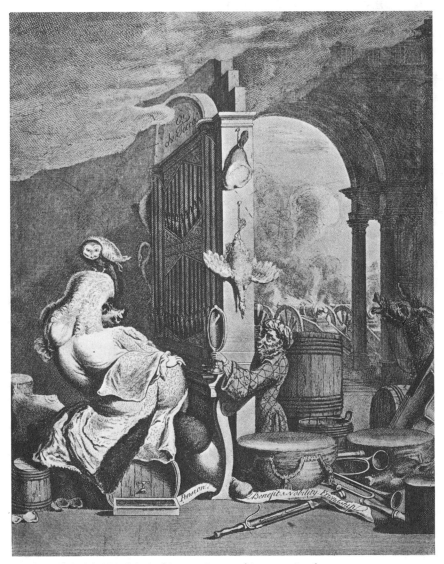

**George Frederick Handel:** As his enemies saw him—a vain glutton.

ceptions, an alternative playwright too good to write bad plays. A pioneer in the Off-Off-Broadway movement, he is completely committed to alternative theater and over the past twenty years has written, directed, and produced more than a hundred productions. Such plays as *Forever After, A Perfect Relationship,* and *The West Side Gang* make him not only "one of a handful of leading contemporary playwrights who deal frankly with the gay experience," but a satirist of the first order whose targets—hypocrisy, cant, and simple human foibles—are universal.

# 24.

**DORIC WILSON, b. Los Angeles, California, 1939.** It's not entirely uncharitable to say that some gay playwrights write for "alternative theatre" because they *have* no alternative. Wrapped in the rationalization that Broadway sucks, they are actually not good enough to write the bad plays that become commercial hits. Doric Wilson is one of the ex-

# 25.

**RICHARD HURRELL FROUDE, b. Dartington, Devonshire, England, 1803.** No, this is not one of Tolkien's little critters, but an English churchman who was a friend and apostle of John Henry Newman. Sexually, Froude is typical of Newman's Oxford movement: a lot of sighing and groaning, an appreciation of the beauty of youth (male), and no physical sex whatever. Froude's poetry, more homoerotic than Newman's, suggests that if he would've, he could've.

# 26.

**CHRISTOPHER MARLOWE, baptised Canterbury, England, 1564.** Marlowe is gay by default. So little is known about him, so many theories advanced over the centuries to create a persona to match his works, that one can almost pick and choose the characteristics one wishes he might have had. What is known is that he was a young firebrand, an anti-clerical rebel in trouble with the law, and that he was dead at twenty-nine after being stabbed in a tavern brawl. His surviving works, to one degree or another, contain homoerotic passages of unsurpassed beauty, so it is even possible that the report of an early critic that Marlowe was "stabbed to death by a bawdy servingman, a rival of his in his lewde love," may be correct. To Marlowe is attributed the epigram, "All they that love not tobacco and boys are fools," which may very well define what his critic meant by "lewde love." If he were alive today, he might likely be a rock musician singing "Lewd Love/Lude Love" or the like. He appears to have been very much a modern man.

**MABEL DODGE LUHAN, b. Buffalo, New York, 1879.** Mabel Ganson Evans Dodge Sterne Luhan, to give her all her names, was married four times (the last time to an American Indian), had countless lovers, was enormously rich, and virtually originated the idea of "radical chic" by inviting to her salons in New York, Italy, and New Mexico the sort of people usually excluded from

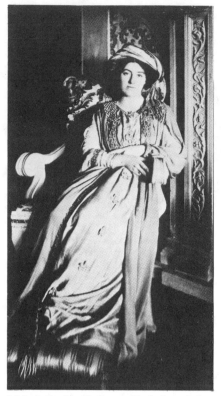

Mabel Dodge Luhan: "I slathered her breast with my dripping lips."

the guest lists of the rich—labor leaders, homosexuals, revolutionary artists, Bolsheviks, *outré* types like John Reed, Margaret Sanger, and D. H. Lawrence. She was also aware of her lesbianism and, more astonishing still, wrote about it for the world to see in a memoir, *Backgrounds,* published in 1933. In every way she was fifty years ahead of her time.

# 27.

**SAPPHO, b. Mytilene on Lesbos, 6th century B.C.** Called "the tenth Muse" by Plato, Sappho was the greatest of all the early Greek lyric poets. Facts about her life are scant, but not scant enough to let stand the nonsense about her having thrown herself into the sea from the Leucadian promontory in consequence of her advances having been rejected by the beautiful youth Phaon. The aristocratic Sappho was completely self-contained in her love for other women. Phaon might have been beautiful, but he was a commoner and a male. For these reasons, Sappho wouldn't have touched him even if he had a ten foot pole. That someone in ancient times decided that what Sappho really needed was a good man, and tacked this phony ending on her story, is only too typical of the male reaction to the fact of lesbianism over the centuries.

# 28.

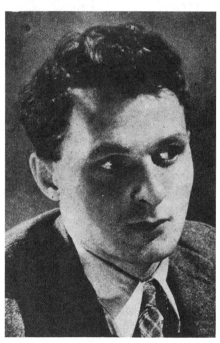

Stephen Spender: Who was the real "Jimmy Younger," his boyhood lover?

**STEPHEN SPENDER, b. London, 1909.** Of the English Trinity, Auden-Isherwood-Spender, only the latter is rarely given his due. Although Spender is mentioned in many biographies and studies of modern

English writers, his appearances are walk-ons, where he delivers his lines and disappears for another hundred pages. Even in Isherwood's *Christopher and His Kind,* where his is a major role, he seems to recede into the background, despite his height and unruly shock of hair. In reading these works one gets the impression that Auden took his virginity and that Isherwood gave it back to him. What is *his* version of their youthful friendships? Since this important poet, editor, and critic's autobiography appeared more than thirty years ago, when one had to talk and write in whispers, we can hardly know.

## Other Personalities Born in February

2. **Mary Anne Talbot,** English sailor known as the "British Amazon," 1778
   **James Joyce,** Irish writer (see his poem "On the Beach at Fontana"), 1882
   **Jonathan Katz,** American writer, 1938

3. **Benjamin Musser,** American poet, 1889

5. **Louis Christophe Lamoricière,** French general, 1806
   **J. K. Huysmans,** French writer, 1848
   **Ricardo Viñes,** Spanish pianist, 1875

6. **Anne,** Queen of Great Britain and Ireland, 1665
   **F. W. H. Myers,** English classicist and poet, 1843

8. **Guercino** (né Giovanni Francesco Barbieri), Italian writer, 1591
   **Jackie Curtis,** American actor, 1947

9. **Jan Ladislav Dussek,** Czech pianist and composer, 1761
   **Digby Mackworth Dolben,** English poet, 1848
   **Robert Hope Jones,** English engineer, 1889
   **Brendan Behan,** Irish writer, 1923

11. **Karoline von Günderode,** German poet, 1780

15. **Bàbur,** Indian warrior and writer, 1483

16. **Bishop C. W. Leadbeater,** American theosophist, 1847

21. **Carl Czerny,** Austian pianist and composer, 1791
    **George Birisima, American actor and playwright, 1924**

22. **Frèdèric Chopin,** Polish pianist and composer, 1810
    **R. S. S. Baden-Powell,** British army officer, 1857
    **Jane Bowles,** American writer, 1917
    **Joanna Russ,** American SF novelist, 1937
    **Lige Clarke,** American activist and writer, 1944
    **Felice Picano,** American writer, 1944
    **Karla Jay,** American activist and writer, 1947

26. **Ferdinand,** King of Bulgaria, 1861

28. **Michel de Montaigne,** French essayist, 1533

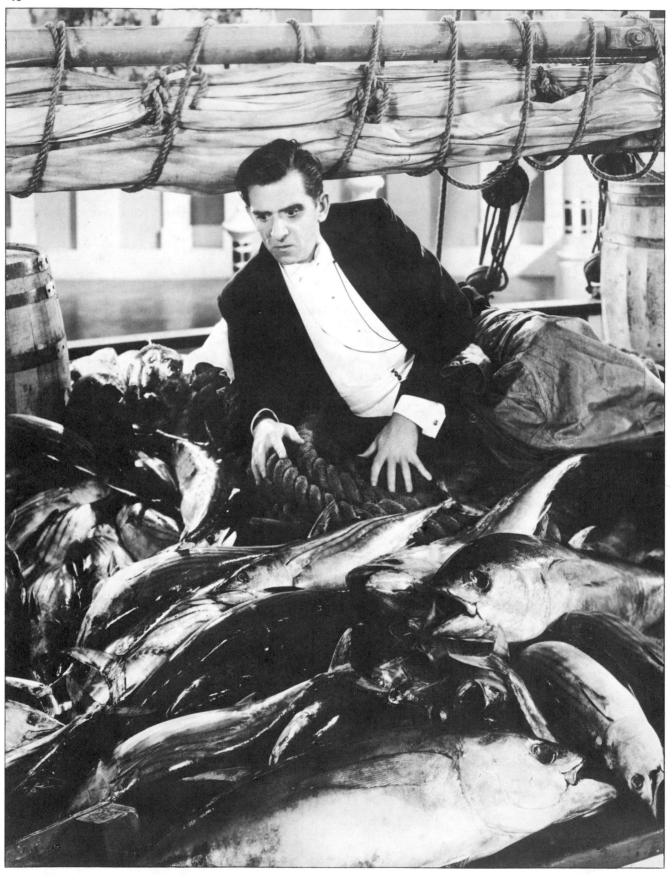

**Edward Everett Horton:** An aversion to fish.

# MARCH

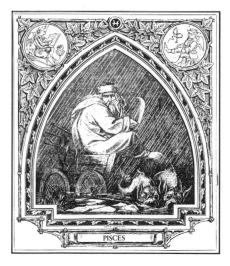

Pisces (February 19th to March 20th), a mutable watery sign, possesses the Jupiterean intellect, but is passive in personality, generally reacting to situations and people rather than imposing himself on them. But, as a child of Neptune, he has the Neptunian qualities of sensitivity and nervousness and tends to live in a world of dreams and imagination. For this reason, many Pisceans are poets, novelists, musicians, artists, and dancers. The strength of the typical Piscean lies in his ideals and aspirations rather than in his actions. He has little or no worldly ambition, cares nothing for rank or power, seldom succeeds in making money, and rarely holds on to it when he has it. His chief weakness, therefore, is that he is almost invariably a burden and a worry to his friends.

## 1.

**LYTTON STRACHEY, b. London, 1880.** Strachey is not only the author of *Eminent Victorians,* one of the most popular books of its day, but also of one of the liveliest rejoinders in gay history. As a conscientious objector during World War I, he was asked what he'd do if a Hun were to rape his sister. "I'd throw myself between them," he replied, with uncharacteristic generosity. (His sister Dorothy, incidentally, was a lesbian.) Because he was such a wit, and because of his battles with John Maynard Keynes over Rupert Brooke, Duncan Grant, and other young men, Strachey is sometimes seen as a bit of an effete twit. But he was experienced enough to tell E. M. Forster that the sexual relationship between the two central characters in *Maurice* was "rather diseased." All

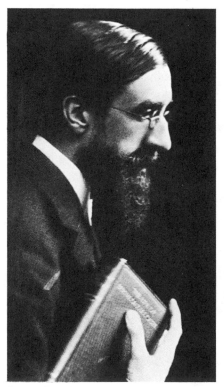

**Lytton Strachey:** Lytton loved Duncan who loved Maynard who loved Duncan. . . .

they ever did, he complained, was masturbate together (all that their creator knew to do, by the way). Strachey thought that there were more interesting things to do, and one of the people with whom he did them was Alan Searle, who eventually became the companion of W. Somerset Maugham. Strachey called young Searle his "little Bronzino," and passed him on to Maugham. Years later, when Searle was sent for to live with the elderly writer, Maugham took one look at what twenty years and pounds had done to Searle and said, "My dear, you used to be quite a dish; now you're quite a tureen."

## 2.

**MARC BLITZSTEIN, b. Philadelphia, Pennsylvania, 1905.** Combining a love of music and theater with

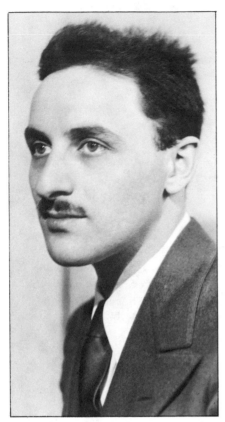

**Marc Blitzstein:** In spirit, a one-man Brecht and Weill.

the social principles of the American left, Marc Blitzstein composed the definitive Depression opera in *The Cradle Will Rock* (1936), the closest work of art produced in America to the genius of Brecht and Weill. It's hardly surprising that Blitzstein's English version of Brecht and Weill's *Three-Penny Opera* ran for years on Broadway and sparked the recent Weill revival. In 1968 the composer was murdered by a hustler in Fort-de-France, Martinique, while at work on an opera about Sacco and Vanzetti.

# 3.

**BEVERLEY NICHOLS, b. London, 1899.** At the age of twenty-five, Beverley Nichols was famous, his

successful book, appropriately called *Twenty-Five,* praised as representing the spirit of the twenties. Ted Morgan's thumbnail sketch in his biography of Maugham is letter perfect: "Beverley was pretty—he looked like a faun escaped from the woods. Beverley was amusing. While at Balliol he had convulsed the Oxford Union with the facetious remark that 'women should have the courage of their complexions.' . . . Beverley was facile, and could write a two-thousand-word interview based on a two-minute meeting. Beverley was flamboyant, like young Byron minus the talent. Beverley was homosexual. . . ." Still, Nichols's books are well worth reading. He may be la-de-da, but he's frequently quite funny and his books on gardening, in particular, are quite lovely.

# 4.

**MERCEDES DE ACOSTA, b. Paris, 1893?, 1900?** What is one to make of this long-forgotten writer? In old age she still affected jet-black hair slicked down with brilliantine, and her autobiography, *Here Lies the Heart* (1960), is just as slippery. An account, in part, of her friendships and amours with famous women, it manages to say everything without saying anything, and its cast of characters is dazzling: Eva Le Gallienne, Poppy Kirk, Claire Charles-Roux, Marie Laurencin, Malvina Hoffman, Alice B. Toklas, and many others. The best scenes, and the most hyperventilated, are those with Marlene Dietrich and Greta Garbo. They have to be read to be believed.

# 5.

**PIER PAOLO PASOLINI, b. Bolo-**

gna, 1922. The renowned poet, novelist, essayist, philologist, translator, and filmmaker (*Salo, or the 120 Days of Sodom*) was open about everything: his homosexuality, his communism, his great compassion for the agonies of the poor, the delinquent, and the young. He once wrote a poem for the dying Pope Pius XII which read in part: "How much good you could have done!/And you/didn't do it:/There was no greater sinner than you." This intelligent and humane man was murdered one night while cruising, but many believe that the murder scene was a set-up to mask a political assassination.

# 6.

**MICHELANGELO BUONAROTI, b. Caprese, Tuscany, 1475.** Everyone knows that Michelangelo was gay. Even Dear Abby who said as much in one of her columns. Poor Abby wound up being gently chewed out by none other than Irving Stone, who insisted that all this queer business was started by that jealous old queen Aretino. After all, would Charlton Heston ever play a fag? Abby stood corrected, although no one even bothered to mention Tommasso Cavalieri, to whom Michelangelo merely wrote his exquisite love sonnets.

# 7.

**COMTE ROBERT DE MONTESQUIOU-FEZENSAC, b. Paris, 1855.** This poison-tongued, poison-penned, aristocrat dandy, poetaster, aesthete, and party giver, some of whose aspects Marcel Proust was to put into his Baron de Charlus, en-

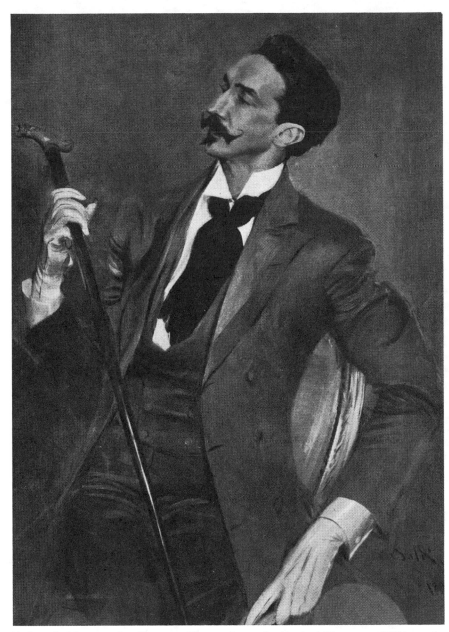

**Robert de Montesquiou-Fezensac:** The aesthete who inspired Huysmans, Wilde, and Proust.

RELIUS ANTONINUS), b. Syria, c. 205. Heliogabalus, the boy emperor of Rome, appears to have been totally madcap, if not completely mad. His great love of swishing ceremony, inherited centuries later by church acolytes, can only be suggested here. Since even mad gay emperors were expected to produce an heir, a suitable bride was chosen for him, and he went through the motions of consummation, finding it all rather futile. But he was impressed with the ceremony itself and later went through it again twice in one night, choosing as his "husband" a well-hung charioteer named Gorianus, and as his "wife" a boy named Hierocles. His wedding night with both was consummated in full public view. He had the makings of a great theatrical producer and virtually invented the casting call by sending out his agents to round up for audition the men with the largest penises in the Roman empire. Eventually his enemies dispatched him with a sword up his bum and dumped his body in a sewer. He was just sweet seventeen.

# 9.

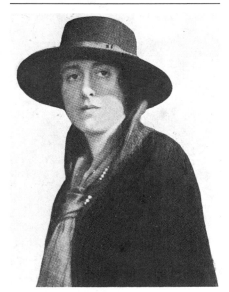

**Vita Sackville-West:** Woolf's Orlando.

dowing his invented character with more flesh and blood than the original, was actually only half an aristocrat, since his mother was merely the daughter of a stockbroker. But, even as an old man, he had his moments. Outraged that the young Jean Cocteau was modeling himself after him, he refused ever to acknowledge the presence of the twenty-year-old upstart. Whenever anyone would attempt to introduce the fawning Cocteau to him, he would pretend to confuse him with the actress Pavlova and say, "I know her well."

# 8.

**HELIOGABALUS (MARCUS AU-**

**VITA SACKVILLE-WEST, b. Knole, Kent, England, 1892.** The story of her marriage to Harold Nicolson—she a lesbian writer and he a gay diplomat—and of her passionate but disastrous affair with Violet Trefusis, is too beautifully told in their son Nigel Nicolson's book, *Portrait of a Marriage,* to require any comment here.

# 10.

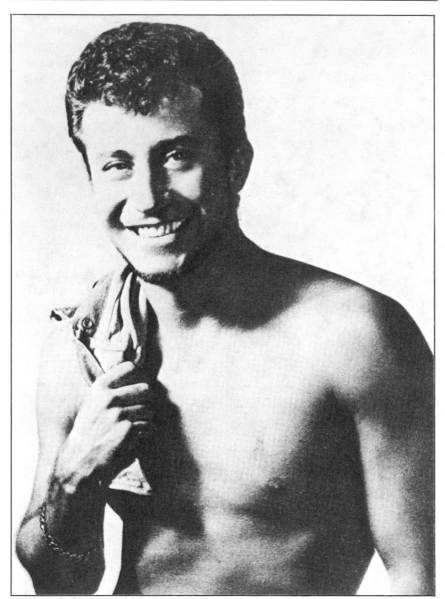

John Rechey: A "sexual outlaw," bodybuilder, and hustler, whose well-wrought prose makes hims an American Jean Genet.

**JOHN RECHY, b. El Paso, Texas, 1934.** *City of Night* (1963) now seems so dated after twenty years that it is hard to remember how enlightening it was in its time as an exploration of the underside of contemporary gay life. An outspoken activist and "sexual outlaw," proud of both his years as a hustler and (like Mishima) his physique, he is not without a sense of humor about both. He reports that he was once told by an irate transvestite at whom he had sneered, "Your muscles are as gay as my drag."

# 11.

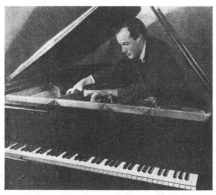

Henry Cowell: Jailed for "sodomy" and abandoned by many of his friends.

**HENRY COWELL, b. Menlo Park, California, 1897.** A great admirer of the music of Charles Ives long before that composer enjoyed any public recognition, Cowells experimented with new musical resources: In his piano compositions he introduced the tone cluster, played with the arm or the fist, and wrote pieces to be played directly on the piano strings. In the mid-1930s, Cowells's career was interrupted by his imprisonment on "morals" charges, during which time, to his eternal shame, Charles Ives completely turned his back on the man who was to prove his sympathetic biographer.

# 12.

**VASLAV NIJINSKY, b. Kiev, Russia, 1890.** His love affair with

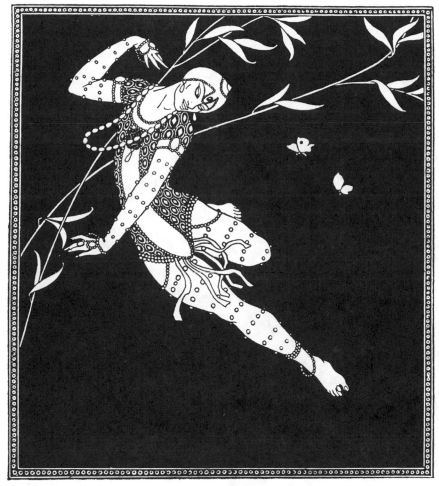

**Vaslav Nijinsky:** Cocteau wrote that "He upsets all the laws of equilibrium, and seems constantly to be a figure painted on the ceiling. . . ."

James responded with "darling Hugh" and "my belovedest little Hugh." Little Hugh, the story goes, once attempted to seduce the virginal James, who promptly broke into tears and cried, "I can't . . . I can't!" Of the many who could, and did, Walpole's greatest loves were the Danish tenor Lauritz Melchior and a married Cornish constable named Harold Cheevers who had once been revolver champion of the British Isles. Like E. M. Forster's London bobby, Cheevers was brawny and masculine and stayed with Walpole until the day the writer died.

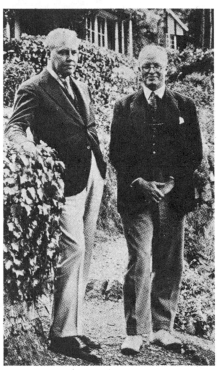

**Carl Van Vechten and Hugh Walpole:** Just good friends.

Diaghilev, his marriage, his madness are known to everyone. But of the thousands of descriptions of the famous Russian dancer, only Jean Cocteau's suggests the "mortal god" that was Nijinsky. Cocteau alone observed "the contrast between the Nijinsky of *Le Spectre de la Rose,* bowing and smiling to thunderous cheers as he took his fifty curtain calls, and the poor athlete backstage between bows, gasping and leaning against any support he could find, half fainting, clutching his side, being given his shower and masssage and rubdown by his attendant and the rest of us. On one side of the curtain he was a marvel of grace; on the other, an extraordinary example of strength and weakness. . . ."

# 13.

**HUGH WALPOLE, b. Auckland, New Zealand, 1884.** As a young man, the future dean of English letters who could make or break literary careers and reputations hero-worshiped Henry James, more than forty years his senior. Walpole called him "my very dear Master," and

# 14.

**STANISLAUS ERIC, COUNT STENBOCK, Estonia, 1860.** In the London of Oscar Wilde, Count Stenbock was the only aesthete who could out-aesthete the great Oscar himself. One never knew what one

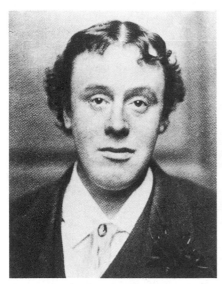

**Count Stenbock:** His "True Story of a Vampire" blends gayness and death.

would find at his house, where he wrote opium-induced poems and stories and where he kept a pet toad named Fatima and a lover picked up on a London bus. Visiting Stenbock one day, Oscar Wilde dared to light a cigarette at the votive lamp before the bust of Shelley that his host venerated. This sacrilege caused Stenbock, in true dandy style, to fall to the floor in a dead faint. The unperturbed Wilde, in even truer form, exhaled a puff of smoke, stepped over the prostrate body, and took his leave.

# 15.

LIONEL JOHNSON, b. Broadstairs, Kent, England, 1867. Johnson was an influential literary critic in his time and wrote, among other books, the first critical study of Thomas Hardy (1894). He was also the victim of one of the oldest ironies in the history of love. He introduced his young lover to a friend who promptly walked off with him. The young lover was Lord Alfred Douglas; the friend, Oscar Wilde. Johnson's poem "The Destroyer of a Soul" ("I hate you with a necessary hate . . .") is, naturally enough, directed to Wilde. Johnson lived only long enough to see Oscar get his and, at thirty-five, died of a fractured skull after falling off a barstool.

# 16.

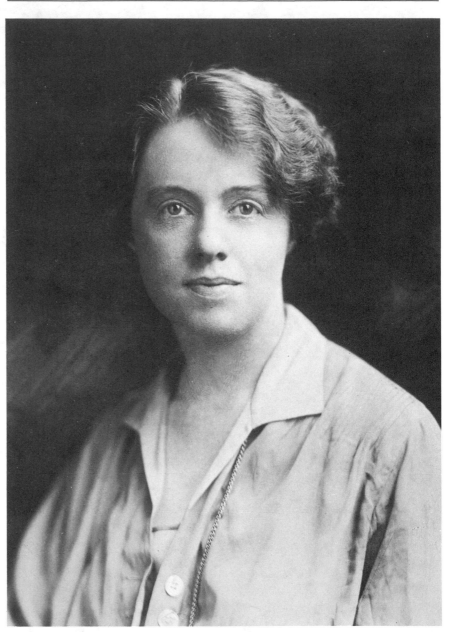

**I. A. R. Wylie:** In love with a woman named George.

I. A. R. WYLIE, b. Melbourne, Australia, 1885. In 1940 novelist I. A. R. (for Ida Alexa Ross) Wylie published a book, now little read, called *My Life with George.* What was unusual about it was not merely its honest treatment of a life shared with someone other than a husband, a lover with whom she had lived for twenty years, but that "George" was in fact another woman—Dr. S. Josephine Baker, a pioneering public health specialist who was famous for having captured "Typhoid Mary." Anyone interested in learning more about Wylie's George, ironically, will have to look Dr. Baker up in old editions of *American Men of Science.* That's right, *Men.* You've come a long way, baby.

# 17.

**RUDOLF NUREYEV, b. Ufa, East Siberia, 1938.** Rudolf Nureyev became the most famous male dancer in the West before he was thirty— and the most publicized. That he partied everywhere and was photographed partying everywhere was as clever a manipulation of the press as Diaghilev's successful attempts to get the public to concentrate on Nijinsky's crotch. "We want Rudi," the fans screamed, "especially in the nudi." It was all part of the show. So when Dave Kopay, an athlete of a different sort, casually mentioned in his best-selling autobiography that

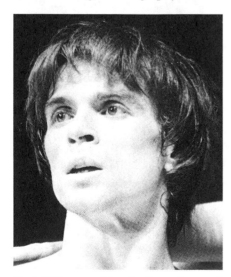

**Rudolf Nureyev:** Muscle, dynamism, and incomparable grace.

Nureyev visited gay bars, no one particularly cared. *The Celebrity Register* had already printed the peculiar warning of an English friend: "I told Rudi, he can be as naughty as he likes, but if he isn't more careful, they're going to find him . . . some morning in an alley in Soho, his head laid open with a lorry driver's spanner." To which the great dancer responded: "I'll die on exactly the day I want." Considering the determination written on his extraordinary face and muscular body, who can possibly doubt that he is right?

# 18.

**EDWARD EVERETT HORTON, b. Brooklyn, New York, 1886.** There's no way to think of the comedies of the '20s, '30s, and '40s without recollecting this lanky, bushy-browed Nervous Nellie. Of all the sissified comedians of the past, he was unquestionably the best, certainly the most eccentric and humanly complicated. Watch him in comic support of Astaire and Rogers in *Top Hat* (1935), where his attempts at getting out of the clutches of Alice Brady provide small gems of gay sexual innuendo and perfect timing. In private life he lived with his mother on a large estate named "Belly Acres." One can almost hear him arguing, in that firm but nervous way of his, "Now, mother. I *like* that name, and I don't *care* that you find it undignified. Belly Acres it *is,* and Belly Acres it *stays.*"

**EDWARD ALBEE, b. Washington, D.C., 1928.** Hailed as the most compelling playwright since Tennessee Williams and Arthur Miller, Albee enjoyed something like instant success as a dramatist. His most powerful work, *Who's Afraid of Virginia Woolf?,* was the most talked-about

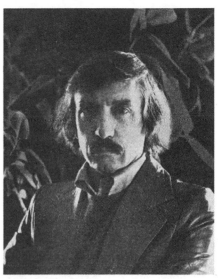

**Edward Albee:** His plays tell us that we are uneasy, without comfort, unhinged.

play of the 1962-63 season. The evening-long argument between a married couple is a strong denunciation of modern marital relationships, amusingly bitchy on the surface but murderously vicious underneath. More than twenty years later, Albee's homophobic critics still insist that George and Martha are actually a male couple in straight drag. What "normal" couple, they insist, would behave so viciously? These critics have apparently not read the divorce statistics lately. In 1963 Albee was denied a Pulitizer Prize for his electrifying play. Wonder why.

# 19.

**OCTAVE THANET (née Alice French), b. Andover, Massachusetts, 1850.** One of the most popular novelists of the late 19th century, Octave Thanet is no longer read, and with good reason. Her stuff is unredeemably dreadful by any standard. (In one novel, for example, the heroine falls in love with a young woman and proceeds to tell her so, nonstop, for twenty-two pages, not

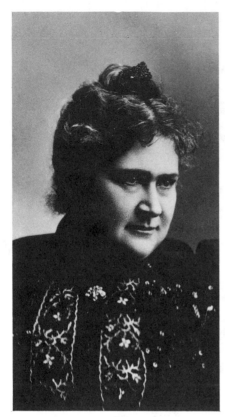

**Octave Thanet:** One of her fans was Calvin Coolidge. It figures.

counting heaves and maidenly sighs.) For fifty years Thanet, a 200-pound six-footer, lived together with petite Jane Crawford at their mansion "Thanford" (for Thanet and Crawford), a name which, one has to admit, does sound better than "Crawet."

**SERGEI DIAGHILEV, b. Novgorod, Russia, 1872.** One cannot underestimate the influence of Diaghilev's Ballets Russes on the development of 20th-century art. But the importance of his homosexuality to Diaghilev's creative art is sometimes overlooked. Had he not been gay, had he not attracted to his cause the great homosexual writers and artists of his day, the stream of 20th-century art might have flowed in a different direction. As Martin Green writes in *Children of the Sun*, "He made the dancer Nijinsky first

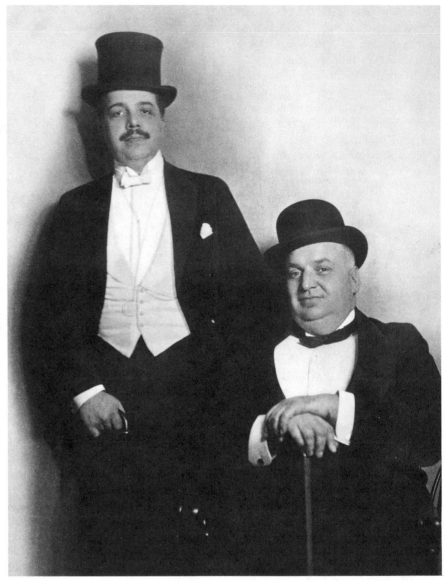

**Diaghilev (with his manager Salisburg):** Svengali to Nijinsky's Trilby, Massine's Trilby, Lifar's Trilby, Dolin's Trilby. . . .

his lover and then his choreographer, slyly displacing Michel Fokine and inspiring Nijinsky to become the company's chief ballet-creator. Diaghilev's superb taste . . . was made manifest in this new Nijinsky, the choreographer, and in the ballets

he created. These works of art were the children of Diaghilev's sexual passion. The same thing happened later with Leonide Massine and Serge Lifar. . . . These men created ballets under the spell of Diaghilev's passion, and he created through them."

# 20.

**LAURITZ MELCHIOR, b. Copenhagen, Denmark, 1890.** The famous

Danish Heldentenor was virtually a household name in the 1930s and

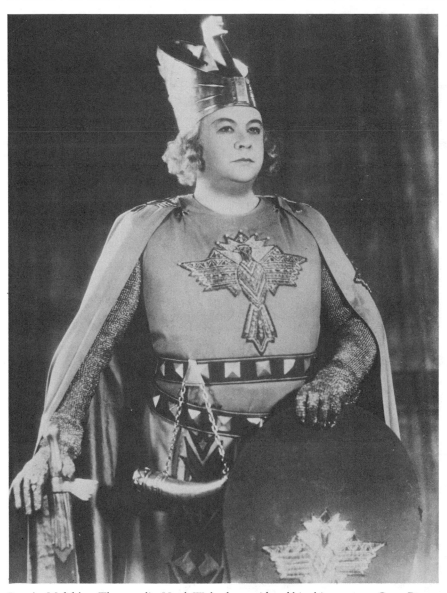

**Lauritz Melchior:** The novelist Hugh Walpole considered him his very own Great Dane.

## 21.

**GAVIN ARTHUR (né Chester A. Arthur III), b. Colorado, 1901.** Gavin Arthur, the grandson of President Chester Arthur, awakened to the fact that he was gay, dropped his all-too-memorable name, and headed out on his own at an early age. Working his way around the world in the merchant marine, he managed through his strong and attractive personality to make the acquaintance of the great gay gurus of his youth —Edward Carpenter, Havelock Ellis, Magnus Hirschfeld. An early apologist for the gay life, and a forerunner of today's gay activists, he collaborated for several years with Hirschfeld, as he later did with Kinsey. His own philosophy is explained in his book *The Circle of Sex* (1966). Arthur is a key figure in what has come to be called the gay "apostolic succession" from Walt Whitman to Allen Ginsberg: Whitman slept with Carpenter, who slept with Arthur, who slept with Neal Cassady (Jack Kerouac's "Dean Moriarity"), who slept with Ginsberg, who slept with Burroughs, etc. It's a quaint idea, this "Whispered Transmission, capital W, capital T," as Ginsberg calls this phenomenally egoistic shtick. Let's hope that Whitman, first on the cosmic daisy chain, didn't have capital V, capital D.

## 22.

**ROSA BONHEUR, b. Bordeaux, France, 1822.** Writers used to explain Rosa Bonheur's penchant for dressing in men's clothing by saying that the famous painter of animals needed a disguise in order to paint unmolested in the markets she fre-

'40s, first because of his Tristan played to Kirsten Flagstad's Isolde at the Met, and later for his appearances in some of MGM's very worst musicals in which he was to opera exactly what José Iturbi was to classical piano playing. One wonders what clean-thinking Louis B. Mayer would have throught had he known that the former opera star, now solving the adolescent love problems of Jane Powell, had once been the lover of novelist Hugh Walpole. Walpole, in fact, had been Melchior's patron (in return for services rendered) and reputedly became hysterical when the singer left him, claiming that he liked women better, after all. Melchior's new persuasion, however, did not prevent him from regularly sharing the shore leaves of an American sailor with his spiritual brother, poet Hart Crane. Is this what Mayer had in mind by good family entertainment?

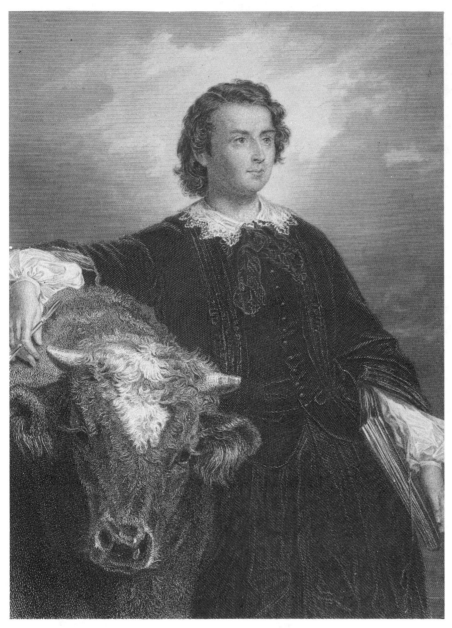

**Rosa Bonheur:** On one of the rare occasions when she dressed as a woman, she was arrested by a gendarme who thought her a male transvestite.

# 23.

**J. C. LEYENDECKER, b. Montabour, Germany, 1874.** Leyendecker was one of the most successful commercial artists of the 20th century, best known, perhaps, as the creator of the Arrow Collar Man. Almost seven decades after the height of his vogue, the Arrow Collar Man still appeals. Blond, classically handsome, patrician, somewhat aloof, probably a bit of a shit, he is definitely more interested in himself than he is in any of the beautiful women pictured with him. When he first appeared in magazine ads, the Arrow Collar people received carloads of fan letters from adoring women eager to discover the identity of the sexy artist's model. Some proposed marriage. Little did they know that the Arrow Collar Man was the artist's lover, Charles Beach, blond, handsome, patrician, vain, and very much a self-interested shit.

# 24.

**CONRADIN, b. Wolfstein, Bavaria, 1252.** Conradin was the last legitimate Hohenstaufen, the son of the assassinated Conrad IV. While he was still a child in Germany, his uncle Manfred made himself king of Sicily (1258), but when Manfred died eight years later, the kingdom was seized by Charles of Anjou. Conradin was persuaded to come to Italy to recover his kingdom, and, accompanied by his lover, Frederick of Baden, titular duke of Austria, he gained the support of several Italian cities. In the end, however, Conradin was captured by Charles, tried as a traitor, and beheaded. His lover, at his own request, was executed with him. Conradin was just sixteen;

quented for her subjects. It's a nice thought, but untrue. Rosa Bonheur, who lived together with Nathalie Micas for most of her life, dressed as a man because she wanted to. She drank, she smoked, she became one of the most popular painters in the world and a member of the French Legion of Honor. She was, in short, very much her own man. As she once said to a male friend who was concerned about her movement through the world of men unchaperoned, "Oh my dear Sir, if you knew how little I care for your sex, you wouldn't get any ideas in your head. The fact is, in the way of males, I like only the bulls I paint."

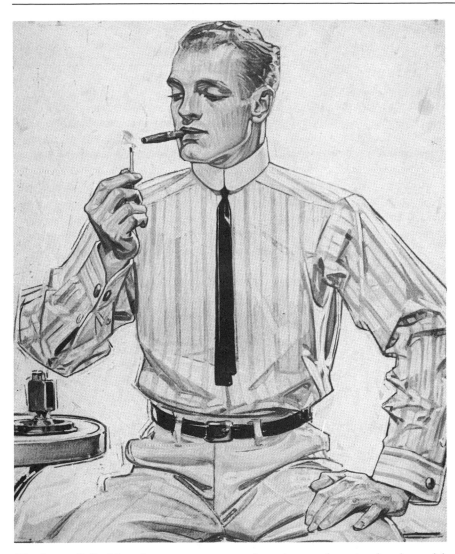

**The Arrow Collar Man:** Some women proposed marriage not knowing that the model was the illustrator's lover.

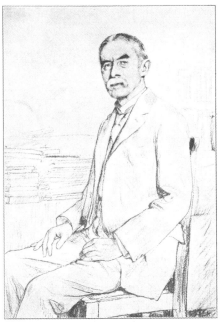

**A. E. Housman:** He sent *A Shropshire Lad* to Oscar Wilde in Reading Gaol.

Frederick, twenty-one. To this day gay lovers make pilgrimages to the church of the monastery of Santa Maria del Carmine at Naples, where the two young men were laid to rest together.

# 25.

**ELTON JOHN, b. Pinner, Middlesex, England, 1947.** You've got to hand it to Elton. Coming out publicly in *Rolling Stone* when he was at the top of the charts took guts. Not many rock stars would have dared to take the risk. But everything's worked out just fine. Elton has a new look and a sharp wit. "Ever since I had that interview in which I said I was bisexual," he grins, "it seems twice as many people wave at me in the streets."

# 26.

**A. E. HOUSMAN, b. Fockbury,**

**Worcestershire, England, 1859.** Alfred Edward Housman was a classical scholar and poet of note. He was once viewed as a great grey presence, divorced from the flesh and married to the mind. Young men read *A Shropshire Lad* and wondered. Was he or wasn't he? There was no way to find out. Later, he was painted as a sad recluse, sighing quiet sighs over a straight friend, Moses Jackson, and jerking off the Muse in unrequited love. In this view, Housman was "in the grip of the 'cursed trouble' that soured the wells of his life, produced his poetry, and urged him to the topmost heights of scholarly renown." Now we learn that the scholarly Cambridge don, far from being "cursed," used to make merry with a string of Venetian gondoliers supplied by his friend Horatio Brown, and was as well a regular patron of the male brothels in Paris. Can it be that the myth of the scholar virgin is just that, a myth?

**TENNESSEE WILLIAMS, b. Columbus, Mississippi, 1911.** Changing his name because he thought

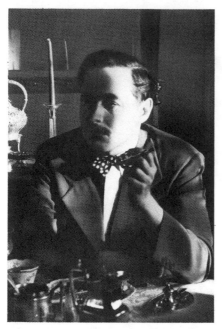

**Tennessee Williams:** His letters reveal him to be the chicken hawk of all time.

"Thomas Lanier Williams" sounded "like it might belong to the sort of writer who turns out sonnet sequences to Spring," Tennessee Williams won the New York Drama Critics Award in 1945 with his first Broadway production, *The Glass Menagerie.* The rest is history. If at times Williams has appeared to be his own worst enemy, he has long lived with the pressure of having been the first publicly-known gay celebrity in America. It cannot have been much fun to watch his great Blanche DuBois undressed in quest for her penis by homophobic critics obsessed with proving that gay men know nothing about straight love. His other heroines have been similarly violated. If all writers pay a price for fame, Williams, being openly gay, has paid more than his share.

# 27.

**MARIA SCHNEIDER, b. Paris, 1952.** The talented actress, who claims to be the illegitimate daughter of French star Daniel Gelin, played opposite Marlon Brando, as it were, in *Last Tango in Paris.* For several days in 1975 there was a great deal of heavy breathing in tabloids all over the world when Schneider, declaring the "right to be insane," checked into a Rome mental hospital so that she could be near her committed lover, American heiress Patty Townsend. Then the tumult died down. And her name started to disappear from most of the standard reference books. Isn't that strange?

# 28.

**JANE RULE, b. 1931.** This Canadian novelist, critic, and teacher has written several acclaimed works of fiction, including *This Is Not for You* and *Against the Season.* But the essential Jane Rule can be seen most directly in her remarkable book *Lesbian Images* (1975) in which she attempts to set down nothing less than what it means to be a lesbian. She realizes this aim beautifully by measuring her own attitudes toward the lesbian experience against the images made by other women writers, including Gertrude Stein, Willa Cather, Radclyffe Hall, Vita Sackville-West, Elizabeth Owen, and Maureen Duffy among others. When Rule's first novel, *The Desert of the Heart,* was published in 1964 a critic, complaining of the lesbian subject matter, wrote: "But all the time you keep turning to the photograph of the author on the jacket and wondering how such a nice looking woman could ever have chosen so distasteful a subject." Read *Lesbian Images* not only to discover why she writes on "so distasteful a subject," but for a compassionate explanation of how any critic could have written anything so terribly, terribly sad.

# 29.

**DIRK BOGARDE** (né Dirk Niven van de Bogaerde), b. London, 1921. Before agreeing to play the role of a blackmailed homosexual barrister in *Victim* (1961), a film that pleaded for the decriminalization of homosexual acts, Dirk Bogarde had specialized in playing leading men in light comedies. "It was a tremendous departure, playing 'my first queer,'" he writes. "The fanatics who had been sending me 4,000 letters a week stopped overnight . . . not because I was playing a homosexual, but because I was playing a middle-aged man." Bogarde, one of the great British film actors, is included in these pages not because of his role in *Victim,* but because of a bizarre childhood experience with a Mr. Dodd that the actor relates in his memoirs. Mr. Dodd, who it seems had a fetish for bandages, picked young Bogarde up in a cinema, took him back to his flat on the pretext of showing him books about mummies, tied him up with bandages, and seduced him. The reader is advised that this story is retold here for the historic record only and that one swallow doth not a summer make.

# 30.

**PAUL VERLAINE, b. Metz, France, 1844.** Did he or didn't he? We know that Verlaine wrote eighteen volumes of verse in alternating moods of sensuality and mysticism, that he wandered over Europe with that strange and perverse young poet Arthur Rimbaud, that he was imprisoned for two years after shooting his lover. But did he in fact write a poem that is almost certain never to be taught in French I—the so-called

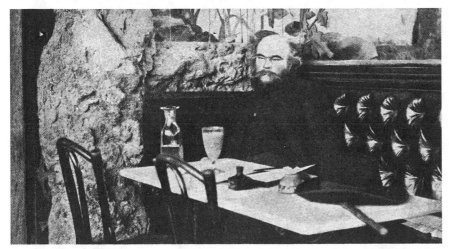

Paul Verlaine: After prison, poverty, and drink—the satisfaction that tourists were seeking him out to stare.

"Sonnet to an Asshole"? The chances are that he did. Even in English translation, the poem reflects the musical quality that was Verlaine's hallmark: "Dark and wrinkled like a deep pink,/It breathes, humbly nestled among the moss/Still wet with love. . . ."

# 31.

EDWARD FITZGERALD, b. Breedfield, Suffolk, England, 1809. In 1851 FitzGerald published a work called *Euphranor: A Dialogue on Youth* in memory of a friend who had died young. In it he recounts how, after the death of his beloved William Kenworthy Browne, he cruised the Suffolk docks "looking for some fellow to accost me and fill a very vacant place in my heart." Whether he was in fact accosted, and whether his vacant place was filled, he does not say. But fifteen years later, now famous as the translator of *The Rubaiyat of Omar Khayyam*, FitzGerald returned to the docks and became part owner of a herring-lugger, *Meum and Teum*. The "You" of the *I and You* was a strapping young fisherman named Joseph Fletcher, whom he called "Posh." Although FitzGerald wrote about being taken with Posh's blue eyes and auburn hair, and although several letters addressed to "My Dear Poshy" have survived, there is no proof that the virile Posh ever actually filled FitzGerald's vacant place. For the sake of love, let us hope that he did.

## Other Personalities Born in March

1. **James Grove Fulton,** U.S. congressman, 1890.
   **Dimitri Mitropoulos,** Greek conductor, 1896.

3. **John Moray Stuart-Young,** English poet, 1881
   **James Merrill,** American poet, 1926

5. **Dr. Louise Pearce,** American medical researcher, 1885

7. **Maurice Ravel,** French composer, 1875
   **Parker Tyler,** American writer, 1907

9. **Samuel Barber,** American composer, 1910
   **Thomas Schippers,** American conductor, 1930

11. **Torquato Tasso,** Italian poet, 1544
    **Joe Brainard,** American poet and artist, 1942

12. **Thomas Augustine Arne,** English composer, 1710
    **Lady Hester Stanhope,** English traveler and eccentric, 1776
    **Jack Kerouac,** American writer, 1922

13. **Janet Flanner,** American writer, 1892

14. **Olive Fremstad,** American opera singer, 1871

18. **Marquis de Custine,** French writer, 1790

19. **Daniel Curzon,** American writer, c. 1939

20. **Friedrich Hölderlin,** German poet, 1770

21. **Giulio Alberoni,** Italian statesman, 1664
    **Modest Mussorgsky,** Russian composer, 1839
    **John Paul Hudson,** American writer, actor, activist, 1929

26. **Benjamin Thompson, Count Rumford,** American-born English scientist, 1753

27. **Perry Deane Young,** American writer, 1941

28. **Mary C. Du Bois,** American writer, 1879

30. **Muhammed II,** Turkish sultan, 1432

31. **Gustaf Mauritz Armfelt,** Finnish-born Swedish statesman, 1757
    **Nikolai Gogol,** Russian writer, 1801

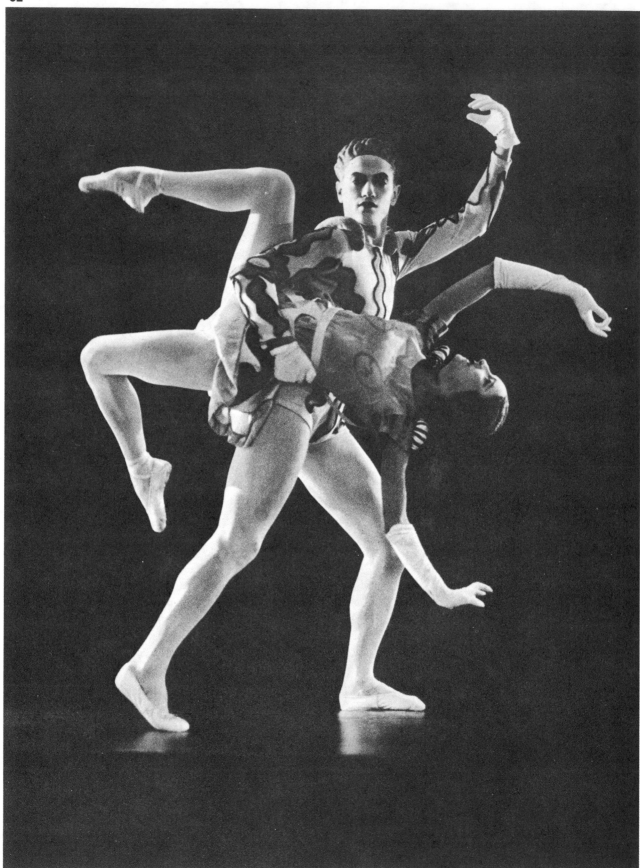

**Sergei Lifar:** He was sexless and felt desire for neither men nor women, but he wanted the attention of Diaghilev and knew just how to get it.

# APRIL

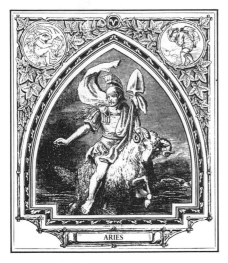

Aries (March 21st to April 20th), a cardinal fiery sign, is ruled by Mars, the planet which is declared to be the chief center of divine energy. The martial type, naturally enough, is always aching for a fight, and the type of fight most congenial to the Arietan is what astrologer Isabelle Pagan calls the "forward charge!" "He is the captain, the leader, the pioneer among men, going out in sympathy to new thought, rapidly assimilating fresh ideas . . . Enterprise and ardor are the characteristics of the type." The ram, after all, is an aggressive, fierce-tempered, wilful sign. Arietans are very social, very lively, and no type is more warmhearted or more affectionate. Because he is so easily befriended, the Arietan can disappoint, since his great energy leads him to outgrow his friends very rapidly.

## 1.

FERRUCCIO BUSONI, b. Empoli, Florence, Italy, 1866. This important musician was torn by several major conflicts. Like Rachmaninoff, he was one of the greatest pianists of his day, yet yearned for more time for composing, his first love. He was an Italian who wanted to contribute to the musical life of his own country, and yet was far more attracted to the musical heritage of Germany, where he settled and spent most of his life. He was married, but apparently liked the fellas, too. At least that's what pianist Egon Petri (1881-1962) claimed—and he was in a position to know. He once walked in on his famous teacher and discovered him in bed with Italian Futurist painter Umberto Boccioni.

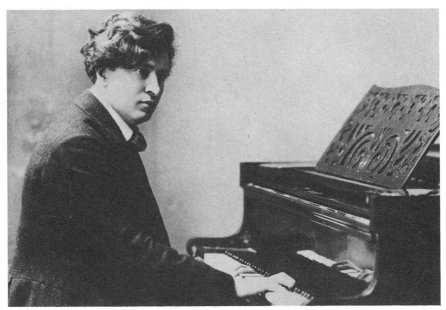

Ferruccio Busoni: His tastes were clear in music and in art: Bach and Liszt are fine, but Futurism sucks.

## 2.

HANS CHRISTIAN ANDERSEN, b. Odense, Denmark, 1805. Forget that silly Danny Kaye movie of yesteryear in which Hans sings to inchworms and measures all the marigolds. Andersen was an odd duck, all right, but odd in ways not even hinted at in that Technicolor atrocity. The *real* story, on the contrary, might actually make a good film. One can already see the scene between his poor parents as they realize that something's a little strange about the lad. When the other kids are out doing masculine things, like circle jerks and pulling wings off flies, all he wants to do is sew clothing for his dolls. Then we can have the scene where he decides to leave his place as apprentice to a tailor to try to make it as an opera singer. He's really torn about leaving, because he just loves being surrounded by all those clothes to sew. Then there's his time of starvation on the road until he's taken in by two gay musicians who see to it that the hungry young man is plenty stuffed. Passed on to a middle-aged poet, and getting a little wiser, he decides that it's much more fun being kept than taking dancing lessons, as he had originally wanted, in return for services rendered. Eventually he makes it big as the greatest fairy-tale writer in Europe, and the entire cast joins in the great production number, "It Takes One to Write One."

**SERGEI LIFAR, b. Kiev, Russia, 1905.** Lifar was the last of Diaghilev's dancer-lovers, and probably the most spiritually faithful. Although he had the talent, the body, and the looks to conform to the great impresario's idea of perfection, one slight fault had to be corrected before their honeymoon—and before the stardom that marriage brought. "Don't sit in the sun, the paraffin will melt," his colleagues teased. But the nose job had its intended results. Lifar, just twenty, was now the lead dancer of the Ballets Russes, and Mme. Diaghilev as well.

# 3.

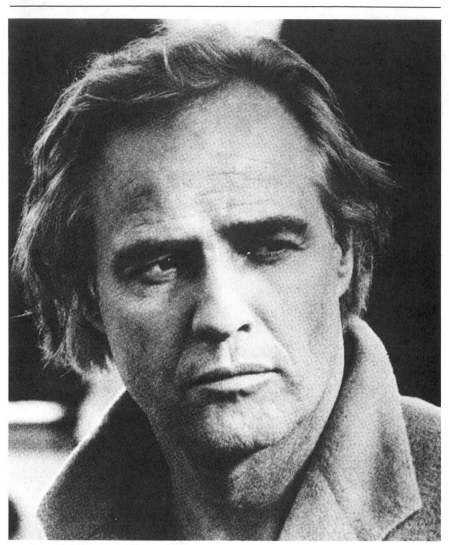

**Marlon Brando:** His raw sexual magnetism made his predecessors look manicured and preened.

**MARLON BRANDO, b. Omaha, Nebraska, 1924.** "Like many men, I too have had homosexual experiences and I am not ashamed." So said the famous actor to the press. No one sniggers at honesty and quiet dignity. So when the news was reported, the sun came up the next day just as it had the day before. Let us hope for an autobiography from Brando before he gets the trash treatment that was Flynn and Power's fate.

# 4.

**ELISABETH (BETTINA) BRENTANO VON ARNIM, b. Frankfurt-am-Main, Germany, 1785.** No one knows exactly what passed between this willowy creature out of Sturm-und-Drang German romanticism and the poet Karoline von Günderode. Bettina devoted one of her books to this intense friendship, but since the

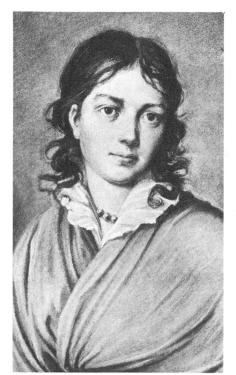

**Bettina Brentano von Arnim:** The essence of romantic *Sturm und Drang*.

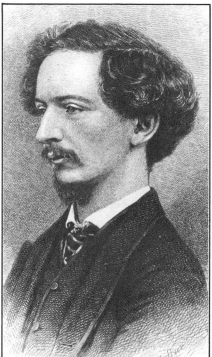

**A.C. Swinburne:** He may also have been D.C. Swinburne.

**Urbino, Italy, 1483.** Almost every Renaissance painter has been thought to be gay by one writer or another over the years, and Raphael, the "divine painter," is no exception. The clues, however, may be purely circumstantial in Raphael's case. (1) As a young man he was exceedingly beautiful. (2) As an adult he lived together with his two favorite students, Giulio Romano, reputed to be bisexual, and Gianfrancesco Penni. (3) When he died at thirty-seven, he left the larger part of his fortune to the two young men. (4) As *The New York Times* would have put it, "he never married." Reach your own conclusions.

letters she published as being from Goethe to herself have turned out to be largely fictitious, how much can we believe? Bettina and Karoline had apparently been lovers. When Bettina overheard a handsome young man talking of his love for Karoline, she jealously reprimanded him for daring to speak of the poet as if he had a right to her love. So pronounced was her outrage that all present were aware that she was speaking as if *she* had a right to Karoline's love. Shortly thereafter the two women quarreled, and Karoline, selecting a beautiful, romantic spot, unobtrusively blew her brains out. She was twenty-six. Ah, love.

language, Swinburne spent much of his life countering charges that his poetry was overly sensuous. Although his defensive critiques were undoubtedly necessary in the Victorian era, he needn't have bothered. His critics were right and he was wrong. His poetry *is* sensuous, and all the better for it. "Fleshly" his poems may have been, but whether he himself was fish or fowl is more difficult to say. He was most certainly a masochist who loved to be flogged, and he was probably homosexual as well. All we know is that he and gay painter Simeon Solomon used to chase each other naked through the poet Rossetti's house, but that's hardly conclusive. Or is it?

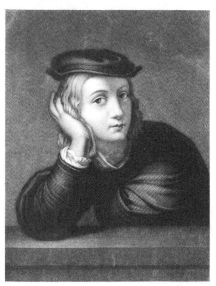

**Raphael:** The "divine painter" in his handsome youth.

# 5.

**ALGERNON CHARLES SWINBURNE, b. London, 1837.** One of the great lyric poets of the English

# 6.

**RAPHAEL (né Raffaelo Santi), b.**

**WILLIAM RUFUS DE VANE KING, b. Sampson County, North Carolina, 1786.** King, a U.S. Senator from Alabama, was the best friend of America's only bachelor president, James Buchanan. And he paid a political price for the closeness of that friendship. Andrew Jackson called him "Miss Nancy," and others referred to him as "her" and "Aunt Fancy." When an attempt was made to check the gossip by shipping King

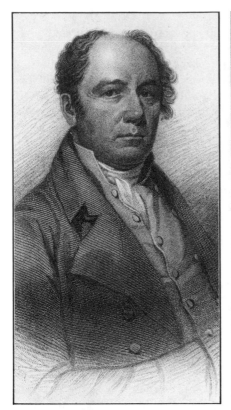

**Rufus De Vane King:** President Buchanan's First Lady.

off as U.S. minister to France, jokes circulated about the presidential "divorce." Washington has always been such a vicious city, hasn't it?

# 7.

**VIOLETTE LEDUC, b. Arras, Pas de Calais, France, 1907.** Violette Leduc was not exactly a jolly old soul. Born the bastard of an orphan serving girl, she saw herself as the evidence of the crime against her mother's sexuality as well as the punishment for it. Her best known book, *Le Bâtarde,* is unfortunately often read as a parable of the condition of all women, rather than as the autobiography of one particularly wretched, albeit brilliant, one. Aside from the women in her life, her great

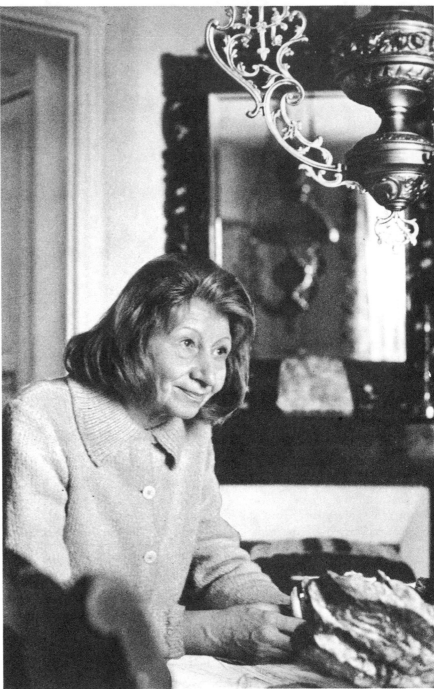

**Violette Leduc:** Of *Therese and Isabelle* she said, "I wrote with one hand, and with the other . . . I loved myself to love them."

passion was the homosexual writer Maurice Sachs, who, to get rid of her, used to urge her to write instead of bothering him. Fond of calling herself "a sort of bluestocking made up mainly of runs," she was so unhappy about being a woman that she fantasized about dressing herself in a light body stocking with a false penis attached so that she could attract the attention of gay writer Jean Genet. She may have know how to pick 'em, but she was hardly your average garden-variety woman.

# 8.

**C.M. BOWRA (Sir Cecil Maurice Bowra), b. Kiukiang, China, 1898.** C.M. Who, you say? Not if you were a whiz in classics or English lit., you don't, for then you'd immediately remember reading any number of books by this renowned English classical scholar and critic. During his long association with Oxford University, he was warden of Wadham College, Professor of Poetry, and vice-chancellor of the university. His many books include *A Book of Russian Verse, The Creative Experiment, Classical Greece,* and *The Oxford Book of Greek Verse.* Given his appearance in A. L. Rowse's *Homosexuals in History,* the title of Bowra's most famous book, *The Greek Experience,* takes on new meaning.

# 9.

**CHARLES BAUDELAIRE, b. Paris, 1821.** Born to a bourgeois family, the author of *Les Fleurs du Mal* for a while lived the modish life of a literary dandy on an inheritance from his father, reluctantly joining the Paris *bohème* when his fortune ran dry. His character, as we view him from the 20th century, is perverse and fascinating. Critics see in him a conflict of many opposites: he was both Catholic and satanist, debauchee and mystic, cynical sensualist and yearner for purity. Unable to excel in virtue, he made himself a legend of vice. He was probably homosexual, or at least Marcel Proust thought so, as did André Gide, Roger Peyrefitte, and many others. The floppy cravat that Baudelaire affected became the rage

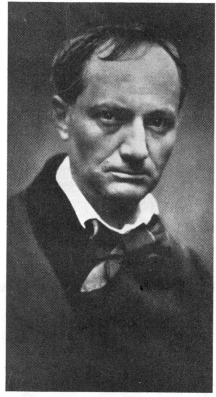

**Charles Baudelaire:** Proust and Gide both thought him gay.

of European dandies during the first decades of the 20th century, gays having adopted him as their very own at an early date.

# 10.

**JOHN WILMOT, EARL OF ROCHESTER, b. Ditchley Manor House, Oxfordshire, England, 1644.** If you've never read the poetry of Rochester, run, don't walk, to the nearest library and, after leafing through the pages, order a copy of your very own. He is easy to read, witty, very funny, and delightfully obscene. He's also proof positive that the world didn't begin with Queen Victoria, his age being almost as unzipped as he. Rochester was an incomparably dissolute rake whose sexual philosophy was clearly "any port in a storm." Consequently his poetry extols the joys of every possible type of human coupling. One poem, possibly unique in the language, is about two men entering a woman fore and aft, but obviously making love to each other. Other poems are about the pleasures of boys: "If by chance then I wake, hotheaded and drunk,/What a coyle do I make for the loss of my Punck?/ I storm and I roar, and I fall in a rage,/And missing my Whore, I bugger my Page." Rochester was once banished from the court of Charles II for smashing the king's clocks and dials when they refused to answer his drunken question, "Dost thou fuck?" He was like that; he was also burned out at thirty-three.

# 11.

**GLENWAY WESCOTT, b. Kewaskum, Wisconsin, 1901.** If you haven't read Wescott's *The Grandmothers* (1927), you're really not civilized. Not that there's anything even remotely gay about it. There isn't. It's simply a beautiful book, well worth discovering. Despite his literary reputation, Wescott has published relatively little—but he has never stopped writing. Having known almost everyone who was anyone in the arts during the past sixty-five years, he has kept careful journals of his observations. The eventual publication of these journals —which take up all the shelf space in a very large room—will be a literary event. They provide one man's record of who was who, and who slept with whom, during a good portion of our century. Perhaps they will also explain the meaning of a spectacular Paul Cadmus painting that hangs in his house. In it, three men, clearly arranged in a triangle, are sit-

## 13.

**ARISTIPPUS, b. Cyrene, North Africa, c. 435 B.C.** There being no one of particular gay interest born this day, all hail the philosopher Aristippus. And with good reason. He held pleasure to be the highest good and virtue to be identified with the ability to enjoy. Wouldn't you know that the founder of hedonism would be gay as a coot, history having recorded the name of his favorite beau, the youth Eutichydes, who assuredly kept Aristippus good and virtuous.

## 14.

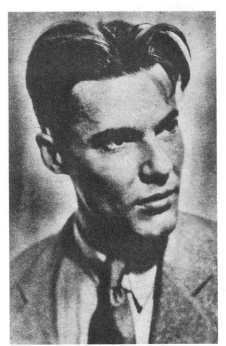

**Glenway Wescott:** What treasures are locked within his journals?

ting on a picnic blanket. The men are the photographer George Platt Lynes, museum curator Monroe Wheeler, and Wescott himself.

## 12.

**MARC-ANTOINE MURET, b. Muret, near Limoges, France, 1526.** It wasn't exactly easy to be a humanist in the 16th century. The slightest misstep and you could see your entrails pop before your very eyes as you wound up burned at the stake. In France in particular, the Church had a couple of effective ways to dispatch those whose views were too liberal. Charge them with sodomy or with Protestantism, much the same abnormality to the official mind. Muret was too liberal, so he was regularly charged with both offenses. Only one of them was true.

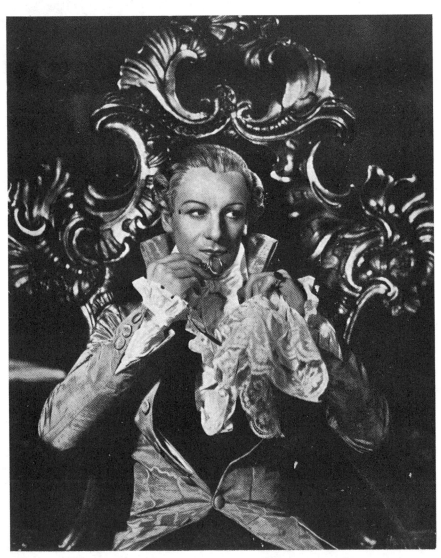

**Sir John Gielgud:** A great tragedian, a great comedian.

**SIR JOHN GIELGUD, b. London, 1904.** Why skimp on superlatives? Sir John has spent a lifetime of hard work earning accolades. Simply put, he is one of the great men of world theater, has the most extraordinarily mellifluous voice of any actor on the English-speaking stage, and remains perhaps the only actor today capable of taking on any role, no matter how slight, and making it play. In his youth his only rival as the most beautiful man on the English stage was Ivor Novello. And he has lost little of this beauty in old age. Try taking your eyes off him when he acts, if you doubt this. Enough said. Let's move from one who has stayed young in old age to someone who was never young at all.

# 15.

**HENRY JAMES, b. New York City, 1843.** In a brilliant series of articles, endorsed by James's biographer Leon Edel, Richard Hall has shown that James was in love with his brother, the Harvard philosopher William James. This finally puts to rest the speculations that have ranged (honest Injun) from a severe lifelong case of constipation to his having been hit in the nuts with a pump handle to explain why the famous writer seems never to have had a sex life. For many years Henry James has been the darling of graduate students and other masochists, almost everyone else being bored to death by his crabbed prose. Here is Maugham on the subject: "I don't think Henry James knew how ordinary people behave. His characters have neither bowels nor sexual organs. [In James's books] people do not go away, they depart, they do not go home, but repair to their domiciles, and they do not go to

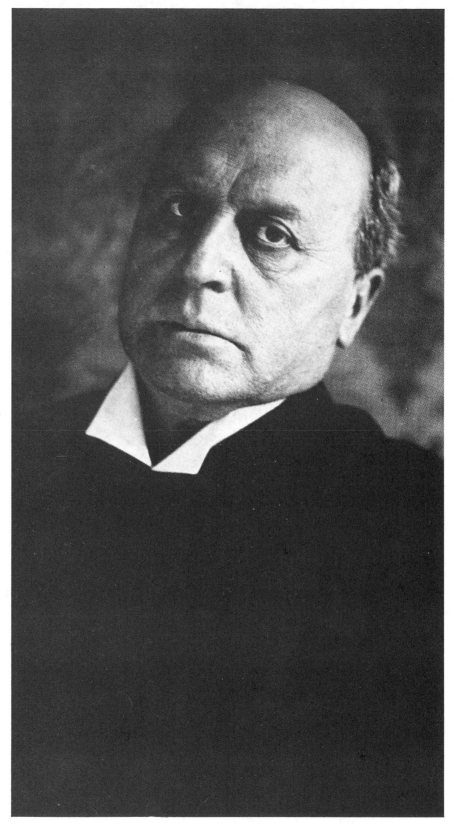

**Henry James:** A genius? Or mannered, pompous, observing life from a window?

bed, they retire." Late in life, James seems to have fallen for a sculptor thirty years his junior, but it is doubtful that anything remotely physical occurred. James was seventy-two when he finally rusted.

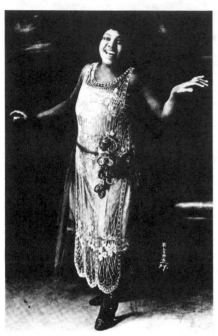

**Bessie Smith:** "I know women that don't like men; it's dirty but good, oh yes."

**BESSIE SMITH, b. Chattanooga, Tennessee, 1894.** When, in "Foolish Man Blues," Bessie Smith sang, "There's two things got me puzzled, there's two things I don't understand;/ That's a mannish-actin' woman, and a skippin', twistin' woman-actin' man," she wasn't the least bit puzzled. She was a good friend of male-impersonator Gladys Fergusson and had been introduced to the world of women-lovin' women by the blues singer Ma Rainey. Among her many gay male friends was composer Porter Grainger. Bessie herself slept with as many female members of her performing troupe as she could. So never believe that the songs an entertainer sings are necessarily true to their own lives. They're just part of the act, that old show-biz scam.

# 16.

**LEONARDO DA VINCI, b. Vinci, near Florence, Italy, 1453.** How much of what is known about the homosexuality of this greatest of history's geniuses is fact and how much speculation? (1) When he was twenty-three and working in Verrochio's workship, Leonardo was accused of having committed homosexual acts with one Jacopo Saltarelli, aged seventeen, and described as a "boy of ill repute." (2) He complained in his notebooks of his attachment to his student Andrea Salaino, whom he nicknamed "Salai" (little devil). Calling Salai a liar and a thief, he was nonetheless sufficiently obsessed with the handsome young man to have left him a good portion of his estate. (3) Francesco Melzi, Salai's replacement as Leonardo's assistant, was left the larger part of the master's estate. These are the only known facts. That Leonardo chose his students for their looks is contemporary gossip. That all his female subjects were painted from young male models is wild speculation. That the *Mona Lisa* is actually a man is a pretty giggly idea. Thirty years ago, the then-daring *Sexology* magazine attempted to prove this assertion by dressing up the famous painting with a boy's haircut and clothing. Without knowing it, *Sexology* actually came up with definite proof that the Mona Lisa is really Julie Andrews

# 17.

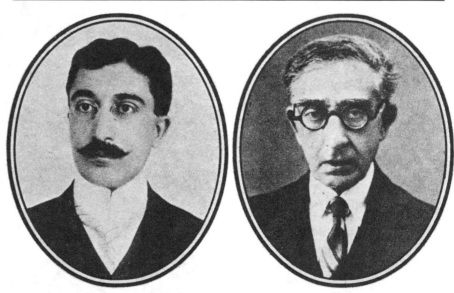

**C. F. Cavafy:** The poet in 1901 and 1932.

**C. V. CAVAFY, b. Alexandria, Egypt, 1863.** During his lifetime Constantin Cavafy was considered *the* poet of Alexandria, and today his name, for those who don't know his poetry, is identified primarily with Lawrence Durrell's characterization of him in the *Alexandria Quartet*.

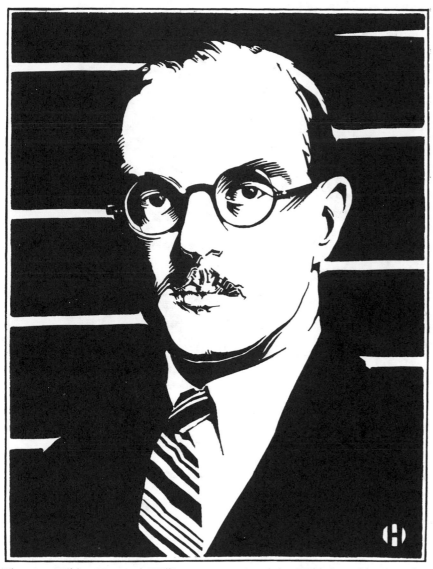

**Thornton Wilder:** Tennessee Williams was convinced that Wilder's problem was that he'd "never had a good lay."

folding chairs on which the dead of Grovers Corners sit, think of Samuel M. Steward (see July 23) who, when Wilder was having difficulties in finishing his play, accompanied the playwright on a long, long walk in the rain. The next day Wilder completed his play. Wilder was a superb craftsman, but now that his homosexuality has been officially recognized, his reputation is almost certain to slip. As we all know, queers don't know how to write plays.

# 18.

**PHILIP II OF MACEDON b. 382 B.C.** Philip was the ancient military genius who defeated the combined Athenian and Theban army and conquered all of Greece, setting in motion the grandiose ambitions of his son, Alexander the Great. After a long, hard day at battle, Philip liked to slip into something comfortable, and, women being an inconvenience in the combat zone, he availed himself of some 800 young eunuchs brought along for his pleasure and his friends'. In the end Philip was murdered by his beautiful teenaged page, Pausanias, who sought revenge after Philip sodomized him in full view of the other guests at a banquet.

# 19.

**WILHELM AUGUST IFFLAND, b. Hanover, Germany, 1759.** Iffland was a powerful force in the German theater of the 18th century, even though his plays are generally unknown outside his native country. He is mentioned here as the only gay personality of note born on this day.

Few know, however, that E. M. Forster was responsible for introducing Cavafy to English-speaking readers, for acting as the poet's unpaid agent, and for promoting his reputation. In return, Cavafy doubted that his mousy benefactor even knew what his poems were about. He was wrong, and others were quick to find out, as well. As Marguerite Yourcenar, his French translator, has remarked: "Cavafy's poems are like Near Eastern cafés—you never see a woman in them."

**THORNTON WILDER, b. Madison, Wisconsin, 1897.** Nowadays, you're supposed to be decidedly middle-brow if you get wet-eyed at the concluding scene of *Our Town*. Well, hell, who wants to be high-brow anyway? So admit it, the end of that play really gets you every time, doesn't it? (Well, *almost* every time. When June Allyson attempted to play the lead many years ago, the perverse among us cheered when Emily died in childbirth.) When you think of that famous closing scene, with its umbrellas and the

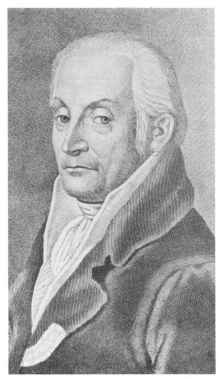

**A. W. Iffland:** At eighteen he ran away from home to learn about men.

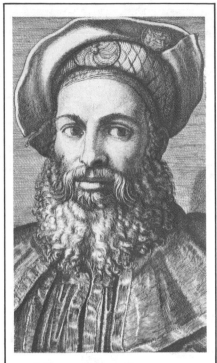

**Pietro Aretino:** He died laughing.

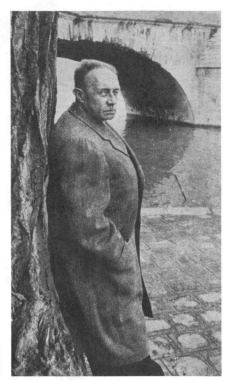

**Henri de Montherlant:** Little read in America, *hélas*.

Enough said. If you'd like to learn more, read Iffland's autobiography, *Meine theatralische Laufbahn*. It has never been translated into English.

# 20.

**PIETRO ARETINO, b. Arezzo, Tuscany, Italy, 1492.** This colorful Renaissance writer and dramatist, described as the first professional writer of his century, was probably the son of a cobbler, although he preferred to claim that he was illegitimate and of noble origin. He had a flair for self-dramatization, a fertile dirty mind, and an uncanny knack of profiting from the politics of his age. He first achieved notoriety for a series of pornographic sonnets, each describing a different position of sexual intercourse, and each illustrated by Giulio Romano. Later he was known and admired for his

*ragionamenti*—dialogues, often audaciously filthy, on contemporary Roman life. Public figures so feared his clever and vicious pen that Aretino became rich from promising *not* to write on certain subjects. He is said to have died from a stroke while laughing at a dirty joke.

# 21.

**HENRI DE MONTHERLANT, b. Paris, France, 1896.** Montherlant is often compared with Ernest Hemingway, with whom he has much in common temperamentally. He is said, in fact, to be the French Hemingway. Do critics know what they are saying? In his novels, Montherlant is exploring the difficult area of his ambiguous sexuality, exploiting his sexual affairs with women while muffling his even more intense affairs with men. What, if

anything, does this tell us about Papa Ernest?

# 22.

**MADAME DE STAËL (née Anne Louise Germaine Necker), b. Paris, 1766.** When old editions of the staid *Encyclopaedia Britannica* say that someone's sex life is "unconventional," it can sometimes mean little more than that the subject enjoyed something other than the missionary position with his clothes on and the lights off. When a woman's sex life is even mentioned, no less described as "unconventional," then, man, you'd better sit up and notice. Madame de Staël liked not only men, but (gasp) women too. In 1798 the French novelist, separated from her husband and living with a male lover, met Juliette Récamier, the most celebrated beauty of her time. Mme. de Staël was thirty-one, Juliette ten

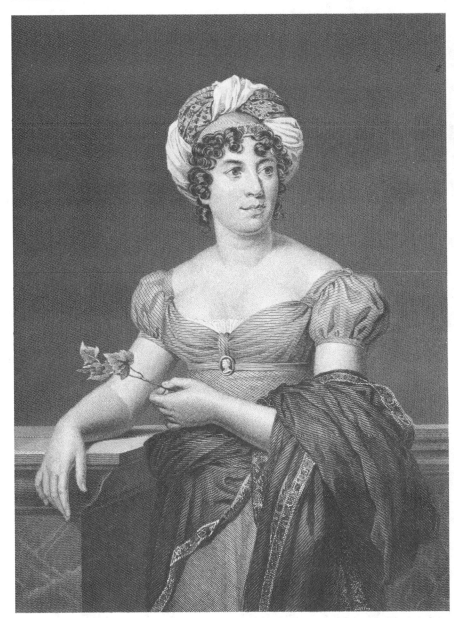

**Anne Louise Germaine de Staël:** "Love is the whole history of a woman's life; it is but an episode in a man's."

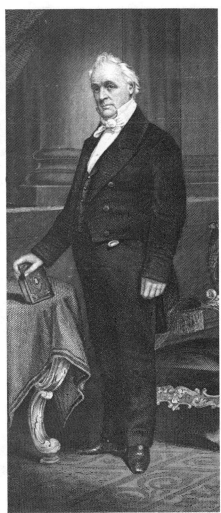

**James Buchanan:** America's only bachelor president.

years younger. 'She fixed her great eyes upon me," wrote Juliette, "and paid me compliments about my figure which might have seemed exaggerated and too direct had they not seemed to have escaped her. From that time on I thought only of Mme. de Staël." They lived together for the next nineteen years, until the novelist died. Her final words to Juliette, to whom she had once written, "I love you with a love that surpasses that of

friendship," were "I embrace you with all that remains of me."

# 23.

**JAMES BUCHANAN, b. near Mercersburg, Pennsylvania, 1791.** The fifteenth president of the United States was the nation's only bachelor

chief executive. If Washington gossips called Buchanan's best friend, Senator William Rufus De Vane King, "Miss Nancy," they did so implying that Buchanan was himself "*Mr.* Nancy." *See April 6.*

# 24.

**DAME ETHEL SMYTH, b. at Sidcup in Surrey, England, 1858.** Ethel Smyth had balls. A composer of note and one of the foremost feminists of her day, she achieved even greater fame as the author of some seven

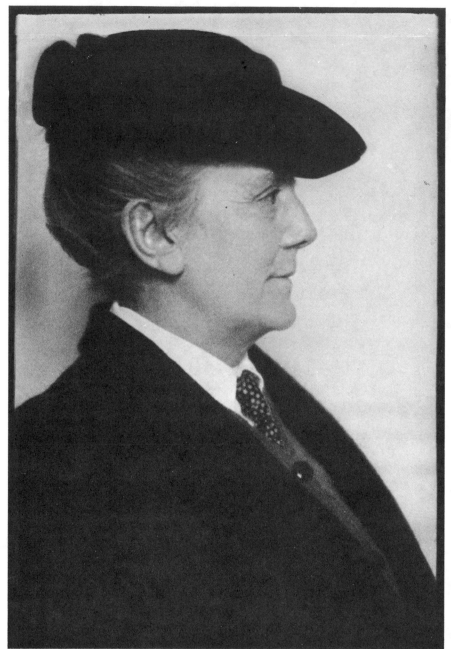

**Dame Ethel Smyth:** Harold Nicolson once described her as "having the profile of Wagner and Frederick the Great at the same time."

# 25.

**EDWARD II, b. Caernavon, 1284.** By the 14th century, as John Boswell has shown in his brilliant, groundbreaking book, *Christianity, Social Tolerance, and Homosexuality,* the Church had radically altered its attitude toward "sodomy." If, in the 12th century, the king of France could elevate his lover to high office and live to tell the tale, such was more than impossible two centuries later. Among the earliest victims of this changed attitude, and certainly the most important, was Edward II, king of England. His love affair with Piers Gaveston, which had begun ten years before his marriage and lasted for thirteen years, ended in the death of Gaveston at the hands of hostile barons. Edward's next friendship, with Hugh le Despenser, resulted in the murder of both lovers. In a grisly application of the punishment fitting the crime, and in a manner clearly revealing the sexual roles of the king and his friend, "Hugh's genitals were cut off and burned publicly before he was decapitated, and Edward was murdered by the insertion into his anus of a red-hot poker."

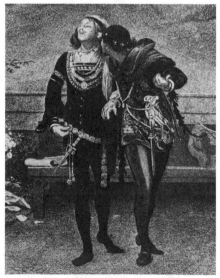

**Edward II and Piers Gaveston:** As the 19th century saw them.

volumes of explicitly candid memoirs. She made no bones about her lesbianism and did not tire of presenting herself as something of a female Don Juan. Dame Ethel had a positive talent for sexual intrigue and specialized in sleeping with the wives of men who wanted to sleep with her. She nursed a strong attraction to Virginia Woolf, but never succeeded in getting it on with her. The fragile novelist was apparently her only major failure. By her own account, Dame Ethel was still going strong in the bedroom in her late sixties. It makes one wonder why, if there's a "y" in 'Smyth," there isn't one in her first name in place of the second "e."

permitting the greatest poet in the English language to be anything but straight as a board. Still, why would a straight poet write sonnets to a man he called the "master-mistress of [his] passion"? And why on earth would he speak of "pricking out" the young man for "women's pleasure"? Does that sound like watching the big game on TV with a can of beer in a hairy paw to you?

# 27.

**MA RAINEY (Gertrude Malissa Nix Pridgett), b. Columbus, Georgia, 1886.** The great blues singer was part of a circle of black lesbians and bisexuals that included Bessie Smith, Jackie "Moms" Mabley, and Josephine Baker. For her relationship with Bessie Smith, see April 15.

# 28.

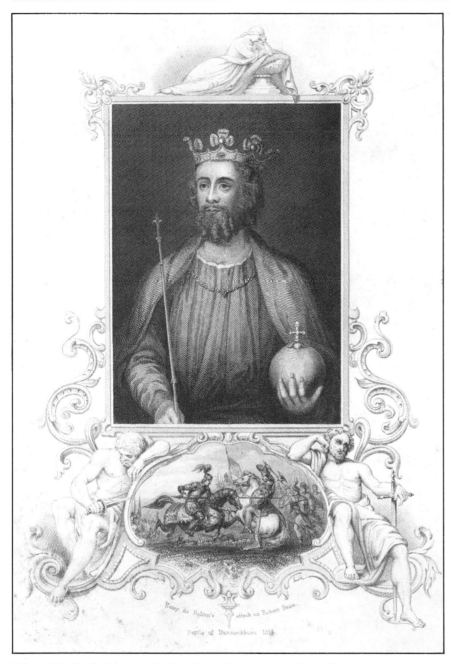

**Edward II:** He died because he loved another more than himself.

# 26.

**WILLIAM SHAKESPEARE, baptised Stratford-on-Avon, Warwickshire, England, 1564.** OK, OK. Let's not get involved in the great debate that erupts each time a new interpretation of Shakespeare's sonnets is published. The "problem" will never be solved, because the "evidence" never changes, only the interpretations. Besides, too much is at stake in

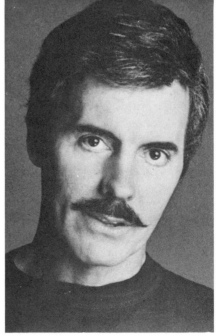

**John Paul Hudson:** An anarchist with a heart of gold.

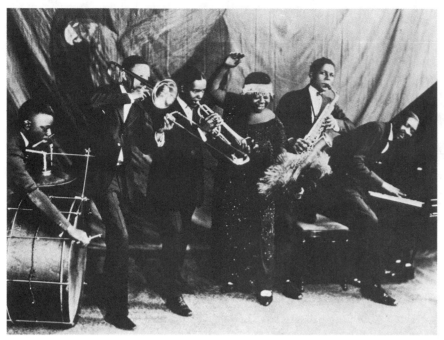

**Ma Rainey:** A woman-lovin' woman.

**JOHN PAUL HUDSON, b. 1929.**
With all the modesty his detractors claim he lacks, John Paul Hudson calls himself "a militant gay journalist of the earliest days of the Gay Liberation Movement." But that description is no more complete than would be calling a laboratory skeleton a living human being. Hudson was a pioneer of the gay press, a contributor to a half dozen of the early gay periodicals, beginning with *Gay* in 1969 and *The Advocate* in 1970, and including *David, Gaysweek, NewsWest, Flash,* and *Vector.* In the years following Stonewall, he was a tireless organizer, his growing radicalism more and more reflected in his writing as he himself became increasingly disillusioned with the "organized gay community" he'd helped to bring about. Like many radicals, he is pure of heart and intolerant of hypocrisy. Unlike most radicals, he is not self-righteous. Like all radicals he is unwilling to allow history the necessary time to catch up with itself, insisting that all social changes must be effected *now.* No wonder he is disillusioned. More than a decade ago, Hudson (as "John Francis Hunter") gave us those eccentric and literate guides, *The Gay Insider* (1971) and *The Gay Insider USA* (1972). Without them there could have been no *States of Desire,* no *Gayellow Pages.*   John Paul Hudson, in short, is an innovator, with a spirit as impatient as his flesh is attractive. Today, incidentally, is not his birthday. (His day is March 21.) But it is the anniversary of his awakening as a born-again radical (1970), and is thus commemorated here.

# 29.

**ROD McKUEN, b. Oakland, California, 1933.** If McKuen is the Edgar Guest of our day, so what? He's never pretended that he writes poetry; in fact, he claims that poetry doesn't even appeal to him. "You have to use a dictionary," he complains. "People don't understand it. It's outdated." What's very much of our time, however, are such verses as "Those of us who walk in light/must help the ones in darkness up./For that's what life is all about/and love is all there is to life." After all, people don't a dictionary need in order a greeting card to buy. McKuen calls himself "a stringer of words," and that seems fair enough. But don't infer that he is insensitive to the *meaning* of words. As he has said, "I have had sex with men; does that make me gay?"

# 30.

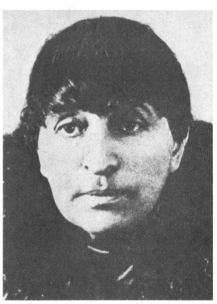

**Alice B. Toklas:** Gertrude called her "Pussy."

**ALICE B. TOKLAS, b. San Francisco, California, 1877.** There are any number of stories that can be told about this unredeemably homely woman, ranging from nasty cracks about her spidery moustache to vicious *bons mots* about the disfiguring hump on her forehead. But there is really only one Alice B., that one very beautiful indeed, who need con-

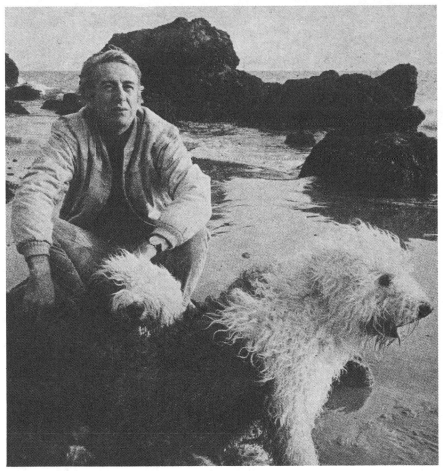

**Rod McKuen:** He risked alienating a million readers by taking a public stand against Anita Bryant.

11. **Ferdinand Lasalle,** straight German gay rights advocate, 1825

12. **William M. Hoffman,** American playwright and editor, 1939

14. **Maximilian Kronberger,** German teenaged inspiration for Stefan George's poetry, 1888

15. **Bliss Carman,** Canadian-born American poet, 1861
    **Dr. Howard Brown,** American public health administrator, 1924

20. **Karl Eitel,** German king of Rumania, 1839
    **David Loovis,** American writer, 1926

21. **Dorothy Baker,** American novelist, 1907
    **James Kirkup,** English poet, 1918
    **Martin Swithinbank,** publisher of literature on boy-love, 1923
    **Charles Silverstein,** psychologist and writer, 1935

24. **Joseph Gallieni,** French general and statesman, 1849
    **A. C. Benson,** English educator and writer, 1862

25. **Gaston de France, duc d'Orleans,** French nobleman, 1608

26. **Eugène Delacroix,** French painter, 1799
    **Charles Shannon,** English painter, 1865
    **Ludwig Wittgenstein,** Austrian-born American philosopher, 1899

27. **Kenward Elmslie,** American composer and librettist, 1929

29. **Jeremy Thorpe,** English politician, 1929

30. **Jacques Louis David,** French painter, 1748
    **Florence Converse,** American novelist, 1871

cern us here. Throughout most of her life, this selfless woman's major occupation was the care and maintenance of Gertrude Stein. She was cook, secretary, manager, nurse, and lover, and in return received a love as faithful and intense as any recorded in the history of friendship.

She was also a highly intelligent woman, whose correspondence reveals her to be a writer and commentator no less brilliant than her more famous partner. She called Gertrude "Lovey." Lovey called her "Pussy." And they lie together, head to head, in Père Lachaise.

## Other Personalities Born in April

4. **Caracalla,** Roman emperor, 188

6. **Charles Jackson,** American writer, 1903

7. **Henry Hay,** English-born American founder of the Mattachine Society, 1912

9. **Ellen Thorneycroft Felkin,** English novelist, 1860

10. **Hans Licht** (né Paul Brandts), German classicist, 1875
    **George Stambolian,** American scholar, 1938

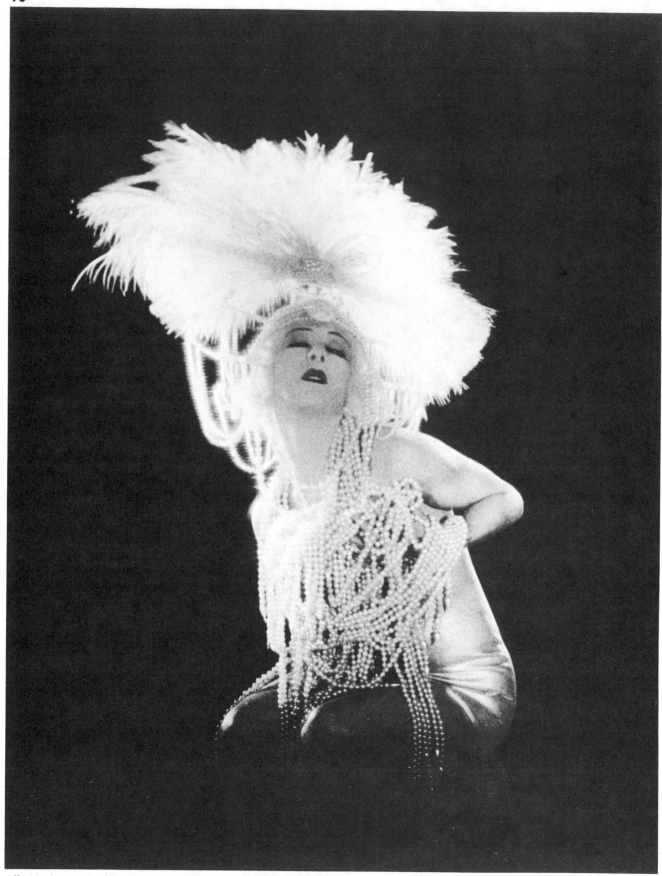

**Alla Nazimova:** In the all-gay version of Oscar Wilde's *Salome* (1923).

# MAY

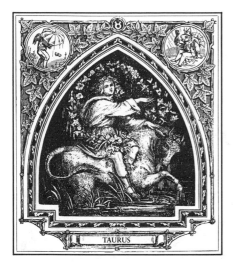

Taurus (April 21st to May 20th) is a fixed earthly sign. The typical Taurean is, accordingly, a down-to-earth, practical person. The rulership of Venus makes the Taurean loving, affectionate, and kind. Normally he is placid and even-tempered, but he can be as terrifying as a bull on the rare occasions when he is roused to anger. The other ruler, Venus, gives the Taurean a loving disposition and a strong sexual instinct. Still, the chief characteristic of the Taurean is his stability of character and purpose. He is steadfast of mind, unshaken in adversity, and quietly persistent in the face of difficulties. He refuses to be hustled or hurried or frightened or pushed into any false position, either mental or physical. As a realist, the Taurean is generally blessed with a good sense of humor.

## 1.

**ROMAINE BROOKS, b. Rome, Italy, 1874.** At the beginning of World War I, when the American heiress Natalie Barney, a free spirit in Paris known as "the wild girl of Cincinnati," had just broken with her lover, the actress Liane Pougy, Romaine Brooks was making a name for herself as a society portrait painter. Romaine, an American, had been briefly married, had had an affair with Gabriele D'Annunzio, and flirtations with several women. When she became the lover of Natalie Barney, both women had just turned forty, and Natalie was known as an adventuress, a reckless seducer of women. Natalie's ideal, what she had always wanted, was a *great* love, enlivened by numerous sexual adventures on the side. Romaine became

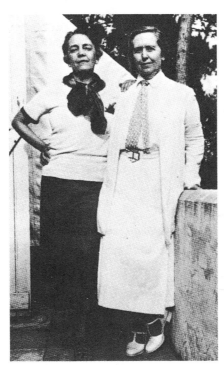

**Romaine Brooks and Natalie Barney:** Barney was "Nattie; Brooks, "Angel Darling."

that great love, and there were, in fact, countless little adventures that would have destroyed a more conventional friendship. Romaine's only condition was that Natalie's affairs had to be mere passing fancies. Their friendship, a very modern marriage indeed, lasted for more than half a century.

## 2.

**LORENZ HART, b. New York City, 1895.** As a composer, Richard Rodgers wrote music that perfectly matched the meaning of his lyricists' words. Before he started writing drippy, sentimental tunes to match the sappy, saccharine sentiments of Oscar Hammerstein II, he composed some of the finest songs of the 1920s and '30s, songs that were snappy, syncopated, witty, cynical. His first lyricist, Lorenz Hart, had been his friend at Columbia University, was barely over five-feet tall, had a razor-sharp wit, and, according to Rodgers, was "a partner, a best friend—and a source of permanent irritation." What was most irritating, perhaps, was Hart's homosexuality, a carefully guarded secret from the public until a biography appeared thirty-five years after the lyricist's death. Amusing, isn't it, that Hart, gay as Ganymede, wrote lyrics that are tough, muscular, and butch, whereas Hammerstein, a six-footer and straight as a tombstone, wrote verses that a marcelled dowager could have submitted to *The Ladies' Home Companion*.

# 3.

**MAY SARTON, b. Wendelgem, Belgium, 1912.** May Sarton has written some of the most beautiful lyric poetry of the 20th century. Her poems are accessible, free of self-conscious experimentation, and divorced from membership in any particular school of poetry. Many of them are pellucid reflections of the lesbian experience, as are her most recent novels. May Sarton's reputation was soundly established before she published her novel *Mrs. Stevens hears the mermaids singing* (1965). She feared, rightly, that writing so stongly about lesbianism would lead to a diminution of the value of her work. "The fear of homosexuality is so great that it took courage to write *Mrs. Stevens hears the mermaids singing*," she says in *Journal of a Solitude* (1973), "to write a novel about a woman homosexual who is not a sex maniac, a drunkard, a drug-taker, or in any way repulsive, to portray a homosexual who is

neither pitiable nor disgusting, without sentimentality. . . ." Read this remarkable novel, and read the

*Journal,* where May Sarton reveals, not surprisingly, that she is Mrs. Stevens.

# 4.

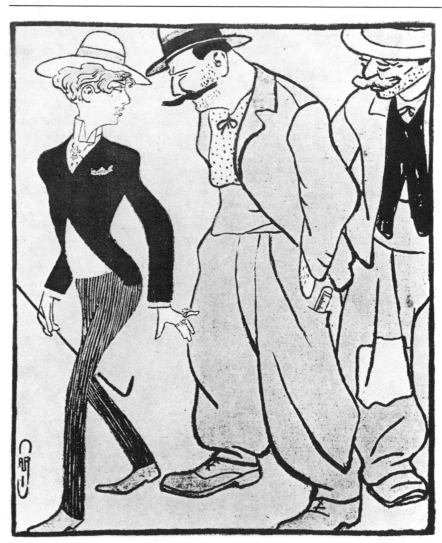

**Count Adelsward Fersen:** A caricature of Fersen with the *real* men of Capri.

**COUNT ADELSWARD FERSEN, b. Sweden, c. 1880.** Today is really the birthday of F_____ Cardinal _____, one of the princes of the Church, and we can't talk about him now, can we? So this is as good a place as any to mention Count Fersen, whose exact date of birth is not recorded in any standard reference work. Fersen, a Swedish count living in Paris, was the momentary darling of the dandy set, his poetry transporting his colleagues into raptures, when he decided—impetuously, of course—to marry and break his ties with Sodom. To celebrate his engagement, he threw an extravagant gay party (a "pink mass"), was arrested for playing with male jailbait, then shot himself, recovered, and lived in exile in Capri with a young Italian hustler. At that time Capri was the world's gay mecca and the home of such writers as Norman Douglas and Compton Mackenzie, as well as the scene of Fritz Krupp's key-club orgies (see February 17). Within a few years the burnt-out Fersen was dead from morphine and opium addiction.

# 5.

**TYRONE POWER, b. Cincinnati, Ohio, 1913.** Tyrone Power wasn't much of an actor, but, oh my, he was handsome. According to the original "under-the-table" version of Kenneth Anger's *Hollywood Babylon,* before it was made respectable for public consumption and tarted up with pretty pictures, Tyrone Power was a coprophiliac. If this was in fact so, it is never mentioned in *The Secret Life of Tyrone Power,* a biography which announces its big secret on the front cover of the dust jacket: "The drama of a bisexual in

the spotlight." It's hard to know whether the biography is dull because the actor was dull (a real possibility) or whether a disservice has been done to an interesting subject by a dull writer (an even greater possibility). Whatever, once you know that

# 6.

**SIGMUND FREUD, b. Freiberg, Germany, 1856.** The next time your brother-in-law suggests that you see a shrink to get yourself "cured," just tell him that dear old Siggy Freud himself was head-over-heels in love with a Berlin physician named Wilhelm Fliess. Physician, heal thyself!

**RUDOLPH VALENTINO (né Rudolfo Alfonzo Raffaelo Pierre**

Power liked it both ways (by page 2), there's really little need to read further. Now, if only Kenneth Anger had been correct, there could have been a perfect marriage between biographer and subject: "The drama of a coprophiliac by Hector Arce."

Filibert Guglielmi di Valentina d'Antonguolla), Castellaneta, Italy, 1895. Valentino was such a slab of packaged beefcake that it's very difficult to know where fact begins and legend leaves off. His undeniable good looks and animal appeal, his foreignness in the land of the WASP, and the very plots of his films made women dream of submitting to the fate worse than death if Valentino would only draw his sword. And

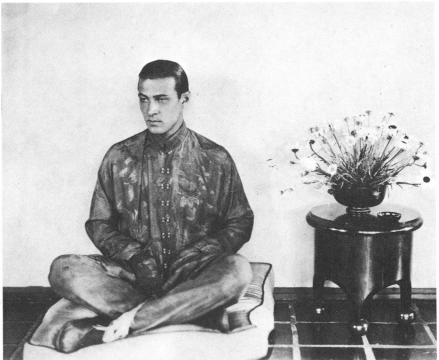

Rudolph Valentino: In 1924 he recorded a one-night stand in his journal: "I went back with him to his home . . . I was wildly passionate . . . We made love like tigers until dawn."

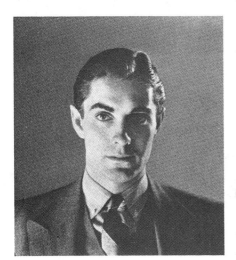

Tyrone Power: In 1937 he was described as "less creamy than Robert Taylor." Was that a compliment or an insult?

rumor had it that he wielded a weapon even longer than his name. But the press, and men in general, would have nothing of this un-American dream. He was ridiculed as a "pink powder puff," and we all know what that means. The consensus is that Valentino was most likely gay. But there are those who disagree. The film historian Kevin Brownlow is one of them. In one of the strangest passages ever written by a serious scholar, Brownlow, who was born many years after Valentino died, tells us that the Latin Lover couldn't have been "that way" since he had a sense of humor. Huh?

# 7.

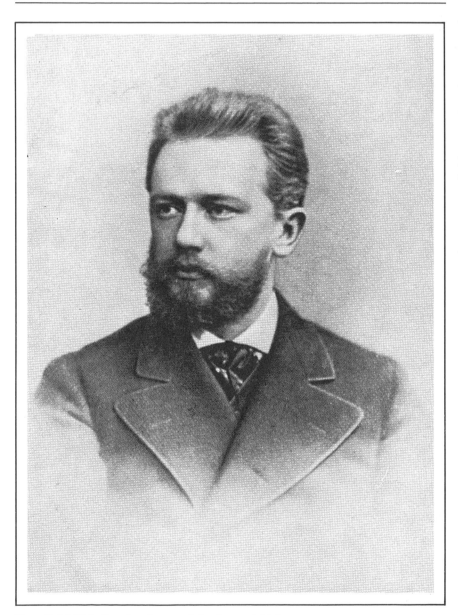

**Peter Ilyich Tchaikovsky:** A natural death or suicide?

**PETER ILYICH TCHAIKOVSKY, b. Votinsk, Russia, 1840.** Perhaps because his music remains popular with concert-goers despite changes in musical fashion, perhaps because all the world loves the romance of unhappy heroes, perhaps because almost every schoolboy knows that he was gay, more nonsense has been written about Tchaikovsky than about any other composer. And the nonsense seems never to end. At the moment, the scholarly world is in a tizzy over the theory that the composer did not die of cholera in 1893, as officially reported, but was forced to commit suicide by the Russian musical establishment because he was gay. A nice fantasy, but not very likely, since in Czarist Russia homosexuality was tolerated and, although hardly condoned, was not punishable by death, no less enforced suicide. Poor Tchaikovsky. First he gets stuck with Ken Russell and now this.

# 8.

**CLAUDE-LOUIS-HECTOR, DUC DE VILLARS, b. Moulins, France, 1653.** The sharp-tongued Charlotte Elisabeth, the second wife of gay Phillipe d'Orleans, left behind a collection of letters, many of which reveal her passion for sniffing out the private affairs of court homosexuals. Of her favorite subject she wrote, "Our heroes take as their models Hercules, Theseus, Alexander, and Caesar, who all had their male favorites. Those who give themselves up to this vice, which believing in Holy Scripture, imagine that it was only a sin when there were few people in the world, and that now the earth is populated it may be regarded as a divertissement. Among the common people, indeed, accusations of this kind are, so far as possible, avoided; but among persons of quality, it is publicly spoken of; it is considered a fine saying that since Sodom and Gomorrah, the Lord has punished no one for such offences." One of the gay "persons of quality" who flit through the duchess's letters is the duc de Villars, one of the greatest generals in French history and marshal of France under Louis XIV.

rie, for example. Her marriage was never consummated and she wasn't particularly happy about it. But, then, Barrie never consummated any relationship with anyone, including his strange friendship with the three Davies boys, whose guardian he became after their parents died. The great love of Barrie's life, George

Davies, was only five years old when the playwright met him one day while walking his dog. The precocious child took him home, and the remainder of this bizarre story is superbly told in Andrew Birkin's *J. M. Barrie and the Lost Boys.* It is one of the oddest closet stories ever told.

# 9.

James M. Barrie: "Do you believe in fairies? . . . If you believe, clap your hands!"

**JAMES M. BARRIE, b. Kirriemuir, Forfarshire, Scotland, 1860.** The diminutive creator of *Peter Pan,* whose whimsical fairy-tale play kept Maude Adams, Jean Arthur, and Mary Martin gainfully employed for many years, was also responsible for other popular plays and novels, including *The Admirable Crichton, Dear Brutus,* and *The Little Minister.* He once wrote a play called *What Every Woman Knows,* which is decidedly not what almost every woman wants. Like Mrs. J. M. Bar-

# 10.

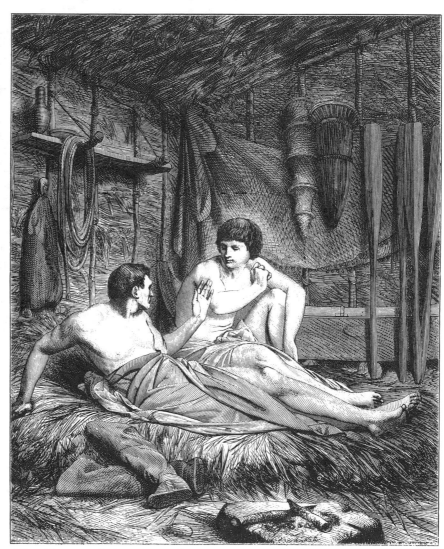

**"The Fishermen of Theocritus":** The poet was particularly fond of chicken of the sea.

**THEOCRITUS, b. Syracuse, c. 320 B.C.** As any student of literature knows, Theocritus developed the verse form known as the pastoral, a stylized and artful poem in which shepherds and cowherds sing of love and friendship. Whereas Greek shepherds really did sing to their flocks, it's doubtful that they were ever quite so philosophical about screwing as Theocritus and his followers pretended they were. In many of his *Idylls,* Theocritus is praising the love of boys, and these poems are really quite beautiful, even in English translation. Theocritus's pastoral was widely imitated in the Renaissance, but, by the 18th century, a few wiseacres were already beginning to see the form as inherently silly. Jonathan Swift, bless his cantankerous hide, once lampooned the pastoral mercilessly. In his poem, the shepherd boy takes his fair shepherdess into the fields to do more than merely philosophize about love. Before he mounts her, the shepherd, a realist like Swift, spreads plenty of paper around so as not to roll, as he puts it, in the sheep shit. And he warns his true love to take care that she doesn't get any rocks up her ass. So much for the joys of nature. Not too long after Swift's poem, the pastoral died a merciful death.

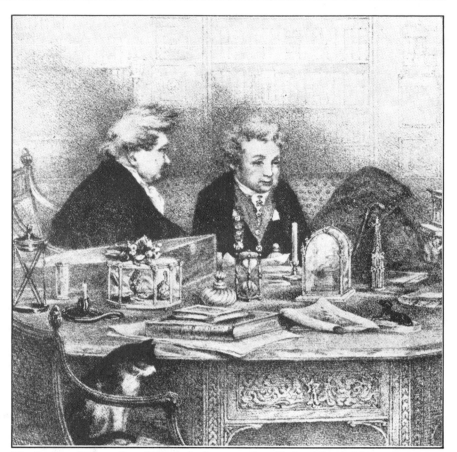

**The Ladies of Llangollen:** With their short powdered hair, riding habits, waistcoats, and cravats, they looked like little old men.

# 11.

**THE LADIES OF LLANGOLLEN,** **Eleanor Butler (1739-1829) and** **Sarah Ponsonby (1755-1831).** In the 18th century, a polite euphemism for lesbianism was coined—"romantic friendship," a term occasionally invoked in our own time whenever the press wants to touch on such delicate matters as Eleanor Roosevelt's friendship with Lorena Hickok. The 18th-century press was particularly fond of attacking "romantic friendships," which they called "the latest unnatural vice," and singled out for cen-

sure Marie Antoinette and her court of "Sapphists," the sculptor Mrs. Damer, the comedienne Miss Farren, and especially the infamous Ladies of Llangollen. Butler and Ponsonby, Irish ladies of quality, ran off together to Llangollen, Wales, where, together with their servant Mary Caryll, known as "Molly the Bruiser," they set up house and lived together in domestic tranquility for half a century. That theirs was a physical relationship is clear from Lady Eleanor's journal, written in an easily decipherable code. That the modern vulgarism "bush" is hardly modern at all may be seen in the journal's constant references to shrubbery—even in the dead of winter: "My beloved and I spent a delightful evening in the shrubbery." Fifty years of gardening is a long time, and the two women are well

worth reading about in any of several full-length books about their life together.

# 12.

**EMMA LYON HAMILTON, b.** **Great Neston, Cheshire, England,** **1765.** The bare outline of this famous beauty's life is well known. She was the mistress of Charles Greville, then of Sir William Hamilton, ambassador to Naples, whom she married. And she was, of course, the mistress of Horatio Nelson, who risked career and reputation to live with her. Less known, and the reason for her inclusion here, is her liaison with Neopolitan Queen Marie Caroline,

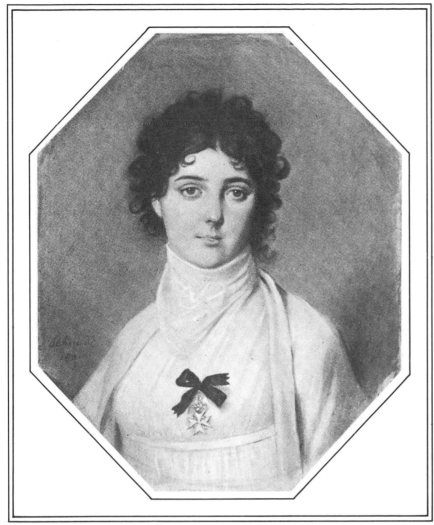

**Emma Lyon Hamilton:** As independent as her men allowed.

—from poor eyesight to a big nose—found or invented for never marrying, and by references in his journal to intense suffering each time one of his pretty young men married. If you weren't brought up on Lear, you've missed one of the joys of childhood; if you still don't know him as an adult, get out there and start reading. "How pleasant to know Mr. Lear!/Who has written such volumes of stuff:/Some think him ill-tempered and queer,/But a few think him pleasant enough." That's Lear to a T. Queer, pleasant, and very funny.

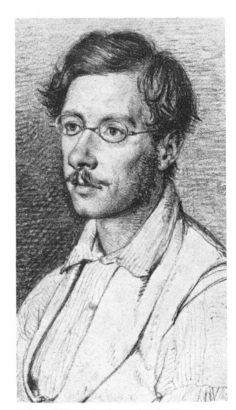

**Edward Lear:** Author of "The Dong with the Luminous Nose."

# 13.

SIR ARTHUR SULLIVAN, b. London, 1842. Like the later partnership of Rodgers and Hart, the musical

over whom she exercised considerable influence. This affair, aided and abetted by the queen's lesbian sister, Marie Antoinette, was well known to Sir William Hamilton, who found his wife's lesbianism an invaluable aid to his diplomatic mission in Naples. Ironically, no matter how "modern" and independent a spirit Lady Hamilton appears to us today, her every nonconforming move was made possible only by its profitability in flesh or influence to powerful men.

**EDWARD LEAR, b. Highgate, near London, England, 1812.** Whether

Lear was gay or not is of little consequence. His nonsense poetry has never been equalled, nor have his whimsical illustrations. No one who reads his limericks, a form that he virtually perfected, can doubt that he was anything other than a comic genius on the order of Lewis Carroll, his contemporary. Still, all the signs of probable homosexuality are present. What he called his "natural affinity for children" went well beyond garden-variety naturalness and beyond affinity. His entire life is characterized by close friendships with handsome young men many years his junior, by dozens of reasons

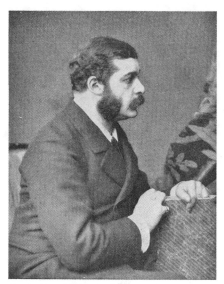

**Sir Arthur Sullivan:** A secret as quiet as the lost chord.

marriage of Gilbert and Sullivan was one of temperamental unequals —Gilbert straight and Sullivan gay—perfectly matched in the art they created jointly. Sullivan's homosexuality, though widely known to his contemporaries, was practiced discreetly. He played by the rules that permitted the upper classes their "vices" so long as there was no threat of public scandal. That Sullivan, unlike his straight partner, was knighted shows how well, and how prudently, he played the game. Hypocritical? Perhaps. But the Irish Oscar Wilde might not have died quite so young had he understood the English character as well as Sullivan.

**HALL CAINE (né Thomas Henry Hall Caine), b. Runcorn, Cheshire, England, 1853.** As a novelist, Hall Caine was the English Octave Thanet (see March 19), immensely popular in his own time and almost completely forgotten today. Whereas Thanet was tall and gargantuan, Caine was diminutive and slight. Both, however, are equally impossible to read today, their language so stilted, their plots so melodramatic,

as to be rendered unintentionally hilarious to modern readers. Caine's novel *The Deemster* (1887) resets the biblical David-Jonathan story in contemporary England. The chapter called "Passing the Love of Women" is of particular interest, not only for its significant title, but for its Victorian heavy breathing thought to simulate men in love. Its pages fairly flicker like a silent-movie melodrama.

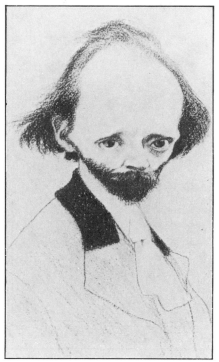

**Hall Caine:** Among the worst "serious" novelists in history.

# 14.

**JULIAN ELTINGE (né William Dalton), b. Newtonville, Massachusetts, 1883.** Eltinge was the most successful female impersonator of his day, if not of all time. Although long a star on stage, he was known throughout the world primarily because of the popularity of his many silent films, a fact almost completely ignored in modern film histories. Just

how popular he was may be seen by this wonderful footnote to history: During the Korean War a troop ship was named in his honor. One wonders how many of our boys realized that they were climbing on board a female impersonator each time they sailed the *Julian Eltinge?*

# 15.

**ALEXANDER THE GREAT, b. 356 B.C.** In his time, no one ever dared ask Alexander if he could whistle. King of Macedon and conquerer of most of Asia, Alexander was unquestionably one of the greatest generals of all time and one of the most powerful personalities of antiquity. He influenced the spread of Hellenism and instigated profound changes in the history of the world. A full-time general, Alexander, like almost every other high-born Greek, was a part-time homosexual, reproducing his kind by loving women, and reaching a "higher good" by loving boys. His love for his friend Hephaestion is the stuff of legend, his grief at his friend's death resulting in the order to crucify the physician who failed to save him. And his pleasure with the eunuchs Medius and Bagoas is equally well known, Alexander having ordered the death of the satrap Orsines for mocking Bagoas by saying that he would not talk to a man who prostituted himself like a woman. Throughout the centuries, whenever anyone attempted to "justify" homosexuality by listing the names of famous practitioners, Alexander always headed the list. Since he was once the most powerful man in the world, it hardly hurt the cause to invoke the name of someone who most certainly never ate quiche.

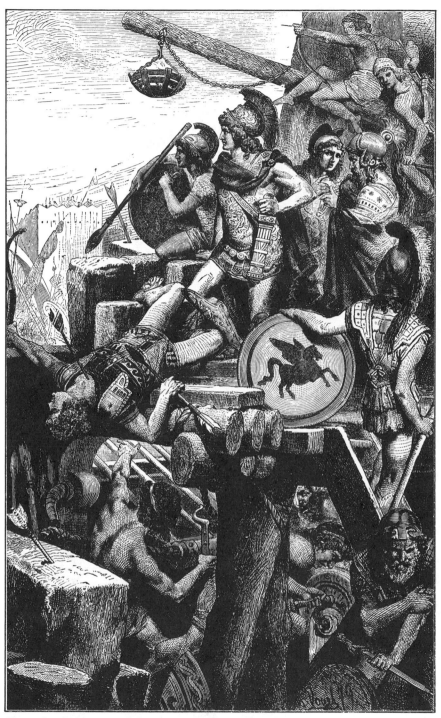

**Alexander the Great:** A full-time warrior and a part-time homosexual.

# 16.

**PATRICK DENNIS** (né Edward
Everett Tanner III), b. Chicago, Illinois, 1921. Listing Patrick Dennis
here is very much like discussing Paul

Whiteman as a black jazz musician.
Patrick's genius lay in cleverly
packaging gay camp for public consumption so that the audience could
congratulate itself on discovering
something "new" without vaguely
suspecting its origins. Anyone who
puts down Dennis's accomplishment
doesn't appreciate just how hard it is
to write for the public taste, no less
create it. The author of *Auntie
Mame* holds the record as the only
author ever to have had three novels
on *The New York Times* best-seller
list at once [for eight weeks in 1956].

# 17.

**ERIK SATIE, b. Honfleur, Calva-
dos, 1866.** Any way you look at it,
Satie was a character, a bona-fide eccentric. Dissatisfied with the compositions of his youth, which were
overshadowed by the music of
Debussy, he went back to school to
study music formally at the age of
forty, the resulting compositions all
but completely overshadowed by the
music of the young Stravinsky.
Together with Cocteau and Picasso,
he created the ballet *Parade* for
Diaghilev. He is thought to have
been gay because of the company he
kept, but his private life was so hidden from his contemporaries that no
one really knows whether he was
straight, gay, bisexual, or nothing at
all. He was known to enter a room
and sit down without ever removing
his hat, coat, or gloves, and he was
rarely seen in public without a brand-
new umbrella, which would never
leave his hands no matter where he
was. He lived in a tiny Parisian room
that no one was ever permitted to
enter. After he died, great curiosity
centered on the contents of that
room. In it were found hundreds of
unbrellas, many of them still in
wrapping paper, and little else.

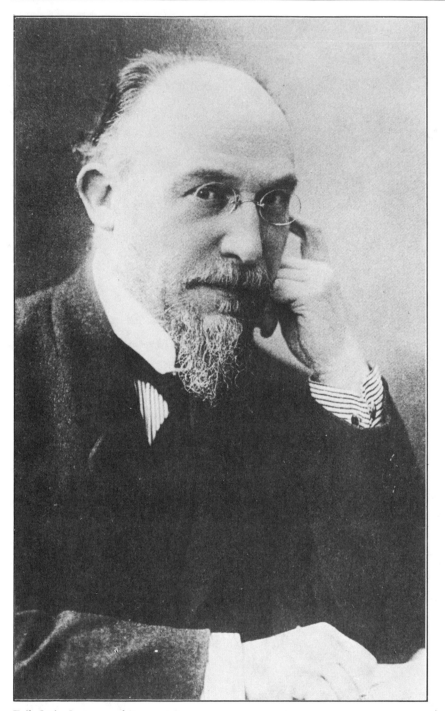

**Erik Satie:** Just a wee bit eccentric.

themselves not open to criticism, given the incestuous nature of the publishing racket to begin with. It's the stories he tells, the family secrets, that don't always hold water. Like, for example, that well-told story of how Uncle Willie arranged to have his lover Gerald Haxton screw the innocent young Robin until he was black and blue. A nice yarn, and, given the good looks of Haxton not exactly a fatal experience for a young homosexual to have endured. Only it's not true, as Maugham's latest biographer has shown. Apparently, Robin Maugham was a novelist even when writing autobiography.

# 18.

**ARTEMISIA ABROTANUM.** What? A plant? How can a plant have a birthday? Well, in *this* book it can, especially on a day when no one of any gay interest was born and *something* had to fill up the space. *Artemisia abrotanum,* commonly known as "Ladslove," was frequently used as a symbol in gay poetry of the 19th and early 20th centuries. Just as Walt Whitman used the erect leaves of the Calamus as a sexual symbol, English writers of the same period used Ladslove in the same way—not only because of its erect habit and its appropriate name, but because its smell was thought similar to that of human semen. Happy birthday, *Artemisia abrotanum.*

# 19.

**JOHN VERNOU BOUVIER III, b. New York City, 1891.** Jackie's father? Yup, Jackie's father. A well-known womanizer throughout his life, and an elegant narcissist (his

**ROBIN MAUGHAM, b. London, 1916.** The nephew of W. Somerset Maugham, Robin Maugham was a decent enough novelist in his own right, with or without the influential help of his Uncle Willie. *The Servant,* of course, requires no apology for

literary nepotism. That Robin was gay, and a chip off the old Maugham block in that respect, goes without saying. It's his memoirs of the senior Maugham, however, that are slightly suspect, although his two attempts to cash in on his uncle's celebrity are in

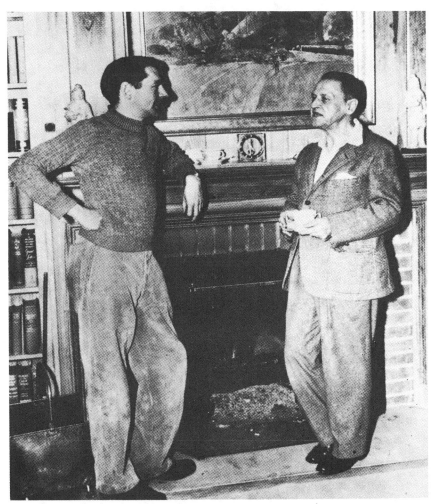

**Robin Maugham with Uncle Willie:** A chip off the old block.

and novelist who was one of the leading figures of the Harlem Renaissance of the 1920s and '30s, was the author of such works as *Color, Caroling Dusk, The Ballad of the Brown Girl, The Black Christ,* and *One Way to Heaven.* With the gay subculture within black society only beginning to be explored, notably by Eric Garber, many studies will undoubtedly appear in the future. Cullen, Garber reports, enjoyed a "lifelong relationship with Harlem schoolteacher Harold Jackman. . . . Arna Bontemps would later remember Cullen and Jackman as the 'Jonathan and David of the Harlem Renaissance.' "

# 21.

**HAROLD ROBBINS (né Francis Kane), New York City, 1916.** What? Harold Robbins? Author of some of the best-selling blockbusters in publishing history? Say it ain't so, Danny Fisher. It seems that while he was writing *Dreams Die First,* a novel which features a bisexual hero, Robbins did a little research, as any good writer should, and "experimented" to see what bisexuality was like. Or so Robbins said in *People* magazine in 1977. This, one supposes, is what a writer refers to as "getting inside his character."

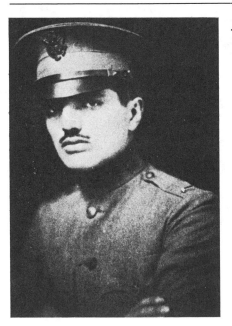

**John Vernou Bouvier III:** Yes, you're right. The spitting image, but without the moustache.

apartment was decorated from wall to wall with pictures of himself), "Black Jack" Bouvier was nonetheless one of Cole Porter's many lovers. The aristocrat of Broadway was reputedly infatuated with him. And why not? His biographer claims that *every* woman found him irresistible.

# 20.

**COUNTEE CULLEN, b. New York City, 1903.** Cullen, the black poet

# 22.

**ALLA NAZIMOVA, b. in the Crimea, Russia, 1879.** Best known for her famous stage portrayals of Ibsen heroines, Nazimova made a series of American films after World War I, including *Camille* (1921) and *A Doll's House* (1922). By the time she produced and starred in the all-gay version of Oscar Wilde's *Salome,* with sets modeled on the well-known illustrations of Aubrey Beardsley, she was already the doyen of Hollywood's lesbian community, which included, among others both temporary and permanent, Natacha Rambova (neé Winifred Shaunessy of Salt Lake City), director Dorothy Arzner, and Dolly Wilde, Oscar's niece, who was a chip off her uncle's block except for the fact that she was the only Wilde who preferred to sleep with women. Considering her fame as an actress and the extraordinary circles in which she moved, it is astonishing that a biography of Alla Nazimova has never been written.

# 23.

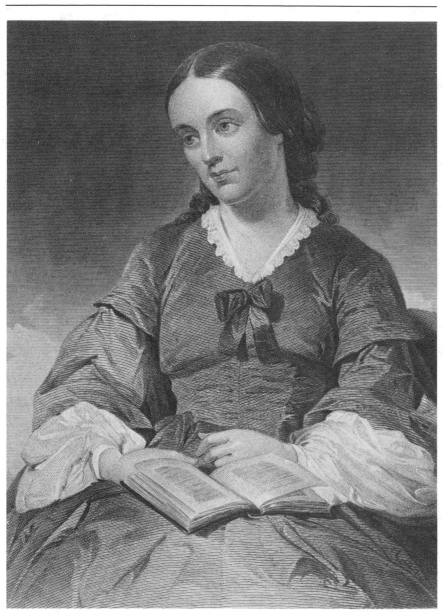

**Margaret Fuller:** Why did Emerson attempt to launder her "dirty" linen?

**MARGARET FULLER, b. Cambridgeport, Massachusetts, 1810.** Margaret Fuller was one of the most influential personalities of her day in American literary circles. An ardent feminist, she was the most prominent woman among the American transcendentalists and, with Ralph Waldo Emerson and others, edited *The Dial,* a quarterly journal of that philosophical movement. That she was bisexual is clear from her surviving writings, even though these were severely bowdlerized by Emerson, W. H. Channing, and J. F. Clark after Fuller's death. Unfortunately for history, her editors, intent on protecting her "reputation," destroyed the original documents after whitewashing the contents for publication. The full story of this desecration is told by Fuller's biographer, Mason Wade, and is excellently summarized in Jonathan Katz's *Gay American History.*

# 24.

**ELSA MAXWELL, b. Keokuk, Iowa, 1883.** It is hard to believe that any age, no less the recent past, could have invented Elsa Maxwell. With no money of her own, and without the proper family background or breeding, this immense woman became the *arbiter elegantiarum* of the international set during the 1920s and '30s. Her social contacts as broad as she was, she was in demand as the planner of the most extravagant society parties of the era and included among her contacts not only wealthy people, but institutions and entire nations. She was in the employ of Monaco to promote Monte Carlo and of Italy to promote the Lido, and she went through life with a rent-free suite at the Waldorf and check-less meals at Maxim's, among other bows to her social influence. Where Elsa went, so did the idle rich. That she was a lesbian bothered no one, especially her best pal, Cole Porter. Together they were the oddest couple of the day—she butch and blubbery, he slight and effeminate.

# 25.

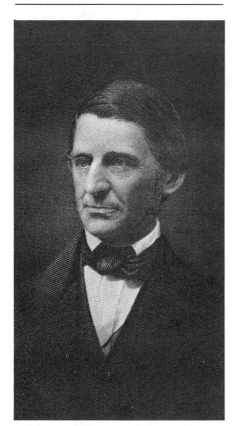

**Ralph Waldo Emerson:** In love with Martin Gay.

**RALPH WALDO EMERSON, b. Boston, Massachusetts, 1803.** The great 19th-century American essayist, poet, and philosopher is included here because of a wild crush that he had on a classmate at Harvard, the exquisitely-named Martin Gay. The entries in Emerson's journal over a period of two years record his growing infatuation (and obsession) with the handsome young man and provide an almost classic case study of adolescent homosexuality. In later years Emerson attempted to obliterate all references to Martin Gay in the journals, succeeding in far too many instances. But his modern (1960) editors were able to salvage or reconstruct enough passages to provide a rare view of the future philosopher in the thrall of same-sex love.

# 26.

**DONALD MACLEAN and GUY BURGESS, 1951.** No, both spies were not born on this day. In fact, neither was. But it *is* the day that the two British Foreign Office officials defected to Russia, setting in motion an English witchhunt as vicious as America's contemporary McCarthy investigations. Unfortunately for their gay brothers, and especially for their old Oxford classmates, Maclean

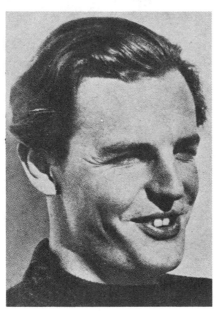

**Donald Maclean:** Guy Burgess, his "cruel master," said he looked like Nelly Melba.

and Burgess were homosexuals. Their actions brought new meaning to the dreaded term "security risk" and cost numerous innocent gay men and women their livelihoods and, in some cases (as the mathematician Alan Turing) their lives. No, Virginia, not all gays are good guys.

# 27.

**WILD BILL HICKOK (né James Butler Hickok), b. Troy Grove, Illinois, 1837.** Wild Bill Hickok? You must be joking. I mean, what about all those old movies with cute Guy Madison? And what about Calamity Jane? Weren't Jane and Wild Bill a team in the Old West? What? Calamity Jame was that way, too? You mean, Doris Day and Howard Keel were playing homosexuals without knowing it? What's that you say? That Wild Bill and Jane used each other as fronts for respectability? What is this world coming to? The next thing you'll be claiming is that the American flag is gay. What do you mean, see September 13?

# 28.

**PATRICK WHITE, b. London, 1912.** Born in England of Australian parents, the Nobel Prize-winning novelist has spent time in both countries. But his heart and his genius are Australian. "Whatever has come since, I feel that the influences and impressions of this strange, dead landscape of Australia predominate." What has come since, and most recently, is White's autobiography, *Flaws in the Glass: A Self-Portrait,* a work of such beauty and importance that it must be read by anyone who would understand how the gay experience, in the hands of a master craftsman, can be transformed into great art.

# 29.

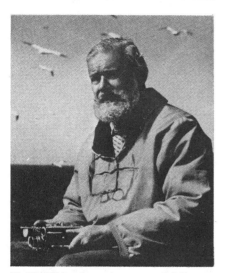

**T. H. White:** Learning as a painkiller.

**T. H. WHITE, b. Bombay, India, 1906.** Terence Hanbury White, known to his friends as Tim White, and to his readers as T. H. White, may be said to have spent most of his life fleeing from his homosexuality, which he feared. "The best thing for being sad is to learn something," said Merlin in *The Sword in the Stone,* the first of White's Arthurian books. Throughout his life he armed himself against his gayness by exploring new fields of knowledge and endeavor—whether it was painting or plowing a field, hunting or Irish history, the Arthurian legends, flying or falconry—all of which became the raw material for his many books. The author of *The Once and Future King* (which became the Lerner and Lowe musical *Camelot*) allowed himself to love without reserve only once, and the recipient of that love was his red setter. Sad.

# 30.

**JOAN OF ARC, d. at Rouen, 1431.** Since the story of Joan was not written down until more than three centuries after she was burned at the stake, how certain can one be that the male attire and short hair that the Maid of Orleans affected did not grow out of her essential nature rather than as the result of her religious visions? And what is one to make of her friendship with Gilles de Rais, the model for Bluebeard, who murdered not wives, but boys he had sodomized? Were they both the victims of Church tyranny that all too easily attached the stigma of "unnaturalness" to any of its enemies, or is there a degree of truth to the darker sides of their legends? What an extraordinary novel, or even opera, their joint stories would make.

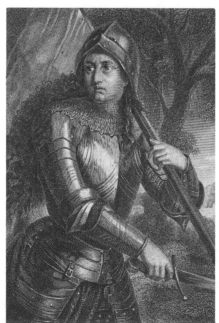

**Joan of Arc:** Medieval drag?

**CHRISTINE JORGENSEN (né George Jorgensen), b. 1926.** "I didn't start the sexual liberation movement," says Christine thirty years after the operation that shook the world, "but I was part of it when it was ready to start." Strictly speaking, Christine is not gay, since having never considered herself male, she could not possibly have been attracted to the "same sex" just because she was interested in men. But she rejects the term "transsexual," believing that sex never really had anything to do with her decision to undergo surgery in Denmark. The problem, as she puts it, was "gender identification." She always conceived of herself as a woman, and a woman is what she determined to become. That she has endured three decades of bad jokes and finger-pointing is more than compensated for by the life she has led, and continues to lead, as an entertainer and as a popular lecturer on college campuses. Then there is the realization that her life has required a degree of courage that would make a soldier or professional athlete pale. "Life has been good to me," she says. "I have no regrets."

# 31.

**WALT WHITMAN, b . West Hills, Long Island, New York, 1819.** The great debate is over. Old Walt has finally been declared gay. Who can believe that it has taken our scholars close to a century to write this footnote to the obvious, or that the battle over whether or not Whitman was gay was ever waged at all? But through the years our eggheads toiled, hoping against hope that Walt's lies about his mistresses and illegitimate babes would somehow turn out to be true, and ignoring

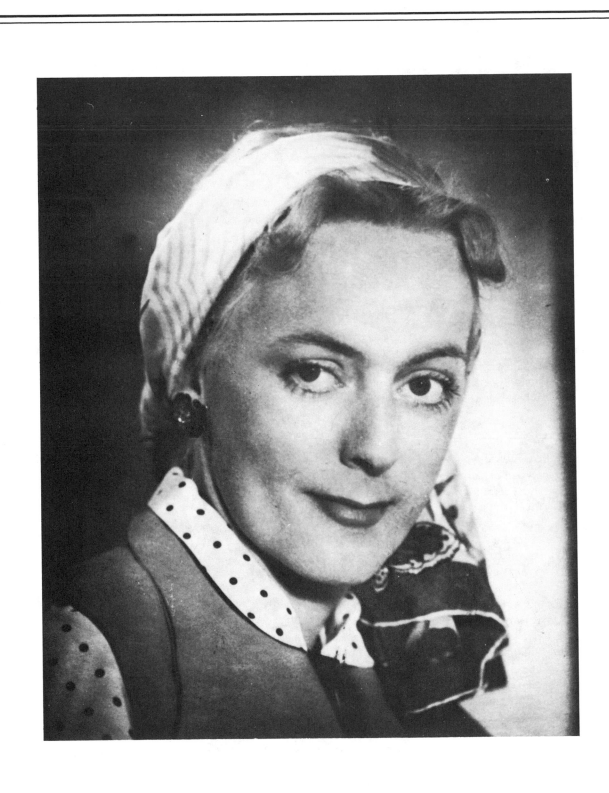

**Christine Jorgensen:** "I didn't start the sexual revolution, but. . . ."

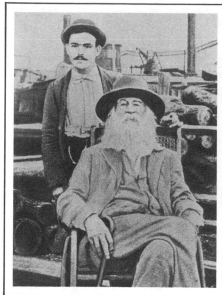 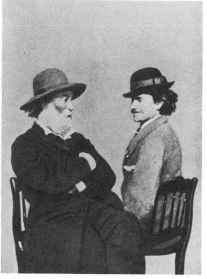

**Walt Whitman:** With his male nurse and with Peter Doyle.

## Other Personalities Born in May

1. **James Mills Peirce,** American mathematician, 1834
   **Calamity Jane (née Martha Canary),** American sharpshooter, 1852

2. **Edith Anna Oenone Somerville,** Irish writer (half of "Martin Ross" writing team), 1858

3. **Niccolò Machiavelli,** Italian political philosopher, 1469
   **Charles XV,** king of Sweden, 1826
   **William Inge,** American playwright, 1913

5. **Angelo d'Arcangelo (né Joseph Busch),** American writer, 1933

6. **Maximilien François de Robespierre,** French revolutionist, 1758

7. **Thomas Sergeant Perry,** American literary critic, 1845

12. **Justus von Liebig,** German chemist, 1803
    **Florence Nightingale,** English nurse, 1820
    **George E. Woodberry,** American poet, 1855
    **Sasha Gregory Lewis,** American writer and activist, 1947

13. **Modest Tchaikovsky,** the Russian composer's brother, 1850

16. **Elizabeth Peabody,** American educator and feminist, 1804

what was apparent to even the city fathers of Philadelphia sixty years ago when they fought against naming a bridge for that white-haired faggot poet. But it's official now. The word has come down from the mountain. Walt Whitman was GAY. Shee-iiit. What else is new?

**RAINER WERNER FASSBINDER, b. Bad Wörishofen, Germany, 1945.** A genius? Or just a competent filmmaker who has been generously overpraised? It's much too early to know. A few things, however, are certain. Fassbinder revitalized the modern German cinema. His homosexuality, worn as a badge for the world to see, did not discourage critical enthusiasm for his films. There are some very lovely touches in his works: In *The Bitter Tears of Petra von Kant,* a film about lesbians, the only men on the screen are the nudes in the huge Correggio mural beside the main character's brass double bed. But there are also excesses: the pathetic death of Fox (played by Fassbinder himself) in *Fox and His Friends.* Fassbinder's own life was a continuous excess, as well—sadomasochistic sex, alcohol, drugs. That he died young did not surprise the gays of Munich, who knew him all too well.

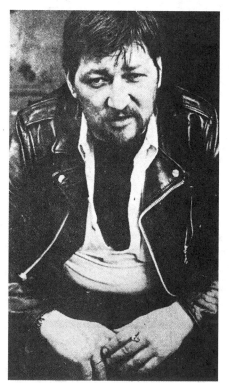

**Rainer Werner Fassbinder:** A burned-out case.

17. **Frederic Prokosch,** American novelist, 1908
    **Merle Miller,** American writer, 1919
    **Jill Johnston,** American writer, 1929
    **Ronald Tavel,** American playwright, 1940

19. **Peter Fisher,** American writer and activist, 1945

20. **Antoinette Brown Blackwell,** American feminist, 1825

**Parker G. Rossman,** American writer on boy-love, 1919
**Charles Reich,** American writer, 1928

21. **Alexander Pope,** English poet, 1688
    **Franklin Kameny,** American astronomer and activist, 1925

25. **Coleman Dowell,** American writer, 1935
    **Michael Lally,** American poet, 1942

27. **Sasha Alyson,** American publisher, 1952

28. **William Pitt the Younger,** English statesman, 1759

29. **Anne Marie Louise d'Orleans, Duchesse de Montpensier,** 1627
    **Louise Michel,** French anarchist, 1830

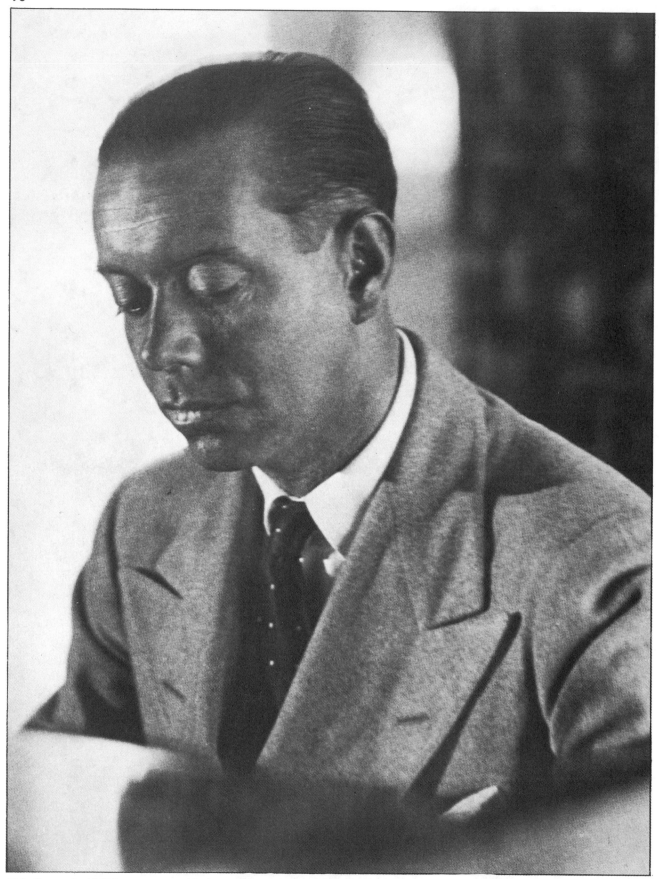

**Cole Porter:** In 1941 he got away with these ambiguous lyrics: "Don't inquire of Georgie Raft/Why his cow has never calfed,/ Georgie's bull is beautiful, but he's gay!"

# JUNE

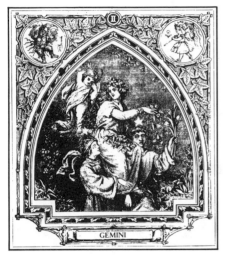

GEMINI

**Gemini** (May 21st to June 20th) is a mutable airy sign. The main characteristics of Gemini are self-expression, eloquence, intellectual energy, and versatility. Mercury, the ruler, is the planet of the mind, and Gemini represents Mercury in his capacity as an artist and agile manipulator of ideas. The versatility of Gemini can become a fault by diffusing the Geminian's energies over too wide a range of activities. The Geminian can often be vacillating and indecisive as well. But the craving for diversity and an impatience with sameness and repetition leads Geminians to brilliant careers in science, literature, and art, for the true function of the type is to make life better for themselves and others. At their worst, they can combine an overly sensitive disposition with cold-blooded selfishness verging on cruelty.

## 1.

**MARILYN MONROE (née Norma Jean Baker), b. Los Angeles, California, 1926.** Poor Norma Jean. Packaged and sold around the globe as a male wet dream, exploited even after death by necrophilic writers great and small, vilified in a gross and pompous play by her former husband, is it any wonder that she once found a rare moment of comfort in an affair with a female drama coach? Of the mountains of words written about her, this one nugget, mined from an otherwise useless book by her personal maid, seems to make good psychological sense. And isn't it interesting that the incident should be related in the only book written about her by another woman?

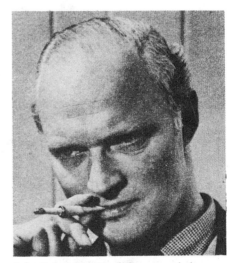

John Lehmann: He did more to help young writers than any contemporary editor.

## 2.

**JOHN LEHMANN, b. Bourne End, Buckinghamshire, 1907.** The editor responsible for first publishing in England such authors as George Orwell, Stephen Spender, Christopher Isherwood, Jean-Paul Sartre, C. Day Lewis, Boris Pasternak, Louis MacNeice, Bertolt Brecht, Lawrence Durrell, Edith Sitwell, and Theodore Roethke, was by no means the most distinguished member of his family. His sister Beatrix was one of the great English actresses, and his sister Rosamund an outstanding writer whose first novel, *A Dusty Answer,* incidentally, is not without its relevance to the present book. Their father, Rudolph Lehmann, wrote for *Punch* for thirty years and

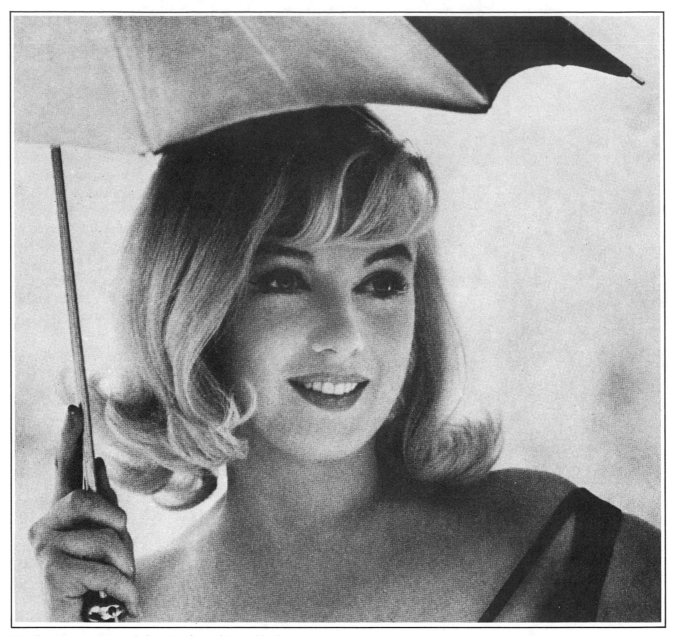

**Marilyn Monroe:** A needed respite from the world of men.

regularly included his children's writings, misspellings and all, in his column. Having grown up surrounded by books, it is hardly surprising that John Lehmann became one of the most influential editors and publishers of modern literature. A list of some of the American authors that he introduced to England is instructive: Tennessee Williams, Gore Vidal, Truman Capote, Carson McCullers, Paul Bowles, the very best post-war gay writers. Lehmann's poetry, much of it quite beautiful, is sometimes unabashedly gay. Some of it appears, with the author's permission, in Ian Young's pioneering gay anthology, *The Male Muse.*

# 3.

**ALLEN GINSBERG, b. Paterson, New Jersey, 1926.** The influence of Ginsberg's poetry on an entire generation has been enormous. How Ginsberg and the other "beats" appeared to readers in the '50s, still wearing flats and dress shields and seven crinolines, is hard to reconstruct. Thirty years later, when today's youth makes yesterday's "beats" look as if *they* were wearing flats and dress shields and seven crinolines, it makes one wonder how the poetry, the pronunciamentos will hold up in the future. The trouble with telling the truth—and Ginsberg is one of the most directly honest writers who ever lived— is that the truth dates much more rapidly than the elegant lie that rarely shows its age. W. H. Auden, who really couldn't stand Ginsberg's poetry, was once visited by the beat poet who had come to Oxford to pay him homage. Auden, to cut the visit short, showed Ginsberg around Christ Church Cathedral, and, in parting, was horrified when the young poet—with the utmost sincerity—knelt and kissed his trouser cuffs. Auden, who knew more than a little about the elegant lie, once wrote that "Sincerity always hits me something like sleep. I mean, if you try to get it too hard, you won't." Of the two poets, it would be interesting to know whose work will survive the longer.

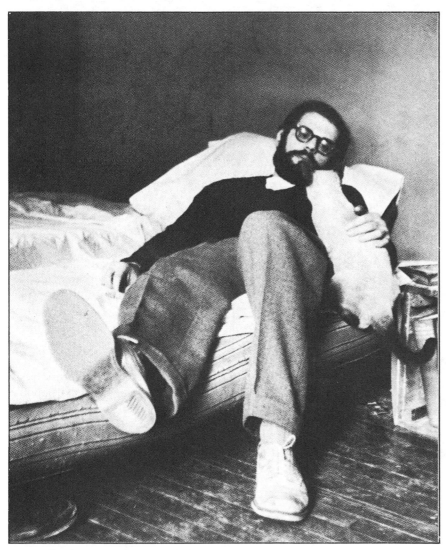

**Allen Ginsberg:** The most important poet of his generation, and the most influential.

# 4.

**GEORGE III, b. 1738.** The first English-born Hanoverian king and the reigning monarch during the American War of Independence, George III was the subject of much gossip during his youth. The gossip is interesting in that the young king actually walked into a preexisting rumor, very much a character in chapter 2, as it were. George's father, Frederick, the Prince of Wales, had been much taken with the charming Earl of Bute, whom he found an agreeable whist companion. When Frederick died, Bute, who had constantly risen in court ranks, stayed on, presumably as the lover of Frederick's widow. Enter the adolescent George, at eighteen very much the opposite of Hamlet. Rumor had it that he not only did not want to drive the usurper from his mother's bed, but that he really wanted to be in her place. Bute's elevation to secretary of state under George only heightened court gossip. How much of this is true, no one knows. That mother and son were both taken with the  handsome Bute is true, but one and one do not always add up to three.

# 5.

**IVY COMPTON-BURNETT, b. London, 1892.** All her many novels, which have been called "morality plays for the tough-minded," are satires of the least attractive aspects of human nature as found among the nobility and landed gentry of the late-Victorian world. They are very strange and very intelligent novels by a very strange and intelligent woman. Compton-Burnett lived most of her life in a "romantic friendship" with

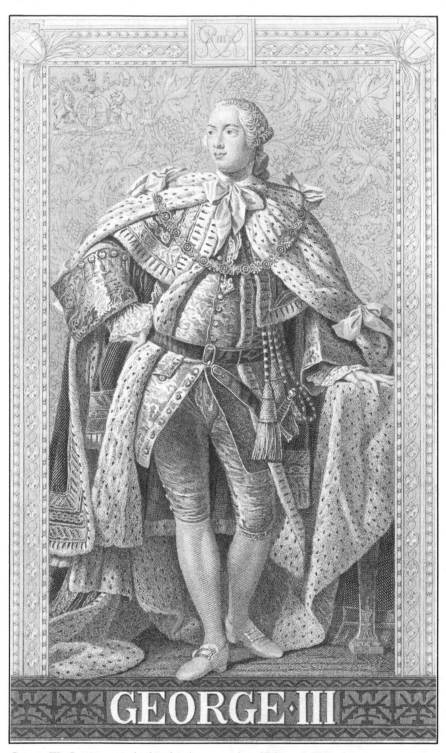

**George III:** Court gossip had it that he wanted to fill his mother's shoes.

when the novelist's fame far exceeded the scholar's, no one entered their *sanctum sanctorum* without paying court to Jourdain alone. They had no sexual contact with each other, nor with anyone else, Jourdain believing that only men experienced sexual desire and Compton-Burnett explaining that they were essentially "a pair of neuters." When Jourdain died, the novelist was almost sixty, but her subservience and dependence never ended. She continued to talk with her friend: "I say 'What do you think? Do you like it? Would you advise me? What shall I do?" Strange. Fascinating. Eerie. Like her novels.

# 6.

**VIOLET TREFUSIS, b. London, 1894.** Violet Trefusis was "the other woman" in the life of Harold Nicolson and his wife Vita Sackville-West. As the daughter of Alice Keppel, the mistress of Edward VII, Violet enjoyed a childhood of mystery and romance in a house where "Kingy" was a regular, if undiscussed, visitor. She and Vita met when they were girls. During World War I their friendship developed into passion. Though they both made conventional marriages, Violet could finally bear her love no longer and instigated the "elopement" that has since become a special chapter in the history of love. When Vita returned to her family and her writing at Sissinghurst, Violet imposed exile upon herself, turning to art and writing and the fantasy world of international society. But the feelings that she and Vita shared never abated. "You are the unexploded bomb to me," Vita wrote Violet in 1940. "I don't want you to disrupt my life." Even after twenty years of separation, she could still write of the love that "always burns in my heart whenever I think of you."

Margaret Jourdain, a woman several years her senior and a well-established scholar and expert in 18th-century furniture. There was no question in the Jourdain/Compton-Burnett household as to who was *numero uno*. Jourdain talked and Compton-Burnett listened. Even

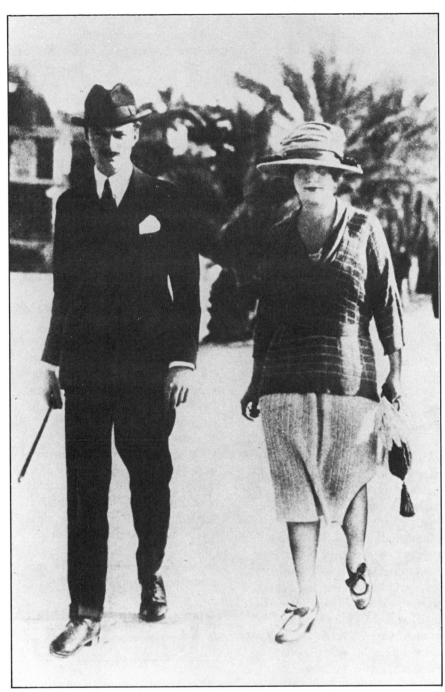

Denys and Violet Trefusis: "The other woman" and her husband.

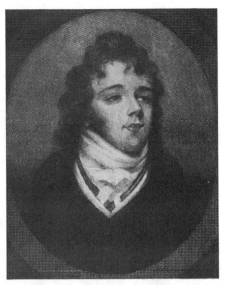

**Beau Brummel:** So refined that he once caught a cold from a damp stranger.

# 7.

**BEAU BRUMMELL (né George Bryan Brummell), b. London, 1778.** Brummell is included here because he epitomizes the dandy, a type that has always characterized *one* aspect of gay life from Oscar Wilde and Ronald Firbank to Waugh's Anthony Blanche and the ubiquitous queen who lives in the poshest apartment in the upper east side of every fashionable city in the world. Brummel loved fine clothes and lived beyond his means to attain them. He was oh so witty and oh so bitchy. So he died in an insane asylum, hounded by his creditors. His *bons mots* have survived him. Asked if he ever ate vegetables, he replied that he "once ate a pea." He also claimed that he once caught a cold from a damp stranger. Clever.

**ELIZABETH BOWEN, b. Dublin, 1899.** Like the outlines of her own life, the novels of Elizabeth Bowen reflect marriage at the center of a woman's life, with the love between women a primal need in adolescence and in widowed middle age. Her earliest novel, *The Hotel* (1928), is about the friendship between a young woman and a middle-aged widow. The character of the younger woman is clearly autobiographical. After her own husband's death, Bowen returned to this theme, switching roles of course. Late in her career, the novelist declared that she could find nothing "unnatural" in love between women. Her writing, she said, was

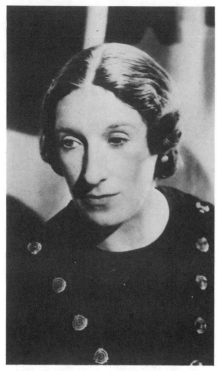

**Elizabeth Bowen:** In her books the lesbian experience brackets the heterosexual experience.

"a substitute for something I have been born without—a so-called formal relation to society."

# 8.

**EDWARD PERRY WARREN, b. 1860.** Warren was a fascinating character who deserves a biography of his own, although he is unlikely ever to have one. Independently wealthy, he left his native America and spent most of his life in England, together with his lifelong "soulmate," John Marshall, whom he had met at Oxford in 1884. Under the pseudonym "Arthur Lyon Raile," he wrote a three-volume *Defense of Uranian Love,* a 60,000-word apologia for pederasty, as embodied in the Greek art that he collected. He also wrote poetry and novels on the same subject, notably *Itamos: A Volume of Poems* and *A Tale of Pausanian Love,* about homosexuality at Oxford. His collection of Greek art, one of the largest in the world, forms the core of the collections at the Boston Museum of Fine Arts and New York's Metropolitan Museum of Art. Whether there are museum plaques fully identifying the background of their original collector is doubtful.

# 9.

**COLE PORTER, b. Peru, Indiana, 1892.** It was typical of the urbane songsmith to have hand-picked Cary Grant to play him in the Hollywood biopic of his life. Grant, then forty-two and at the height of his attractive charms, is what Porter would have liked to look like. The film, *Night and Day,* is an atrocity, but fascinating to watch, not only for its lies and deliberate distortions, but for the wild pleasure of watching Grant, in early middle age, attempt to play a Yale freshman. When, with his faintly absurd Cockney accent, he composes "Night and Day" to the accompaniment of amplified raindrops and a symphony orchestra, it is a moment to treasure, excelled perhaps only by Cornell Wilde as Chopin, addressing Merle Oberon (as George Sand) as if she were the father of her country. Cole Porter thought himself an aristocrat. He was a snob, a bigot, a superficial charmer who was a thoroughly unpleasant person. He also wrote some of the best popular music of the century. Genius and character, after all, are not necessarily correlated.

# 10.

**TERENCE RATTIGAN, b. London, 1911.** Rattigan, whose well-made plays, exceptionally popular in their time, were more or less pushed off the English stage by the works of Osborne, Wesker, Pinter, and Arden, and were considered passé in the 1960s, has never really received his due as a playwright. Yet, his plays have held up very well, even as the reputations of his once-revolutionary successors have begun to decline. Rattigan's *The Browning Version* (1948), an effective and masterly study of failure, may be seen as a precursor of Edward Albee's *Who's Afraid of Virginia Woolf?* The horror of a particular type of marriage, in which the pain inflicted on each partner is ultimately the pleasure of both, is as fully explored in Rattigan's one-act play as it is in Albee's much longer drama. It is not difficult to understand why Rattigan so admired the talent of Joe Orton and was instrumental in helping to get the young writer's early plays produced. A recent review of a New York production of *The Browning Version* implied, snidely, that a more balanced view of marriage might have come from a heterosexual playwright. Until that review, there had probably been no more than three New York theater-goers who had ever even conceived of Terence Rattigan as anything but straight.

# 11.

**GERARD MANLEY HOPKINS, b. Stratford, Essex, England, 1844.** Hopkins, scholar, aesthete, and ascetic of an Anglican family, was received into the Roman Catholic Church while still an undergraduate at Oxford. In 1868 he entered a Jesuit Novitiate and burned all his early poems, resolved to write no more till he should, by ecclesiastical authority, be enjoined to do so. After

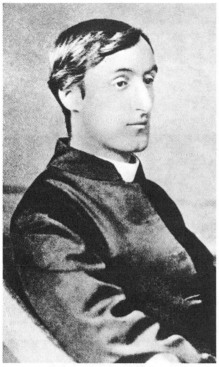

**Gerard Manley Hopkins:** "It is the vice of distinctiveness to become queer. This vice I cannot have escaped."

seven years, the silence was lifted by a superior's suggestion that some member of the community should elegize the five Franciscan nuns who perished in the wreck of the *Deutschland.* The Jesuit poet is a master of word painting, who in freshness of diction and elliptical approach is generally considered the first modern poet. He seems much closer to the 20th century than he does to the Victorians, and, in fact, his poems were only first collected and published in 1918. The constant conflict between Hopkins' desire to be a saint and his desire to be an artist is central to his poetry, but it produced the "nervous prostration" from which he suffered and which led to his failure as a parish priest, teacher, and classical lecturer—his real "occupations." It is now acknowledged that what Hopkins called his "nervous prostration" was in reality his repressed homosexuali-

ty. The poet-priest was completely homosexual in inclination and perfectly celibate in life, a state which resulted in great misery for him and great poetry for us.

# 12.

**HENRY SCOTT TUKE, b. York, England, 1858.** Although a great deal of attention has been paid to the paintings and photographs of naked girl children that were innocently, yet disturbingly, common in the Victorian era (Lewis Carroll's photographs come to mind), almost no attention at all has been paid to the even more prevalent representations in art of prepubescent boys during the same repressive period. In the America of Horatio Alger, the parlors of the fashionable were decorated with the salon paintings of J. D. Brown, whose sentimental studies of newsboys, grocerboys, and street urchins not only prefigure the wide-eyed monstrosities of Keane and the teary-eyed horrors of Woolworth's, but rather perversely transfer the physical horseplay of robust teenagers to the bodies of eight and nine-year-olds. The result was hundreds of male Lolitas in the middle-class parlors of America. In England, the grand master of romantic boy painting was Henry Scott Tuke, whom we know to have been homosexual. Tuke was an athlete who took great pride in his splendid body. He was obsessed with painting nude boys and experimented, and succeeded, in developing a special technique for capturing on canvas the effect of sunlight on naked skin. Interestingly, his name is not mentioned in several multivolume sets of reference books calling themselves "encyclopedias of art," despite the fact that Tuke was enormously popular in his time.

# 13.

**RICHARD BARNFIELD, baptized Norbury, Staffordshire, England, 1574.** There are, as everyone knows, certain inseparable teams: Gilbert and Sullivan, Cheech and Chong, bagels and lox, ham and eggs, Sodom and Gomorrah. In classical mythology, as in ballet, there are Daphnis and Chloë, the Greek shepherd and his lady love—Daphnis and Chloë, as inseparable as yin and yang, gin and tonic, Ron and Nancy. Not in Richard Barnfield, however. His *Affectionate Shepherd* (1594) scandalized Renaissance England by describing in florid detail the love of Daphnis and Ganymede, just a couple of guys foolin' around. What the fuss was all about is difficult to say since, in the absence of Chloë, Daphnis never exercised his shepherdly option of making it with a favorite sheep, choosing a boy instead. "If it be sin to love a lovely lad," wrote Barnfield, "oh, then sin I." He was not quite twenty-one when he wrote his pathbreaking poem.

**PAUL LYNDE, b. Mt. Vernon, Ohio, 1926.** How does one pigeonhole the show-biz persona of Paul Lynde? Perhaps it's not incorrect to say that he was Franklin Pangborn fifty years later, given the license to say what the Hollywood Code prevented Pangborn from ever saying, even though you knew, just looking at his face, that he was capable of saying it. Or perhaps Lynde was Franklin Pangborn crossed with Eve Arden, women always having been given the opportunity for comic bitchery denied men because in women such behavior was seen to be "in character." Whatever he was, Lynde was pretty funny at it. And he was known, on more than one occasion, to have shocked the hair-roller set with his acid queen-like tongue. "Why do motorcyclists wear leather?" he was asked on *Hollywood Squares.* "Because chiffon wrinkles too easily, that's why." That was Paul Lynde in our time. Franklin Pangborn wouldn't have been permitted to know what a motorcyclist was, no less to have known anything about leather. But he might have been seen ironing the chiffon. That's the difference that time makes.

hungry than the legendary Cleopatra, who, nicknamed "Thick Lips," is said to have blown 100 Roman soldiers in a single night. Her reputation notwithstanding, Menken was a manhater whose *Infelicia,* a collection of Sapphic poems, clearly reveals her delight in women. She was for a time the lover of novelist George Sand.

# 14.

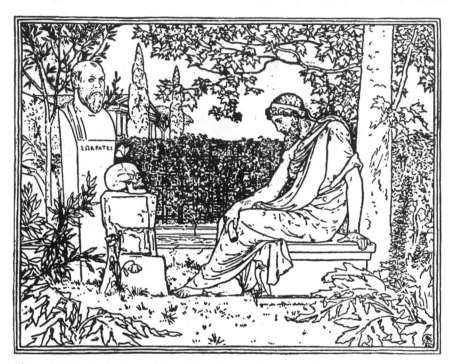

**Plato:** A Victorian setting of the philosopher meditating on immortality.

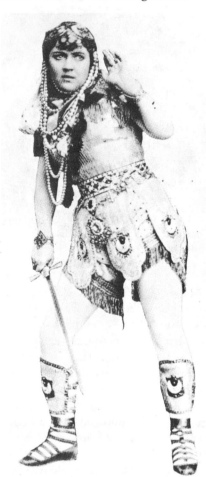

**Adah Isaacs Menken:** Swinburne, who liked to be whipped, considered her his "pitiless goddess."

**PLATO, b. Athens, Greece, c. 427 B.C.** This is hardly the place to summarize the teachings of one of antiquity's greatest thinkers. Suffice it to say that Plato, through his famous *Symposium,* has given his name to the love that dare not speak its name nor show its little fairy wings in public, even though Platonic love has come to mean lately a kind of sexless friendship. That Platonic love before Freud was clearly gay love is evident in *Patience,* Gilbert and Sullivan's devastating satire on the aesthetic movement, in which the effeminate poet Bunthorne sings about "an attachment à la Plato for a bashful young potato and a not too French, French bean!" Plato was born with the name *Aristocles.* He was surnamed *Plato* because of his exceptionally well-developed broad shoulders. Try *that* out on your piano.

# 15.

**ADAH ISAACS MENKEN, b. New Orleans, Louisiana, 1835.** The flamboyant actress got around. She was reputed to be only slightly less man-

**EDVARD GRIEG, b. Bergen, Norway, 1843.** Edvard Grieg? That sweet little guy, the one whose "Anitra's Dance" is always played in third-grade music appreciation class? What's he doing here? In old age he was completely taken with the boyish charms of curly-haired, blond Percy

ography to go on, the slender thread is the drippy *Here Lies the Heart,* Mercedes de Acosta's account of her many lady loves, in which Hoffman is one of the players. Since none of the cast of characters, including Garbo and Dietrich, uttered a public peep when the book was published, we can only assume that the book was either too silly to refute or, sillier still, even true.

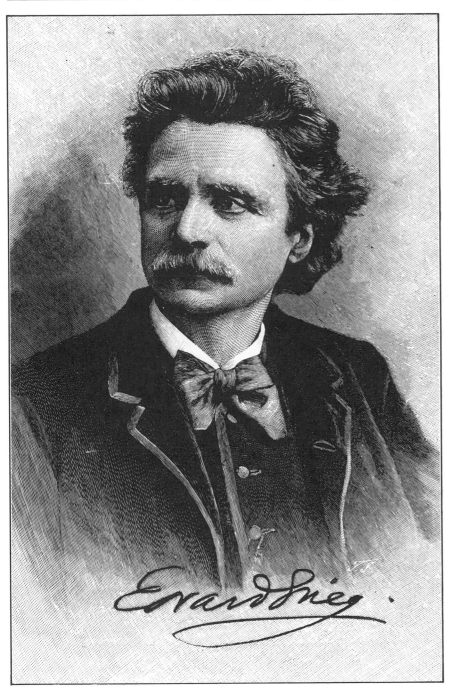

**Edvard Grieg:** Percy, Percy, please have mercy.

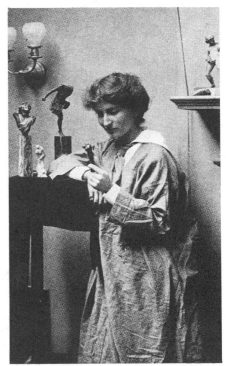

**Malvina Hoffman:** A fascinating life in need of a modern biographer.

# 16.

Grainger, whose "Country Gardens" is inflicted on the same third-grade class of audiophiles. "I love him," Grieg declared. "I love him like I love a young woman." That's odd. That's exactly what poet Vachel Lindsay said about the same Australian Goldilocks. (See November 10).

**MALVINA HOFFMAN, b. New York City, 1887.** The sculptor, who traveled around the world to model the heads of every racial type, is included here on the most tentative "evidence." Since there is no modern biography, and we have only Hoffman's not-too-candid 1930 autobi-

**KING GUSTAVUS V, b. Stockholm, Sweden, 1858.** Before the game became as bloody as a chain-saw murder drive-in movie, tennis was a bit of a joke to red-blooded beer-swilling manly men. The very mention of the phrase "tennis, anyone?" in a play or film meant that the chap in white was as queer as the arrangement of pansies in the English drawing room. Gustaf, as he was called by his adoring subjects, was something of an amateur tennis champion. He is said to have taken up the game to be near the willowy blonds who specialized in knowing how to serve.

# 17.

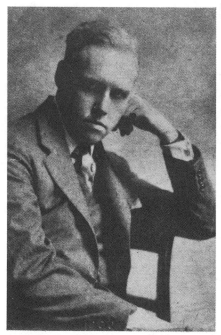

**Carl Van Vechten:** "A thing of beauty is a boy forever."

**CARL VAN VECHTEN, b. Cedar Rapids, Iowa, 1880.** It's funny how these things work. Black pride has led to an exploration of black culture, and the Harlem Renaissance of the '20s and '30s has been rediscovered. The renewed interest in the Harlem Renaissance has led in turn to the de-mothballing of the white man who was at the center of it all, its chief publicist in fact, Carl Van Vechten, photographer and writer, dandy and man about town. In many ways Van Vechten was the American Ronald Firbank, the early Evelyn Waugh from corn-fed Cedar Rapids. Reading Van Vechten is not exactly like eating salted peanuts. But his books have all the flavor of a time when drinks were called cocktails and were served, with fancy little things called canapes, in matching blue-glass shakers, trays, and glasses. Start reading Van Vechten with *The Blind Bow-Boy,* in which a randy duke emblazons his stationery with the motto: "A thing of beauty is a boy forever." You get the general idea.

**MAURITZ STILLER, b. Helsinki, Finland, 1883.** Many of the men in Greta Garbo's life were gay, in-

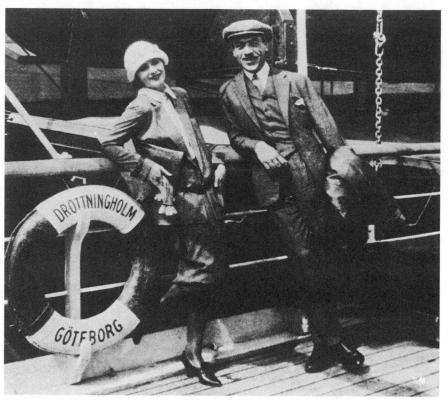

**Greta Garbo and Mauritz Stiller:** Like several other men in her life, her discoverer was gay.

cluding some, still living, whose "affairs" with the film goddess easily threw a naive public off its guard. Stiller, however, really meant something to Garbo. He was her discoverer, her mentor, her friend. The director—tall, lean, gay, with a wild shock of hair and long, expressive hands—was in demand in Hollywood, and his price to MGM to come to Southern California was a contract for pudgy Greta Gustafsson. That his failure as an MGM director was as spectacular as her success is at the heart of Garbo's separation from Hollywood.

# 18.

**ROBERT STEWART, SECOND VISCOUNT CASTLEREAGH, b. Dublin, Ireland, 1769.** Why did Britain's nominal head of state slit his throat with a penknife on the night of August 12, 1822? Was it, in fact, because he had suffered a nervous breakdown after numerous political defeats, as was the official explanation for his death? Or was it the threat of public exposure as a homosexual? If the latter, as many continue to believe, was Castlereagh actually gay? Or was he the victim of an extraordinary scam by a gang of blackmailers who, knowing Castlereagh's weakness for whores, tricked him into a rendezvous with a wench who was actually a boy in female attire? For the answers to these and other questions, don't tune in tomorrow, but turn instead to H. Montgomery Hyde's *The Strange Death of Lord Castlereagh,* a non-fiction mystery as absorbing as any detective story.

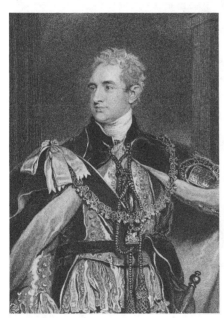

**Viscount Castlereagh:** Why did he slit his throat with a penknife?

# 19.

**KING JAMES I, b. Edinburgh, Scotland, 1566.** The son of a homosexual who was murdered in his bed at twenty-two, together with the page he was buggering, James,

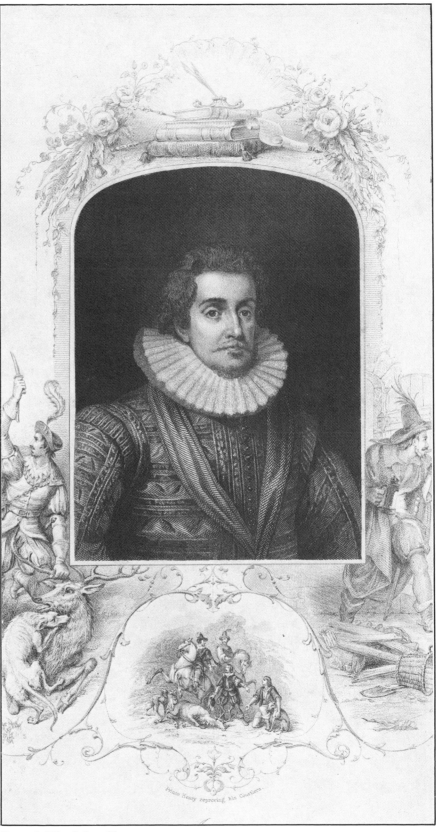

**James I:** Like father, like son.

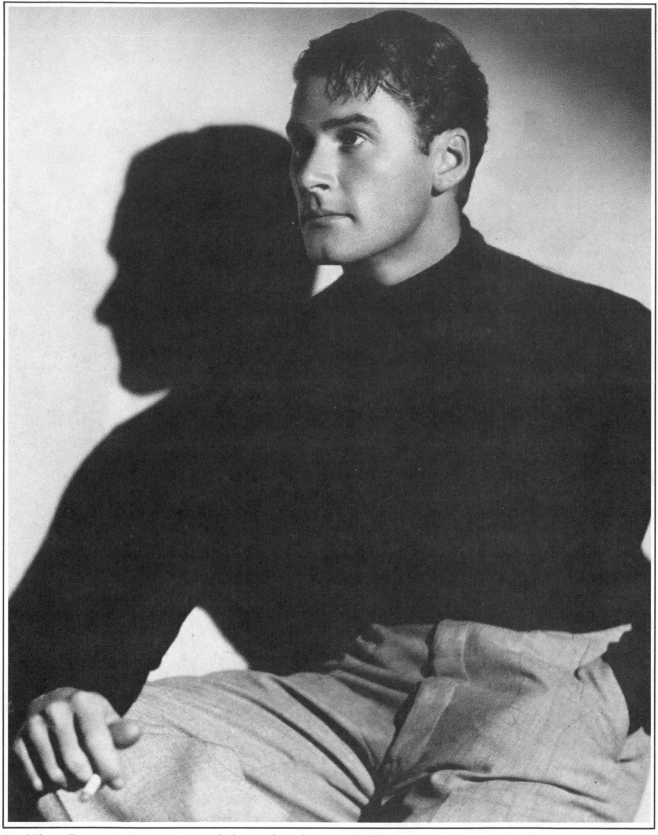

**Errol Flynn:** Trysts with Tyrone Power at the home of gay director Edmund Goulding, who was titillated by the idea of the two stars making it under his roof.

King of Scotland and England, was himself a homosexual, but, understandably, unable to act on his own instincts. All of his great loves were heterosexual men completely unable to return the love that this unhappy man so desperately needed. Fewer heads in history were ever more uneasy in wearing a crown. The joke that circulated about King James in his own day is telling: "*Habuimus regem Elisabetham, habemus reginam Jacobum*" ("We have had King Elizabeth, now we have Queen James.")

# 20.

**ERROL FLYNN, b. Hobart, Tasmania, 1909.** What a surprise to most people when the news broke that this greatest of Hollywood womanizers also slept with men. Flynn, of course, had made his reputation on his body and on his magnificent Black Irish looks, so it made no difference whatever that he couldn't act his way out of his leading ladies' pessaries. When he smiled that dazzlingly wicked smile of his at the camera, he melted panties and B.V.D.'s in darkened theaters all over the world. The actor's trial for rape during World War II only increased his popularity, thanks to the candid details printed in the daily newspapers, even though by modern standards one would be hard-pressed to know whether the two girls in question had actually been raped or whether Flynn had been engaged in building a secret munitions depot for the Allies. ("And then what did Mr. Flynn do?" "He took out this thing." "What thing?" "This big hard thing." "And what did Mr. Flynn do with this thing?" "He told me to close my eyes." "Yes?" "He took his pleasure with me." "You mean you had sexual

intercourse?" "I think so.") Wow, I mean, a stud like that could have whomever he wanted, the cream of the crop, the salt of the earth, the most desirable men and women in the universe. Flynn's biographer, a

# 21.

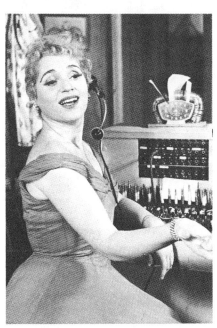

**Judy Holliday:** The bells that rang were belles.

**JUDY HOLLIDAY (née Judith

tease if ever there was one, finally names only three men, two of them, uh, Truman Capote and Howard Hughes. Oh, well. It still gives new meaning to the old phrase, "In like Flynn."

Tuvim), b. New York City, 1922.** Her voice could etch glass, and the blond head that it issued from had the reputed I.Q. of a genius. She stole all the scenes in her first picture from right under the professional noses of Katharine Hepburn and Spencer Tracy, Hepburn having contrived to get her the part in an effort to prove to the monster mogul Harry Cohn that Holliday should be given the starring role in *Born Yesterday,* the play that had made her a Broadway sensation. Her 1950 "Drop Dead" was as famous as Gable's "Frankly, my dear, I don't give a damn" of 1939, but infinitely more funny. Her reign as a top screen comedienne was brief because she died young, of cancer. Judy Holliday is included here because, as her biographer has shown, she was torn between her many affairs with women and her love of men.

# 22.

**PETER PEARS, b. Farnam, Surrey, England, 1910.** It used to be said, politely of course, that the English tenor was the companion of Benjamin Britten. Since "companion" seems to conjure up an image of two old ladies in shawls, let's say, no less politely, but more vigorously, that the tenor and the composer were for many years devoted lovers. As

Poulenc did for Bernac, Britten wrote some of his most wonderful music for Pears, and Pears introduced Britten's songs and operas throughout the world. Together they worked indefatigably toward the creation of the Aldeburgh Festival, their musical child. It used to be said, politely of course, that Pears's is a "quite unremarkable voice." Let's say, no less politely, but more directly, that Pears's voice is pretty lousy, although handled with deft musicianship, and that his place in the annals of music history will rest primarily on his association with Britten.

# 23.

**ALAN M. TURING, b. 1912.** Alan Turing was a British logician, mathematician, and computer scientist. He was the technical genius behind Britain's successful effort to break the German codes during World War II. He designed some of the world's first electronic computers. His 1937 paper laid the groundwork for much of computability theory, and his 1952 paper left a defining test of artificial intelligence. In 1952, Turing was arrested and tried for having had sex with a nineteen-year-old man. He spent a year on probation, including a condition that he receive estrogen injections to kill his sex drive. The conflict between the British government's idea of gayness as an automatic security risk (the idea had begun, of course, in the United States) and Turing's own strong demands for personal liberty was apparently his unsolvable problem. He committed suicide in 1954. As one of his colleagues put it, "All we can do is imagine what it must have been like for a man as sensitive as Turing to be threatened . . . with the loss of everything that mattered to him, his science, livelihood, the esteem of friends. And we must muse on the savage price exacted by a society that without him might not have survived to demand it."

# 24.

**HORATIO HERBERT, LORD**

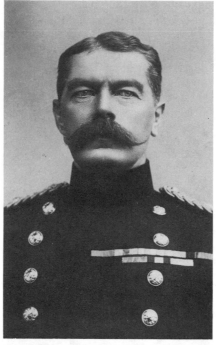

**Lord Kitchener:** He was particularly efficient in giving orders to his military secretary.

**KITCHENER, b. Bally Longford, County Kerry, Ireland, 1850.** A decade after Turing's death, the same Brits who had pushed the mathematician over the precipice, howled in outrage at the publication of Douglas Plummer's *Queer People,* a general history of homosexuality that sought to prove to the English people that gayness was not limited to Oscar Wilde and a few assorted French couturiers. The book named names, among them Lord Kitchener's, one of the great heroes of English Imperialism. No wonder the Colonel Blimps roared.

# 25.

**FORREST REID, b. Belfast, Ireland, 1876.** The Irish novelist was a close friend of E. M. Forster, and their works are in some respects quite similar, even though Reid's are un-

fairly neglected today. As Francis King writes, "Reid led a simple life in the company of his dogs and cats and the boys whom he befriended. An extremely ugly man, he was a pederast who, like many pederasts, perpetually harked back to the lost heaven that had lain about him in his boyhood. He is usually represented as having been happy and uncomplicated; but in fact his was a dark, involuted, troubled nature and in the course of his life he made more than one attempt at killing himself. When, as inevitably happened, the boys whom he loved grew up, had girlfriends and got married, he indulged in scenes of bitter recrimination and maudlin self-pity." While still in his twenties, Reid correctly surmised that Henry James was gay and dedicated his mildly homosexual novel *The Garden God* (1905) to the American writer. James, true to his nature, was not flattered and publicly condemned the book for its "artless portrayal of sinister matters." A later book was dedicated to Forster, who was delighted.

# 26.

**MOTHER CLAP, b. London, c. 1670.** Yes, you've got it. There's nobody of any special note born today, so this is slightly breaded filler, a gay Tuna-Helper, if you will. We don't know Mother Clap's real name, but she did in fact exist. In 1726 she was indicted for keeping a "disorderly house" where some fifty men were found making love, "kissing in a lewd manner and using hands indecently." To these charges she offered this defense: "I am a woman, and therefore it cannot be considered that I would ever be concerned in such practices."

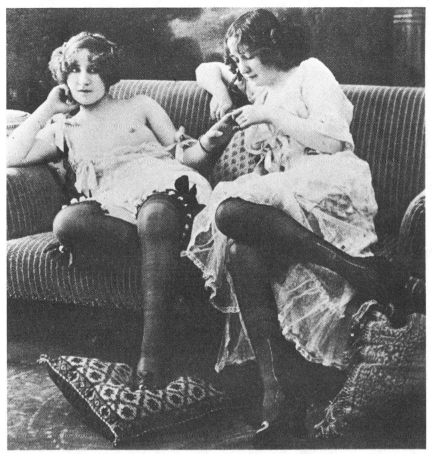

French postcard, c. 1910: No one has yet explained why lesbianism has always been a turn-on for heterosexual men.

# 27.

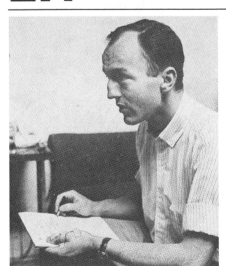

Frank O'Hara: He will emerge at the center of the biographies to be written about his famous contemporaries.

**FRANK O'HARA, b. Baltimore, Maryland, 1926.** This poet, playwright, and art critic died just two days before his fortieth birthday in a freak accident on New York's Fire Island. His talents, diverse but minor, seem to recede with the passing of the years, just as much of the art that he championed when he was with the Museum of Modern Art seems like so such ancient history twenty years after its inception. Frank O'Hara's poetry was published in a collected edition, posthumously, in 1971. In recent years, the painter Larry Rivers, in discussing his own bisexuality, has said that he was for a time one of O'Hara's lovers.

# 28.

**DAVE KOPAY, b. Chicago, Illinois, 1942.** In late 1975, Kopay, a ten-year veteran running back for the San Francisco Forty-Niners, the Detroit Lions, the Washington Redskins, the New Orleans Saints, and the Green Bay Packers, decided to drop his mask and publicly reveal that he was homosexual—the first professional athlete ever to do so. When his story broke in the *Washington Star,* the reaction was as varied as it was unpredictable. Outrage from some sports fans, congratulations from others who respected the athlete's candor. Most unexpected was the hostility from many militant gays who resented the publicity given one man that would have been impossible for them to attain short of a major political assassination. What the stupes missed in those myopic years was Kopay's real accomplishment. In a single stroke he wiped out the stereotypes of centuries, or, at the very least, he raised doubts in the minds of all but the most stupid rednecks. If a running back for the Forty-Niners could be gay, then so could anyone. The old jokes about dippy hairburners suddenly lost their punch.

# 29.

**JEAN LORRAIN (né Paul Duval), b. Fecamp, France, 1855.** The once-famous French journalist worked only because he had to. He preferred to spend his life sleeping with the sailors along the Paris, Nice, and Marseilles waterfronts. "Fucking," he once wrote, "is basically a sport for idle minds. When you work, it's goodbye ass!" Although his works are largely forgotten today, they should be revived and vigorously pursued. How can one ignore an author who, in a fashionable restaurant, once shouted at the top of his lungs the following couplet: "I spent the night between two fellows from the docks,/Who took turns, and cured me of the hots!"

# 30.

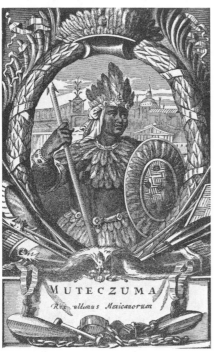

**Montezuma II:** You are who you eat.

**MONTEZUMA II, d. Tenochtitlan, Mexico, 1520.** No one knows the exact date of Montezuma's birth in 1479, but the emperor of ancient Mexico did in fact die on this day in 1520. He is included in these pages only because of a peculiar habit which, the other noble traits of Aztecs notwithstanding, made him a bit less than Rousseau's Noble Savage. In a grisly case of having one's cake and eating it, too, Montezuma is known to have cannibalized the boys he had sodomized. Pass the Pepto-Bismol, please, and goodbye June!

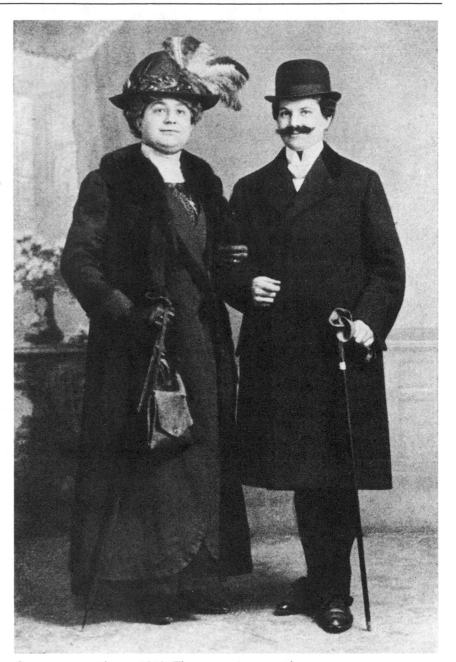

**German transvestites, c. 1910.** The woman is a man; the man, a woman.

## Other Personalities Born in June

1. **Sondra Scoppetone,** American writer, 1936

2. **The Marquis de Sade,** French sexual "philosopher," 1740
   **Alesandro Cagliostro,** Italian adventurer, 1743

3. **Marion Zimmer Bradley,** American writer, 1930

   **Walter Rinder,** American writer, 1934

   **Paul Mariah,** American poet, 1937

5. **Prince Ernest Augustus,** English royalty, 1771
   **John Maynard Keynes,** English economist, 1883
   **Federico Garcia Lorca,** Spanish poet and playwright, 1898

6. **Paul Gauguin,** French painter, 1848

7. **Edward Field,** American poet, 1924

8. **Marguerite Yourcenar,** French novelist, 1903
   **Rev. Malcolm Boyd,** American activist minister, 1923

9. **Peter I the Great,** Russian czar, 1672

11. **Violet Florence Martin,** Irish writer (half of writing team known as "Martin Ross"), 1862
    **George Baxt,** American novelist, 1923

12. **Harriet Martineau,** English feminist, 1802
    **Djuna Barnes,** American writer, 1892

17. **Charles XII,** king of Sweden, 1682

18. **Raymond Radiguet,** Cocteau's adolescent poet-lover, 1903

20. **Rupert Croft-Cooke,** English writer, 1903
    **Audie Murphy,** American war hero and actor, 1924

21. **Robert Bashlow,** American writer, 1939

24. **Theodore Beza,** French theologian and poet, 1519
    **Henry Ward Beecher,** American theologian and reformer, 1813

27. **Charles IX,** king of France, 1550
    **Emma Goldman,** Lithuanian-born American anarchist, 1869

28. **Giovanni della Casa,** Italian poet, 1503
    **Frederick William Faber,** English hymn-writer and theologian, 1814
    **Hunce Voelcker,** American poet, 1940

30. **Reginald Brett,** Second Viscount Esher, English nobleman, 1852

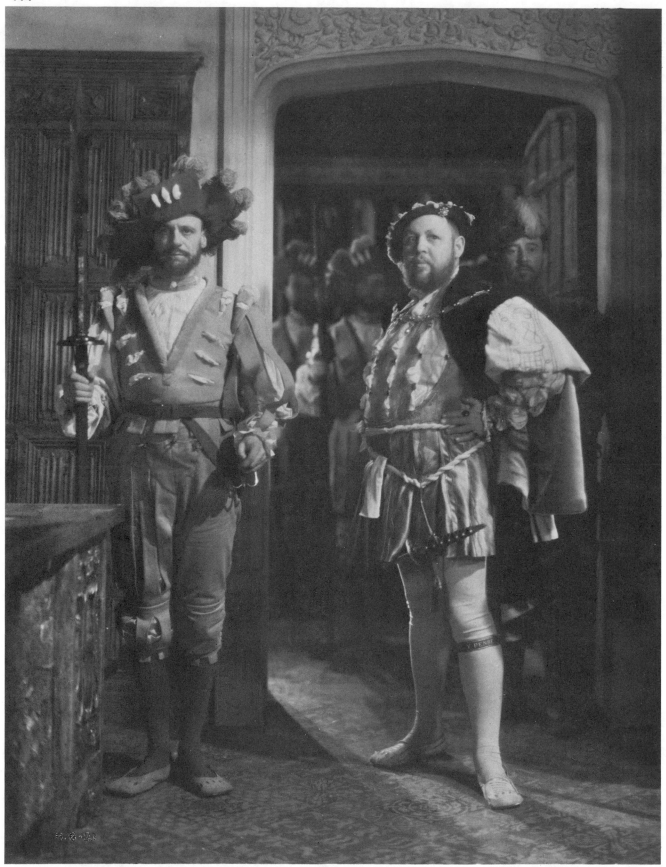

**Charles Laughton:** His face and figure, though he hated them, were his fortune.

# JULY

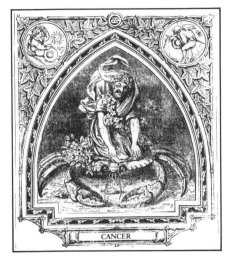

CANCER

Cancer (June 21st to July 21st), is a cardinal watery sign ruled by the moon. The crab is the perfect sign for Cancer since the Cancerian is outwardly hard and unemotional, but inwardly sensitive in the extreme, not only to other people, but also to art, literature, and psychic forces. Another prominent characteristic of the Cancerian is his clannishness and preference for his family and home environment. He is permanently fixed to wherever he puts down roots. The key words in understanding the traits of Cancerians are "adaptability" and "tenacity," which combined mean "patience." Patience is the essential force of this sign and of its ruler, the moon. The moon waxes and wanes, shines in full radiance or suffers eclipse, but in all its varying stages is always *constant in its inconstancy*. When Cancer, the crab, has seized an object and wants to have it, he would rather lose his claw than let go, and having lost it will grow another to take hold again. Cancer is the leader to whose music all the world must dance.

# 1.

**GEORGE SAND (née Amandine Aurore Lucie Dupin), b. Paris, 1804.** Although she dressed as a man, wrote novels under a male pseudonymn, and is known to have had several intense relationships with women (the writer Alfred Vigny referred to her vehemently as "that lesbian"), lesbianism never occurs in the romantic novels of George Sand. Her affairs with prominent men were the talk of Europe and were exploited in her fiction, but she maintained a discreet silence about the friendship of women, even though modern critics are in agreement that her female characters are all independent and dominant women like herself, "masculine" they say with more than a touch of bias. That George Sand chose not to write about lesbianism is understandable.

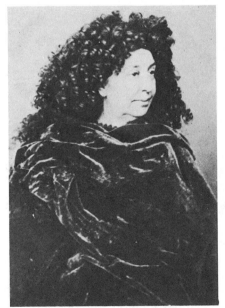

**George Sand:** "What a great man she was, and what a kind woman."

She had sufficient trouble in establishing her independence as a woman to worry about supplying weapons to the enemy. When she died, Turgenev wrote to Flaubert, "What a good man she was, and what a kind woman."

**CHARLES LAUGHTON, b. Scarborough, England, 1899.** Charles Laughton hated the way he looked, hated the face he was born with, and despised his corpulent body. Nonetheless, his face was his fortune and helped to make him the greatest character actor in the history of films, a performer able to portray the most diverse range of personalities with flamboyance or finesse as each part required. No matinee idol could possibly have been assigned the variety of human types that Laughton played in his thirty-year career. As a homosexual he felt cheated because he was not handsome, even though he was blessed with a wife whose love and intelligence allowed her to share him with his gay male friends. Elsa Lanchester's foreword to her husband's biography is a warm and candid document, well worth reading. It is a tribute to the English actor's genius and, unwittingly, to her own.

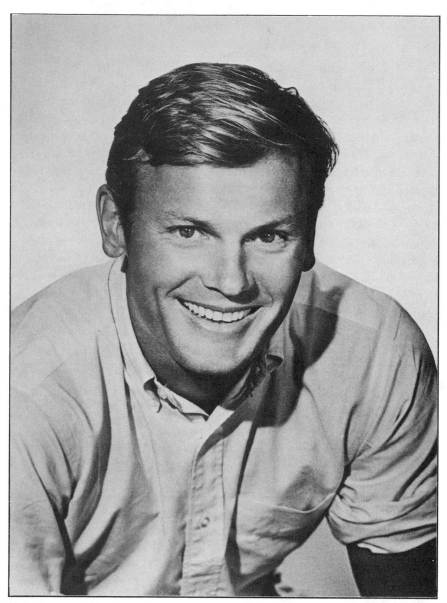

**Tab Hunter:** Golden boy of the '50s and even better today.

**TAB HUNTER (né Arthur Gelien), b. New York City, 1931.** To anyone growing up gay in the 1950s, Tab Hunter was an inspiration. True, the surname assigned him by the Hollywood packagers was a little odd, but that was the day of Rocks and Bricks, and children were beginning to be called Tara and Tammy just as the world was starting to be made of plastic. But he was so handsome, blond, clean-cut, and athletic that every mother's son wanted to look exactly like him, if only their acne would dry up and go away. From the front row of the Bijou or the Gem, he seemed to be so *nice,* unlike the other young actors who always had their moments of being real mean to the ladies, even throwing hot coffee on them or pushing them down flights of stairs. Then he disappeared from the screen and the mean ones continued being mean until, by the 1970s, there were no longer any women to push down stairs since Redford and Newman and the other actors were having too much fun in movies with each other to require actresses for beating up or any other purpose. By the 1980s a miracle occurred. Special effects had totally replaced all leading women on the screen except Divine, and Tab Hunter was back, this time at her side. He is still an inspiration. More handsome and athletic than before, he remains exceptionally nice. He can't possibly imagine how badly he's been missed.

# 2.

**DONALD WINDHAM, b. Atlanta, Georgia, 1920.** Of Donald Windham's novels, the best known is perhaps *Two People,* a lovely book about an affair between a married American businessman and a Roman boy. Despite his own considerable talents, Windham may very likely wind up remembered, like the parts played in endless movies by Ralph Bellamy, as someone else's best friend. The "someone else," in Windham's case, is Tennessee Williams. Windham was nineteen when he met the twenty-eight-year-old Williams. The two had in common their ambitions as young writers, their Southern backgrounds, their lack of money in prewar New York, and their homosexuality. Eventually they decided to collaborate on a play, and, while Windham stayed in New York, Williams wandered between Provincetown, Massachusetts, and other places in search of boys and a quiet retreat in which to write. During these years began a correspondence which Windham collected and finally published in 1977. Although Williams published his own rather disappointing autobiography, the Windham letters, with the novelist's excellent annotations, are the *real,* albeit incomplete, Tennessee Williams memoir. The letters are dazzling, unguarded, racy, funny, and, above all, revealing of every flattering and not-so-flattering aspect of the famous playwright over a twenty-five-year period.

# 3.

**WILLIAM HENRY HURLBERT, b. Charleston, South Carolina, 1827.** Is it the soil? Is it the climate? The American South has produced not only a disproportionate number of Miss Americas, but an equal disproportion of beautiful young men, many of whom, by the way of Princeton University, wander up North, where they settle as innocents, both charming and tantalizing, until middle age hits them like Italian madonnas, if the bottle doesn't get them first. William Hurlbert (né Hurlbut) was one such Southern charmer, a beauty who drove several rather stolid men wild. The minister Thomas Wentworth Higginson, who confessed that "I never loved but one male friend with a passion," found the beautiful Hurlbert "like some fascinating girl" and modeled the hero of his novel *Malbone* (1869) on him. Mrs. Higginson, who took a somewhat dim view of this "romantic friendship," complained after her husband's death that the letters he exchanged with Hurlbert were "more like those between man and woman than between two men." Apparently, at least two other novelists used the handsome Southerner as a lead character in their books, one of these characters a man who, at the end of

the novel, turns out to be a woman! Hurlbert, a writer himself, became the editor-in-chief of *The New York World*. Whether he was merely an innocent bag of gold desired by other men, or actually gay himself, is difficult to say. The record says only that several distinguished men couldn't help falling in love with him.

# 4.

**STEPHEN FOSTER, b. Pittsburgh, Pennsylvania, 1826.** Like Yankee Doodle, the composer Stephen Foster was born on the Fourth of July. His list of sentimental down-home hits— "Oh! Susanna," "Old Folks at Home," "Camptown Races," "My Old Kentucky Home," "Beautiful Dreamer," "Jeannie with the Light Brown Hair," and "Old Black Joe"—make the jingoistic George M. Cohan appear strident and un-American by comparison. Flag waving or no, what made fireworks go off for this star-spangled tunesmith was another composer—George Cooper, a handsome young man who is best known today for his "Sweet Genevieve," a song perhaps best sung as a barbershop quartet when drunk. So taken was Foster with sweet George Cooper that he abandoned his wife and family to run off with him. So, as you put out the bunting to celebrate the glorious Fourth, think of Stephen Foster, grand old American composer, "gwine to Lusiana" with George Cooper, instead of a banjo, on his knee.

# 5.

**CECIL RHODES, b. Bishop's Stortford, Hertsfordshire, England, 1853.**

Like Carnegie, Nobel, and many other multi-millionaires who made their fortunes through the blood of others and are remembered today for the good that has lived on after them in bequests and charities and edifices that their money endowed, Cecil Rhodes is remembered for the scholarships to Oxford that bear his name. Although most people think that Carnegie is a hall and Nobel a prize, it is less difficult to forget Rhodes's South African background, not if one has read a newspaper at any time during the past thirty years. Rhodes was the owner of the Kimberley diamond mines, which he had expanded by expropriating the land of the Matabeles by trickery, and was an active force in South African politics, where, to the chagrin of his native England, he was favorably disposed to the Boers. Many of today's problems in South Africa had their foundations laid during the time that Rhodes was virtual dictator. One of the grounds for selection as a

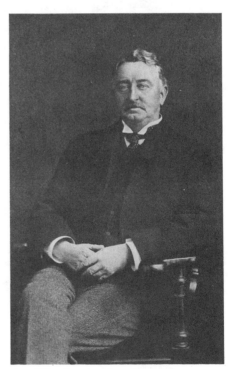

**Cecil Rhodes:** Are the scholars ever told?

Rhodes Scholar that has almost made it impossible for most "grinds" to apply is Rhodes's insistence that a candidate must have a "fondness for and success in manly outdoor sports, such as football and cricket." One wonders whether Rhodes's homosexuality had anything to do with this requirement, or whether such athletic prowess was to be simply another demonstration of the benevolent superiority of the Anglo-Saxon race.

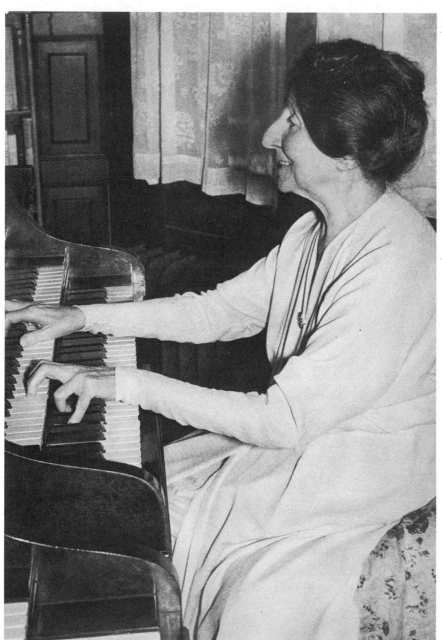

**Wanda Landowska:** Artist, scholar, teacher, wit.

**WANDA LANDOWSKA, b. Warsaw, Poland, 1879.** Landowska is considered responsible for the restoration of the harpsichord to popularity during the 20th century. Not only was she the foremost keyboard artist of ancient music on this instrument, but the first modern works for harpsichord were written especially for her (both of them, incidentally by gay composers, Manuel de Falla and Francis Poulenc). Landowska performed and taught first in Berlin, then in Paris, and finally in New York and Lakeville, Connecticut. She has left behind a legacy of great recordings and scholarly publications. Landowska, though married, was always known in the world of music as a lesbian, although the fact was first recorded by W. G. Rogers in his book about female patrons of the arts, *Ladies Bountiful* (1968). The great harpsichordist apparently had no illusions about the number of homosexuals in music. She is reputed to have startled an American performer who had come to study with her by asking him, without batting an eyelash, *"Et vous êtes un pédéraste, naturellement?"*

**JEAN COCTEAU, b. Maisons-Lafitte, France, 1889.** At ten minutes to four in the morning, just outside of Paris, Jean Cocteau was born with a silver spoon in his mouth. Eighteen years later, according to Harold Acton, this innovator of the arts took the pulse of each of the nine Muses and prescribed the exact regimen she had to follow. Fifty-four years later, Cocteau died in 1963 at the age of seventy-four, after fifty-eight years of kaleidoscopic activity in the arts. The astounding variety of his work, as poet, novelist, playwright, and filmmaker; and the contradictions and paradoxes of his private life, the charm and the nastiness, the generosity and the egotism, the poise and anguish of an opium-addicted homosexual who was equally welcome in the aristocratic drawing rooms of Paris and the raffish waterfront bars of Toulon, and who climaxed an avant-garde life by entering the ultra-conservative

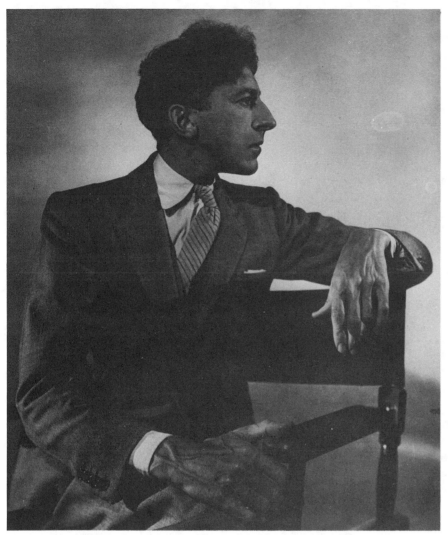

**Jean Cocteau:** Election to the Académie Française was "the final scandal" of a scandalous life.

# 6.

**JÈRÔME DUQUESNOY, b. Brussels, Belgium, 1602.** Like his sculptor brother François ("Il Fiammingo"), Duquesnoy was trained in their father's studio. After a long stay in Spain in the service of Philip IV, he traveled to Florence in 1640 and a year later settled in Rome with his brother. On François's death in 1643, Jèrôme returned to Brussels where he carved several statues of the apostles for the cathedral of St-Michel. He was at work on several projects at the cathedral of St-Bavon in Ghent, where his best sculptures were executed, when he was arrested for sodomy with two acolytes of the church who had served as his models. The brilliance of his work for the church notwithstanding, he was strangled and then burned at the stake, a double death, which, under the circumstances, seems to be a case of clerical overkill and a terrible waste of matches.

# 7.

**GUSTAV MAHLER, b. Kalischt, Bohemia, 1860.** It would be nice to claim Mahler as gay if only because his music is so cosmic, so intensely beautiful, so obviously the work of a genius who somehow understood how to shake the emotions of his listeners until they were overcome with pain or sobs or feeling or something resembling whatever a catharsis is supposed to be. But there's really very little to go on, only Thomas Mann's suspicion that the composer was homosexual, and the homosexual character of Aschenbach that he created in *Death in Venice,* based supposedly on Mahler. It's not much, but enough to have unleashed

precincts of the Academie Française—all this makes him impossible to summarize in a short space. (Fortunately, Cocteau has been well served in a brilliant biography by Francis Steegmuller, which should be read not only for a wonderful retelling of Cocteau's extraordinary life, but for its introduction to the arts and culture of the modern age, Cocteau's age.) Still, some anecdote should be told here that at least, in part, gives some sense of the spirit of the man. Here is one that does not appear in Steegmuller's biography: In the days before the puritanical Yvonne De Gaulle re-

moved the legendary Paris pissoirs, one of the many customs that sprang up regarding polite Parisian pissoir manners was known as the *"privilège du cape."* This custom allowed a Frenchman who could not find a convenient pissoir to approach a gendarme and ask him to extend his cape so that he could take a leak behind it. One of Cocteau's favorite amusements was to choose a handsome young cop and pretend that he was drunk. With luck he could get his trouser buttons undone by the helpful gendarme—and possibly more. Uncooperative victims wound up with wet shoes.

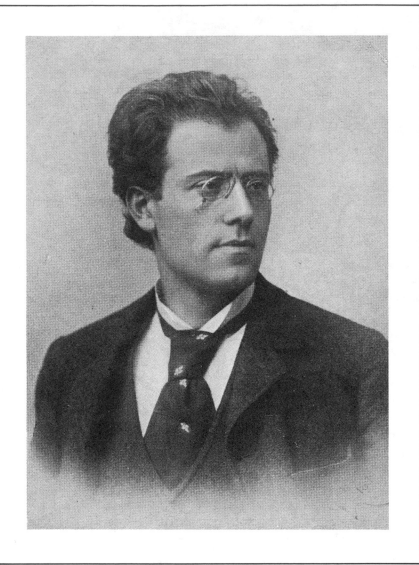

**Gustav Mahler:** Who played Tadzio to his Aschenbach?

and fell in love with the Baroness Hatvany, better known as Christa Winsloe, the author of *Mädchen in Uniform,* the celebrated novel about love in a girls' school. Although Thompson's affair with Winsloe was not her first—she had previously been in love with Gertrude Franchot Tone, the politically-active feminist mother of the movie actor—it was her most intense lesbian attachment and resulted in an outpouring of feeling that she confided to her diary: "I put the incident down here as a record of my own sensibility to this woman. What in God's name does one call this sensibility if it be not love? This extraordinary heightening of all one's impressions; this intensification of feeling? . . . This incredible feeling of sisterhood." Sinclair Lewis was virtually impotent and, knowing of his wife's bisexuality, had just published *Ann Vickers,* a novel about a career woman driven to suicide because of a lesbian relationship. No time could have been better chosen for Thompson's affair with Winsloe, a love affair that her biographer, Vincent Sheean, with little understanding, called "a rather strange interlude."

Visconti to do a job on Mahler *and* Mann in the film version of Mann's unfilmable novella. The Mahler score in *Death in Venice* left no question of Aschenbach's identity. It's Mahler on the Lido putting on makeup to attract the boy Tadzio, not Aschenbach.

# 8.

**DOROTHY THOMPSON, b. Lancaster, New York, 1894.** In the 1930s this newspaper and magazine writer, radio commentator, lecturer, and political analyst became an overnight sensation when Hitler expelled her from Germany because of her critical reports on Nazism. In 1931, when her marriage to Sinclair Lewis was already disintegrating, she met

# 9.

**MATTHEW GREGORY "MONK" LEWIS, b. London, 1775.** Have you ever read an 18th-century Gothic romance? They are incomparably silly, overripe, and, except for their excruciatingly stilted language, great fun to read. Horace Walpole's *The Castle of Otranto (see September 24)* started the literary vogue, and it was quickly followed by Lewis's *Ambrosio, or the Monk* (1795), and, in America, by the novels of Charles Brockden Brown. *The Monk* is the most lurid example of the genre, and Lewis was forced to delete many passages for a second edition that were considered "scandalous," so scandalous, in fact, that Lewis's literary stock skyrocketed and he found himself lionized by high society on the Isle of Hypocrites. *The Monk* combines the supernatural, the horrible, and a little bit of raw sex in its plot about Ambrosio, the superior of the Capuchins of Madrid. (It is essential to the Anglo-Saxon Gothic novel that affairs of the flesh always occur in a Latin clime.) Ambrosio is seduced by Matilda de Villanegas, a woman driven to blind nymphomania by demons, and who enters the monastery and Ambrosio's bed disguised as a boy! After he discovers that the boy is actually a woman, Ambrosio's entire character changes, and he pursues other women with the aid of magic and by murdering. His sins are found out and he is tortured by the Inquisition, finally being sentenced to death. He makes a bargain with the Devil in order to escape, but the Devil destroys him. It seems apparent that had the wild nympho Matilda actually been a boy, none of Ambrosio's problems would have followed. In real life, Lewis at twenty-eight was in love with fourteen-year-old William Kelly, a male incarnation of Matilda, who brought him nothing but misery.

# 10.

**MARCEL PROUST, b. Anteuil, France, 1871.** As almost everyone knows, Proust suffered from chronic asthma and wrote—mostly at night—in a cork-walled room. His vast novel *Remembrance of Things Past (À la Recherche du Temps Perdu)* recounts the life of his hero, virtually Proust himself. It has no plot in the usual sense, but is closely woven together like a symphony by the

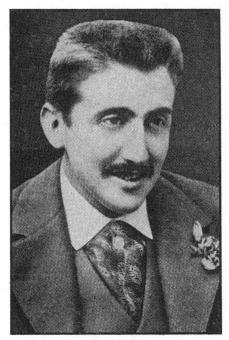

**Marcel Proust:** He set up the footman of a friend as "proprietor" of a male brothel that he owned himself.

recurrence of the same characters and the same themes. Memory plays a large part in the construction, and remembered scenes from boyhood are the device by which the more usual chronological method is replaced. There are many lengthy digressions, ranging from metaphysical dissertations on the flight of time and the timelessness of sensation to beautiful passages on architecture and art. In 1912, when Proust sought to have his manuscript published, it was summarily rejected. The report of a publisher's reader survives. Ironically, the first third of the many-volumed novel, so very rich in aesthetic, scientific, and philosophical learning, and today considered perhaps the most remarkable literary work produced in the first half of the 20th-century, was rejected on the grounds that "one has no idea of what it's all about . . . nothing happens in these 700 pages." One of Proust's major themes, of course, is homosexuality, but the subject is confused because, as Andrè Gide was

the first to point out, Proust made certain characters female when really he meant them to be male. Thus the character of Albertina, for example, is really based on Proust's own chauffer-lover, Alfred Agostinelli, a daring young Italian so in love with the speed of newly invented machines that he died (in 1914) while learning to pilot a primitive airplane. In the past, English and American readers have undoubtedly wondered why so much fuss has been made about Proust, since his famous book seems at times to be insufferably boring. The reason is the Scott Moncrieff translation that is not only dated in its stilted language, but severely bowdlerized to protect the virtue of the Anglo-Saxon reader. Gratefully, the new Terence Kilmartin translation is both modern and unexpurgated. Proust, at long last, is permitted to be gay.

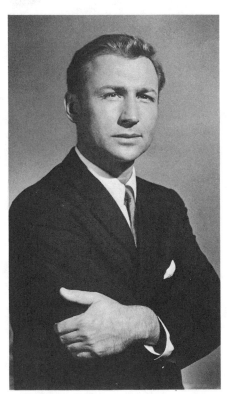

**Nick Adams:** Big things come in small packages.

**NICK ADAMS (né Nicholas**

Adamschock), b. 1932. Nick Adams was a blond, diminutive actor who usually played neurotic or aggressive types and sometimes comic sidekicks (as Andy Griffith's bespectacled pal, Ben, in *No Time for Sergeants*). He died by his own hand at thirty-six in 1968. Hollywood rumor has it that, since big things come in small packages, Adams was a successful hustler while he and his roommate James Dean were trying to break into acting. (In some versions of the story, Dean himself was out hustling as well.) At the time of his death, Nick Adams was the lover of a movie actor who can only be indentified as R_____ C_____.

# 11.

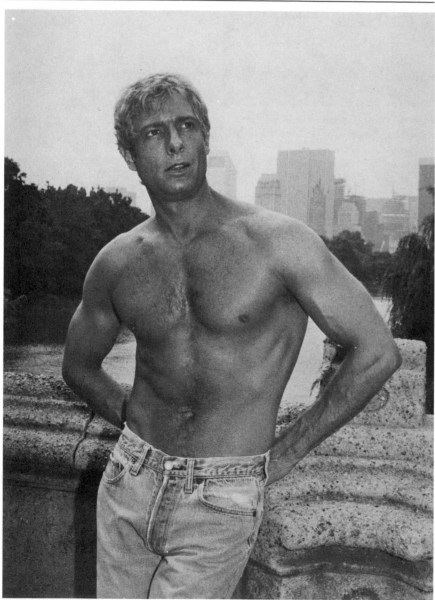

**Jack Wrangler:** He speaks engagingly of his screen persona as "he," as if he and it were mutually distinct.

**JACK WRANGLER, b. Los Angeles, California, 1946.** Jack Wrangler is every inch a star. He has survived the mayfly world of porno flicks, in which the rate of turnover is unusually high, to become a legend in his time. The camera loves him and he loves the camera, and himself, in uninhibited return. Porno-starring is consistently hard work. And if you doubt that such hard labor is difficult to keep up, just think of your own performance in a crowded doctor's office when the army-sergeant nurse bellows loudly that she wants a specimen right this minute in this tiny cup and you spend the next eternity in a narrow cubicle unzipping your fly and looking for it, the poor frightened thing. Would *you* be able to perform on cue in front of three cameras, fourteen arc lights, a script girl, and a crew of six? Porno films are notoriously dumb—dumb plots, dumb faces, dumb music—and uniquely difficult to pull off with any true erotic style. (A spot of acne on a callipygous ass can disconcert.) But the moment the camera focuses on Jack, something magical occurs. He's the real thing, intelligent, alert, alive—the picture stops, and the camera laps him up. The audience rises to a single man and applauds the star. Another standing ovation for Jack Wrangler.

# 12.

**HENRY DAVID THOREAU, b. Concord, Massachusetts, 1817.** In the fall of 1856, when he was thirty-nine years old, the author of *Walden* found "a rare and remarkable fungus, such as I have heard of but never seen before. The whole height [is] six and three quarters inches. It may be divided into three parts, pileus, stem, and base,—or scrotum,

# 13.

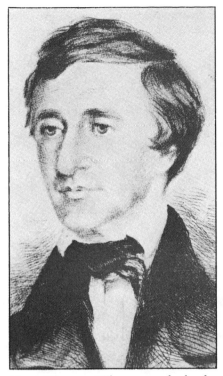

Henry Thoreau: "These young buds of manhood in the streets are like buttercups in the meadows. . . ."

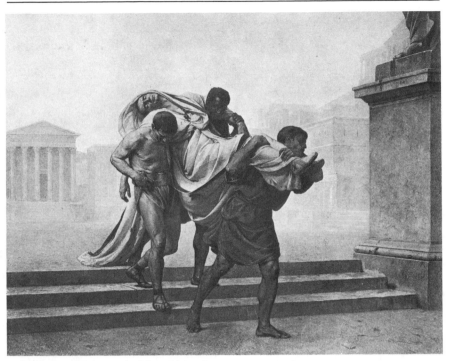

**Julius Caesar:** Beware the Ides of March.

for it is a perfect phallus. One of those fungi named *impudicus,* I think. In all respects [it is] a most disgusting object, yet very suggestive. It was as offensive to the eye as to the scent, the cap rapidly melting and defiling what it touched with a fetid, olivaceous, semiliquid matter. In an hour or two the plant scented the whole house wherever placed, so that it could not be endured. I was afraid to sleep in my chamber where it had lain until the room had been well ventilated. It smelled like a dead rat in the ceiling, in all the ceilings of the house. Pray, what was Nature thinking of when she made this? She almost puts herself on a level with those who draw in privies." Throughout his life Thoreau was falling in and out of love with his male acquaintances. He meditated on the higher meaning of male friendship in his notebooks. He never married. Get to work, you amateur psychologists!

CAIUS JULIUS CAESAR, b. Rome, c. 100 B.C. Although it is by no means the only reason why they carried Caesar out on a slab on the Ides of March, the Roman emperor's reputation as a manly man had once been irrevocably besmirched. The Roman code that permitted men to bugger at their will, allowed only adolescent boys to be on the long end of the stick. In a society where it was considered infinitely better to give than to receive, any male who voluntarily adopted a passive sexual role was forever after considered an inferior being. This Caesar had done in his love affair with Nicomedes, king of Bithynia. Cicero reports that Caesar, acting as royal cup-bearer for Nicomedes, was led, clad in a purple shift, to the royal bedchamber and its golden couch. Nicomedes, he says, was definitely on top. Throughout the remainder of his life, emperor or not, Caesar was taunted by his ene-

mies: Suetonius reports that Caesar was called "the queen's rival"; his partner in the consulship described him in an edict as "the queen of Bithynia"; his soldiers chanted, "Caesar conquered Gaul; Nicomedes, Caesar"; Curio the Elder called him "every man's wife and every woman's husband." "In contrast," as John Boswell writes, "the charge that Augustus had as a *boy* submitted to Caesar in the same way seems never to have done him much harm." Poor Julius Caesar, in so many ways a man in advance of his time! Not long after his murder, the public attitude changed as more and more emperors began to turn the other cheek just for the hell of it. They set the fashion for the glory that was Rome. Or, as an anonymous poet put it, "Rome, which delighted in making love from behind,/Spelled AMOR—love—by inverting its own name."

# 14.

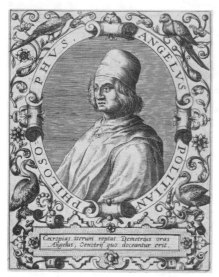

Politian: "The love of boys, I swear, is sweetest, softest, best."

**POLITIAN** (né Angelo Poliziano), b. **Montepulciano, Tuscany, 1454.** The greatest poet of his age, Politian was a friend of Lorenzo de Medici and the tutor of his children. Hailed by his contemporaries as the poetic successor to Ovid, Politian had only one weakness, an obsession with boys, that marred his reputation. But reputation be damned. The poet enjoyed his fame as a poet and cultivated a young following, just as many of our own literary lions do today. The story is told how young men from all over Europe would flock to Politian's lectures and then accompany him, 500 strong, back to his rooms. The storyteller's imagination, Politian's appetite, his quarters, or all three, were apparently a bit outsized. According to legend, Politian died at forty-two after bringing one beautiful youth back to his rooms, a student for whom he nurtured a passion so intense that he immediately broke out into a high fever. Feeling a bit hot under the collar, he took out his lute and began singing a song that he had written for the young man. At the end of the first couplet, he dropped dead. The story sounds like a moral allegory to us, especially the business about the fever and whipping out his lute. All that's certain is that he died at forty-two.

# 15.

**JAMES MIRANDA BARRY, d. Kensal Green, England, 1865.** James Barry (1795-1865) was a woman. What's more, she was a woman who spent her entire life disguised as a man. For over forty years she was an officer and surgeon in the British Army and enjoyed a highly distinguished career without arousing the suspicion of either her superiors or her patients. Much of her medical career was spent in South Africa, Jamaica, Canada, and other outposts of the British Empire. If anything appeared odd about her to her army colleagues it was her slight stature (she stood only five feet tall), but she eventually compensated for this with her own invention of telescoping false heels, antedating Adler elevator shoes by more than a century. Only the South African natives were sufficiently observant to notice another device that she adopted to pass herself off as a man. Because of the elaborately padded shoulders that she affected, the natives called her "the Kapok Doktor." Dr. Barry, over the years, developed a reputation as quite a rake and was known to "flirt openly" at balls with the "best-looking women in the room." She apparently did more than flirt, as well. She carried on an affair with a Mrs. Fenton, although it is not known at what point (if ever) Mrs. Fenton learned that her lover was a woman. Still, Dr. Barry's reputation as an army officer was never sullied since she was known as "a perfect gentleman who did not swear in the presence of women." When she died at seventy, she would have gone to the grave with her secret unknown had it not been for a charwoman who was preparing the body of the female Major General for burial. It must have been quite a surprise.

# 16.

**ANTINOUS, b. Bithynia, c. 110.** Antinous, the favorite of the emperor Hadrian, may have been a male whore when Hadrian met him, but his origins are obscure. All that is known is that Hadrian was immediately smitten with the beautiful fifteen-year-old. From that time on, Antinous was with the emperor constantly until on a journey to Egypt he was drowned in the Nile. Some say that Antinous, knowing that a prophecy had declared the death of Hadrian unless a living sacrifice were to be offered in his place, died so that his lover might live. Others believe that Antinous, growing into young manhood, was ashamed of playing

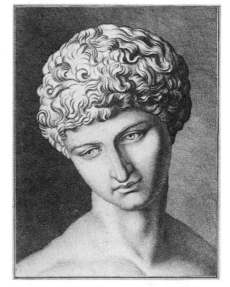

Antinous: Why did he drown himself in the Nile?

mistress to the emperor. The most poignant story is that the boy killed himself because he couldn't bear the idea of growing old. Hadrian's grief at the death of Antinous was uncontained. He had him deified, founded the city of Antinoöpolis in Egypt in his honor, and renamed the youth's birthplace Antinoöpolis as well. A cult was inaugurated in his honor, coins were struck with Antinous's head on them, and many busts and statues were made to commemorate the beautiful youth.

# 17.

ERNEST RHYS, b. London, 1859. There was a time when almost every reader knew the name of Ernest Rhys because he was the editor of the Everyman Library, those matched sets of small cloth-bound books that brought the classics of world literature to the average reader at low cost. By the time he retired, the series numbered 967 volumes. Rhys, who was gay and lived until the ripe old age of eighty-eight, made it a point to know everyone in the world of letters and had a fine wit. When he was a young man and heard that John Addington Symonds was writing his memoirs, he reported in the press, rather snidely, that readers could look forward to learning everything racy about the '90s and Oscar Wilde. Symonds took him to task, saying that he intended telling no anecdotes about people he had known and that gossipy anecdotes had no place in serious autobiography. Rhys apologized to the older man, but, when an old man himself, wrote the delicious *Everyman Remembers,* in which he committed to paper every anecdote he felt that Symonds should have told, plus hundreds of his own. His autobiography, therefore, chronicles the bizarre behavior of Oscar Wilde's gay contemporaries and, though embroidered with anecdotes of suspicious origin, is nonetheless a participant's testimony and a very entertaining one at that.

# 18.

LAURENCE HOUSMAN, b. Fockbury, Worcestershire, 1859. It might have been genetic, or perhaps there was something in the water at Fockbury, or maybe it was the splendid name itself, but the three children of Mr. and Mrs. Housman of Fockbury were all gay. There was the poet and classicist A. E. Housman, whom we've already met, the playwright Laurence, and sister Clemence, who was a wood engraver and a lesbian. Laurence Housman began as a well-known book illustrator, working, in part, together with Clemence who turned his fine designs into wood engravings. Occasionally Clemence wrote books of her own, like *Werewolves,* that were illustrated by her brother. Eventually Laurence became even better known as a playwright of some repute, a career he undertook at about the time that he was known about London as one of Oscar Wilde's most intimate friends. Housman's one great triumph occurred when he was close to eighty years of age, and this was the production of his play *Victoria Regina* (1937), which made household words of his and Helen Hayes's names. It is the play that gave the American actress a new first name, "Miss," a title that has stuck to her like a moray eel ever since.

# 19.

EDGAR DEGAS (né Hilaire Germain Edgar de Gas), b. Paris, 1834. In *Gay Geniuses,* a strange book published several years ago, the author W. H. Kayy comes to the conclusion that the great Impressionist painter and sculptor Degas was gay because he was obsessed with buttocks, both of ballet dancers and of horses. Moreover, Kayy repeats the old canard about Degas as a woman-hater because he painted his ballet dancers in tortured poses. Now any woman-hater who also likes tushies is, according to Kayy, *ipso facto* homosexual. There are of course, several things wrong with this theory. In the first place, more than a few straight studs have been known to refer to a woman as "a piece of ass," and, what's more, seem pretty obsessed by buttocks themselves. Second, most dance positions are pretty tortuous in and for themselves and are hardly dictated by the artist who paints or sculpts merely what the choreographer creates. And, if you don't believe that most dance poses are painful, try a couple if your body is not in perfect shape. Third, why are homosexuals automatically deemed woman-haters? Are the victims of battered-wife syndrome all married to gay men? Yes, Degas painted many ballerinas bending down to tie a slipper, massage a leg, but these are common scenes in the backstage world of dance. Why does this make the artist buttock-crazy? It seems to us as if Degas has been given a bum rap.

# 20.

**ORPHEUS.** It was said that the music of Orpheus's lyre was so beautiful that when he played wild beasts were soothed, trees danced, and rivers stood still. Orpheus married the nymph Eurydice. When Aristaeus tried to rape her, she fled, was bitten by a snake, and died. Orpheus descended to Hades searching for her. He was granted the chance to regain Eurydice if he could refrain from looking at her until he had led her back to sunlight. Orpheus could not resist and Eurydice vanished forever. Grieving inconsolably, he became a recluse and wandered for many years. This much of the legend of Orpheus is fairly certain. It's the final days of Orpheus, however, that are the subject of varying stories. One such version justifies Orpheus's inclusion here. The celebrated Thracian musician became a follower of Dionysius and soothed the Argonauts with means other than his melodies, thus introducing homosexual love into Greece. As a result, Orpheus was soundly hated by Aphrodite who considered him a competitor and rival. Orpheus met his end at the hands of the women of Thrace who, because the handsome hunk refused to pay them any attention, tore him to pieces. The myth of Orpheus is a good yarn, psychologically sound, and perfect for a day on which no one of any gay significance was born.

# 21.

**HART CRANE, b. Garrettsville, Ohio, 1899.** The poet, who killed himself at the age of thirty-two, has been called "a Dionysian ecstatic from Cleveland, drunk on meta-

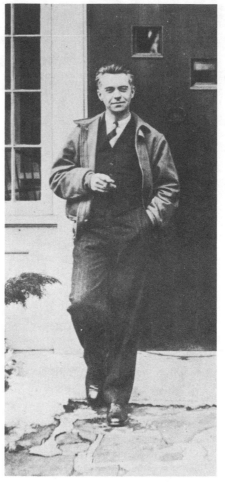

**Hart Crane:** He wrote about, and died within, "this fabulous shadow only the sea keeps."

physics and cheap red wine, a self-educated, self-tortured, self-destroyed homosexual visionary with a lavish gift of words strangled by a profusion of inchoate thought." Hart Crane was evidently the stuff of which legends are made. And they have been. Some of them dead wrong. Most wrong is the idea perpetuated by Crane's biographer that the poet's love for other men was "that open, generous affection we call Platonic love." That may be what John Unterecker wanted to call it in 1969, but that's as sure as hell what it was not. Here we go again! Just as it has taken a century to acknowledge that Whitman actually slept with men, it may take a while

longer before the keepers of the academic flame are ready to acknowledge that Hart Crane was not a shepherd piping songs of love on the Brooklyn docks. He cruised the docks for an entirely different reason.

# 22.

**FREDERICK ROLFE, b. London, 1860.** How many of you have read A. J. A. Symons's *The Quest for Corvo?* Raise your right hands. Hmmmm. That's what I thought. Since Symons's book is one of the great works of literary detection and should not be left gathering dust on library shelves, here's enough basic information on Rolfe to get your juices flowing. Rolfe, who liked to call himself Frederick Baron Corvo, although this was only one of his aliases, was a novelist, more than just a bit of a crook, a terribly sweet fellow, and the self-styled head of the Roman Catholic Church. (His most famous work of fiction is *Hadrian the Seventh,* a fantasy about himself as pope.) In reality, Rolfe's near-surreal life is much more interesting and funny than his writing. So what are you waiting for? Read *The Quest for Corvo* and find out why.

# 23.

**CHARLOTTE CUSHMAN, b. Boston, Massachusetts, 1816.** Said to be America's first great actress, Charlotte Cushman began as an opera singer, but, losing her voice, turned to the drama where in 1835 she first played Lady Macbeth, the role in which she was said to be unequalled. Her portrayals of male characters such as Romeo and

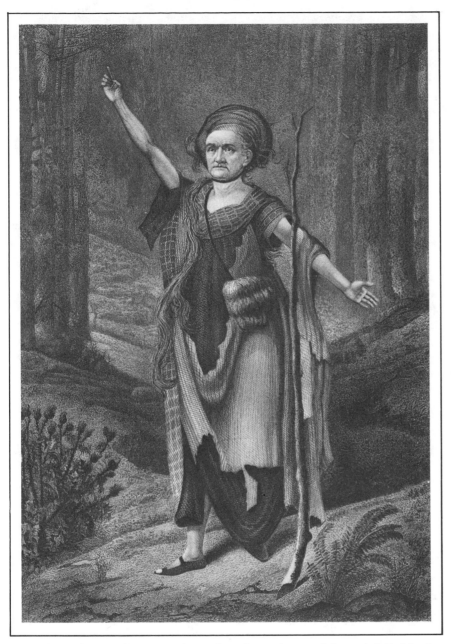

**Charlotte Cushman:** The muses of comedy and tragedy weren't her only lady friends.

**SAMUEL M. STEWARD, b. Woodsfield, Ohio, 1909.** People leave university teaching for many reasons—boredom, dislike of students, dislike of faculty, dislike of the entire academic racket—but Sam Steward is probably the only professor of English ever to have left the university to become a tattoo artist. And what a tattoo artist. "Phil Sparrow," one of several of his professional aliases, was not only among the best known tattooists in America, but the only one in regular contact with Alfred Kinsey, feeding the good doctor sexual information about everything from graffiti on Chicago elevated train stations to classifications of the types of people who are tattooed. A professor of English and a tattoo artist, Sam has led several other lives as well. In his youth he made the acquaintance of André Gide, Thomas Mann, Thornton Wilder, the elderly Lord Alfred Douglas, among other celebrated writers, and earned the friendship of Gertrude Stein and Alice B. Toklas, whom he memorialized in *Dear Sammy,* the only book that presents them as two women who loved each other simply and deeply. If Sam is known as a particularly fine writer because of this book and his *Chapters from an Autobiography,* he is now even better known for an accomplishment quite different. For almost thirty years, readers have been aware of a pornographer named Phil Andros, whose books are vastly superior to any other male pornography ever written. Phil Andros, whose stories, told in the first person singular, occur in such literary places as the John Keats House in Rome, whose hero is capable of quoting Shakespeare while screwing someone black and blue, whose descriptions of the sex act are among the most realistic and beautiful in the language, is of course none other than Samuel M. Steward. Once this identification was made

Hamlet also won her popular favor. Cushman's affairs with other prominent women of her day have long been acknowledged and are all described in intimate detail in her diaries. Among her friends and lovers were Rosalie Kemble Sully, the painter's daughter; Fanny Kemble, the actress; Eliza Cook, an English poet; Matilda Hays, an English ac-tress; Geraldine Jewsbury, an English feminist; Sara Jane Clarke, an American journalist who wrote under the pseudonym "Grace Greenwood"; and the American sculptors Harriet Hosmer, Emma Crow, and Emma Stebbins. Whew. The actress finally settled down with Stebbins, with whom she lived for nineteen years until her death.

public just a short time ago, Sam was lionized not only by his fans of many years, but by a whole new generation of young men discovering the Phil Andros stories for the first time. No, this valentine does not imply that Sam Steward is perfect. He does not know how to make his characters

laugh. In *Dear Sammy,* Gertrude Stein "chuckles" about 173 times, and Phil Andros "grins" until you want to shake the grinning son of a bitch. Even Sam Steward, good as he is, still has something to learn about writing.

# 24.

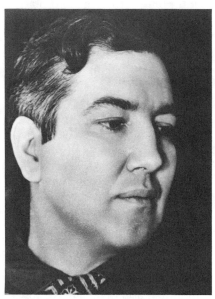

**Robert Graves:** He calls his novels his "dog show," and writes them in order to maintain his "cat," poetry.

**ROBERT GRAVES, b. London, 1895.** The Anglo-Irish-German-Danish poet, novelist, critic, and mythographer has maintained a macho stance for so many years that it is perhaps unfair to list him here at all. His autobiography avoids any mention of homosexuality having touched his life in any way at all. Yet the past has a way of catching up with one, and A. L. Rowse saw fit to correct the record in *Homosexuals in History,* in which he mentions both Graves's gay youth and his early play about homosexuality, *But It Still Goes On.* When he was a student at Oxford, the dandy of dandies,

Harold Acton, clearly saw his young classmate's dual nature. Given to declaiming poetry through a megaphone from the balcony of his rooms, Acton would occasionally read Graves's early poetry aloud. Acton decided that the poetry was old-fashioned in its masculine stance, like the poems of the previous generation, and that it lacked the proper fey spirit of the young Oxford dandies. What Graves needed, he said slyly, was "a Mediterranean holiday."

**AMELIA EARHART, b. Atchison, Kansas, 1898.** In the years since her plane vanished somewhere over the Pacific in 1937, two things have added to the legend of Amelia Earhart. First, numerous books and articles have been written to "prove" that she did not die in 1937, that she was captured by the Japanese, that she was on a secret government spying mission, that she is in fact still living somewhere in the Orient. Second, she is no longer called an "aviatrix." The former is the fate of any celebrity for whom an appropriate corpse cannot be found, especially since there's money to be made from speculating that she really is the dotty old lady in the Victorian house around the corner, where she is shacked up with old Judge Crater. The latter, however well meaning, is unfortunate. "Aviatrix" suits Amelia Earhart to a T. It suggests her flying

costume, the helmet and goggles, the jodhpurs and boots that made flying something akin to riding to hounds. Moreover, it suggests making it in a man's world which was what her accomplishments were all about. She was the first woman "to do this," the first woman "to do that" in the history of aviation. She was adored by millions. If she has always been adopted by lesbians as their own, controversy notwithstanding, this has been on circumstantial rather than actual evidence. That she was a tomboy is true, as was her preference for men's clothing, and her independent frame of mind. But at the heart of the mystery of Amelia Earhart is her relationship with men. Before her marriage to George Palmer Putnam when she was thirty-two, she wrote him an extraordinary letter: "You must know again my reluctance to marry, my feeling that I shatter thereby chances in work which mean so much to me. I feel the move just now as foolish as anything I could do. I know there may be compensations, but have no heart to look ahead. In our life together I shall not hold you to any medieval code of faithfulness to me, nor shall I consider myself bound to you similarly. If we can be honest I think the difficulties which arise may best be avoided . . . Please let us not interfere with the other's work or play, nor let the world see our private joys or disagreements. In this connection I may have to keep some place where I can go to be by myself now and then, for I cannot guarantee to endure at all times the confinements of even an attractive cage. I must exact a cruel promise, and that is you will let me go in a year if we find no happiness together. . . ." The letter is both beautiful and ambiguous, and we are likely never to know its full meaning. One lingering thought: Have you ever noticed the astonishing resemblance between Amelia Earhart and the young Charles Lindbergh?

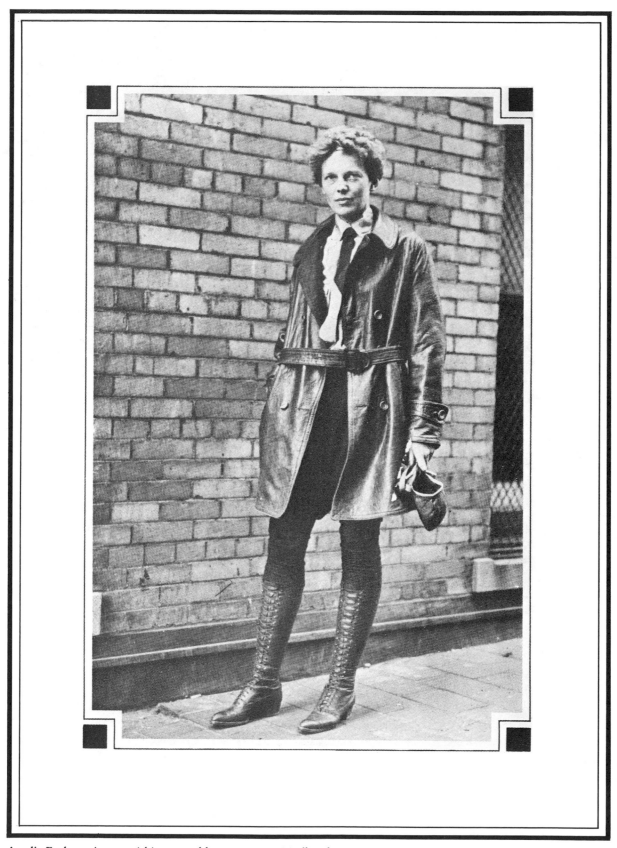

**Amelia Earhart:** An astonishing resemblance to young Lindbergh.

# 25.

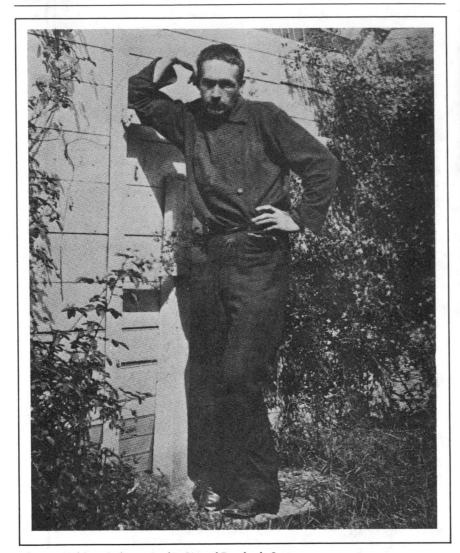

**Thomas Eakins:** At home in the City of Brotherly Love.

**THOMAS EAKINS, b. Philadelphia, Pennsylvania, 1844.** That the great American artist specialized in painting muscular, nude male models, nude male athletes, and nude male bathers doesn't mean anything, now, does it? Naaw, of course not.

# 26.

**MICK JAGGER, b. Dartford, Kent, England, 1944.** Whether authentic or a pluperfect put-on, the androgynous, gender defiant, and ambisex-

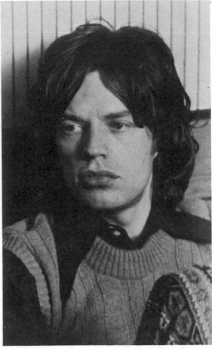

**Mick Jagger:** Androgyny recapitulates phylogeny.

ual rock star has come to symbolize the stylish androgyny of the '60s and '70s. His look-alike ex-wife, Bianca, once claimed that he married her because "he wanted to achieve the ultimate by making love to himself." Rock legend has it that the Mick is as famous for the contraband "Cocksucker Blues" as Auden was for his poem on the same subject.

# 27.

**MURAD IV. b. Turkey, 1611.** Considerations of space, and a weak stomach, force one to mention this monster and move on as quickly as possible to more pleasant people. The Turkish sultan's very name was synonymous in his time with such cruelty, torture, and unspeakable horror that he makes the Ayatollah Ruholla Khomeini appear as sticky sweet as all the members of the Trapp family combined. His reign was so bloody—the armless, legless, tongueless victims of his tyranny so numerous—that he would sicken even the spittle-chinned cretins who cheer each bucket of gore in today's gratuitously violent movies. Murad's great love was a boy named Musa, who, in a period of political turmoil, had been entrusted to the care of two of Murad's aides. To save their own skins, the two surrendered the boy to the enemies of the sultan, who promptly killed him after sharing his favors with the multitudes. What Murad did to avenge the death of Musa, what happened to the two palace aides, could not possibly be described in a book that prides itself on providing wholesome family entertainment.

# 28.

**THEOGNIS, b. Megara (between Athens and Corinth), c. 600 B.C.** This Greek elegiac poet was an aristocrat who apparently lost his wealth and property during one of the many conflicts between the aristocracy and the lower classes that are characteristic of this period in the Greek states. Embittered by these losses and convinced that all virtue resides in aristocracy, Theognis expressed in a number of poems his hatred for the plebeians and his nostalgia for the past when the power of the aristocracy was unquestioned. The poems are really moral precepts addressed to his young boyfried, Cyrnus. Given his reactionary daydreams, if Theognis were reincarnated today, he'd probably be one of those highly moral Republicans who are arrested in Washington men's rooms every now and then.

# 29.

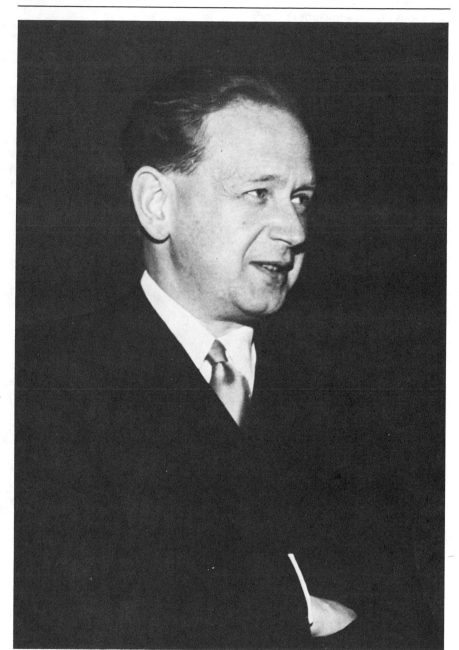

**Dag Hammerskjöld:** Yes he was, no he wasn't.

**DAG HAMMARSKJÖLD, b. Jonkoping, Sweden, 1905.** During the turbulent years that he was secretary-general of the United Nations, rumors circulated that Dag Hammarskjöld was homosexual. His acquaintances say that he was, instead, merely sexless, a workaholic, an intellectual, whose only indulgence was his love of gourmet food and flowers. The secretary-general dealt with the rumors by writing a haiku: "Because it did not find a mate/they called/the unicorn perverted." His official biographer writes that "stupid or malicious people sometimes made the vulgar assumption that, being un-married, he must be homosex-ual. . . ." Stupid, malicious, vulgar? Perhaps some were merely wishing the Swedish unicorn a modicum of pleasure and happiness.

# 30.

**JOHN DOS PASSOS, b. Chicago, Il-linois, 1896.** The famous novelist, author of the trilogy *U.S.A.* (1929-31), was probably not in the slightest bit gay, but warrants men-tion in these pages because the poet E. E. Cummings was convinced (to use the parlance of the day) that Dos Passos was a pansy. The novelist, who had a slight lisp, was asked by Cummings, who believed in the sex-ual meaning of dreams, what he had dreamed of the night before. Dos Passos's reply convinced the lower-case poet that the novelist was a screaming homosexual: "Why I dweamed I had a bunch of aspawa-gus and I was twying to give it to you."

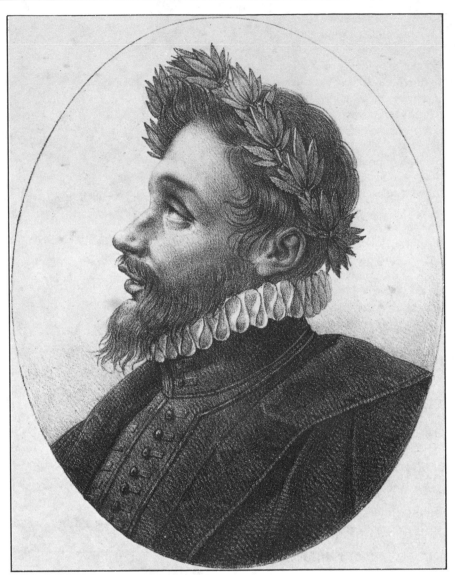

Ètienne Jodelle: Born to be queen.

# 31.

**ÈTIENNE JODELLE, b. Paris, 1532.** Jodelle—properly Seigneur de Limodin—was a member of the circle of poets, under Jean Daurat, that sought to reform the French language and literature in imitation of the classical writers of ancient Greece. The group called itself *La Pléiade* in emulation of the seven Greek poets of Alexandria. Jodelle's first play, *Cléopâtre captive,* was presented before the court of Reims in 1552,

with the effeminate playwright in the title role. By all reports he was a smash hit and every inch a queen. In honor of the play's success, his friends organized a gay little fête at Arcueil, where a goat garlanded with flowers was led in a procession and presented to the delighted Jodelle,

himself decked out in laurel leaves and other frou-frou. These green-room frolics seriously damaged Jodelle's reputation, and, after two more plays, he more or less folded on the road and died in abject poverty long before the days of the Actors' Fund.

## Other Personalities Born in July

1. **Louis-Joseph de Bourbon, Duc de Vendôme,** French soldier, 1654

**Naomi Jacob,** English novelist, 1889

Hans Werner Henze, German composer, 1926

Domingo Orejudas, physique artist known as "Etienne," 1933

2. Valentinian III, Roman emperor, 419

David Webb, American jewelry designer, 1925

4. Harold Acton, English writer, 1904

6. Harold Norse, American poet, 1916

8. Percy Grainger, Australian pianist-composer, 1882

Peter Orlovsky, American poet, 1933

9. David Diamond, American composer, 1915

Henry Geldzahler, Belgian-born American art connoisseur, 1935

David Hockney, English artist, 1937

10. Don Clark, American psychologist, 1930

12. Stefan George, German poet, 1868

Max Jacob, French poet, 1876

13. Pierre de Suffren de Saint-Tropez, French admiral, 1729

Almeda Sperry, American anarchist, 1879

14. Jules Cardinal Mazarin, French statesman, 1602

Comte Claude de Bonneval (Ahmed Pasha), French soldier, 1675

James Purdy, American novelist, 1923

17. Charles XII, king of Sweden, 1682

18. Rudolf II, German emperor, 1552

19. Joseph Hansen, American novelist, 1923

21. Pope Sixtus IV, 1614

23. Hubert Selby, Jr., American novelist, 1928

25. Rev. Al Carmines, American minister and composer, 1936

26. Marcel Jouhandeau, French writer, 1888

Danny La Rue, English female impersonator, 1928

27. Rev. Troy Perry, American minister and activist, 1940

30. Jacques-Louis David, French painter, 1748

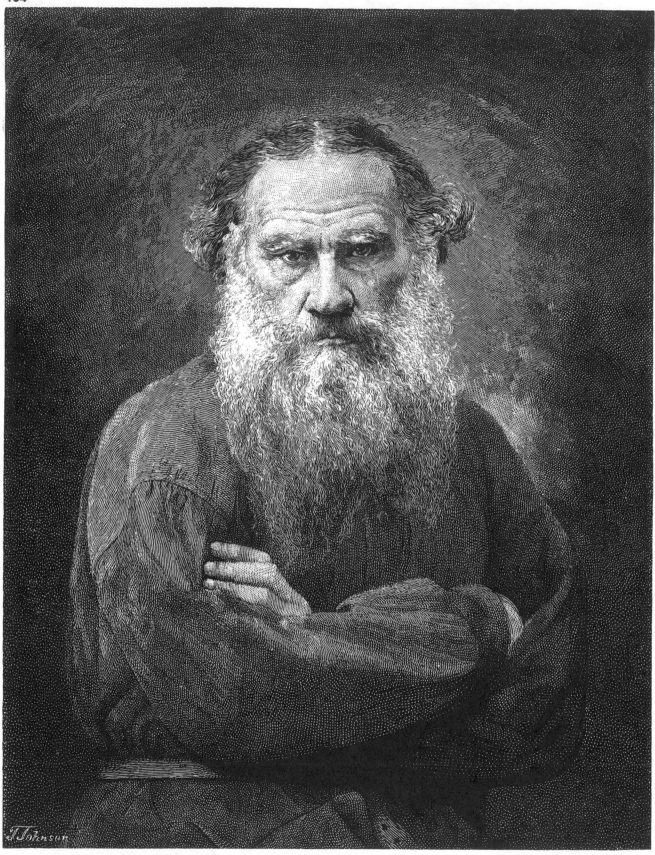

**Count Leo Tolstoy:** His wife thought him gay, but who knows?

# AUGUST

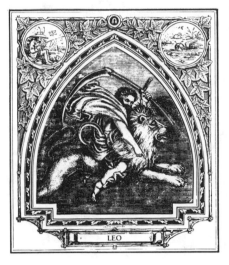

Leo (July 22nd to August 21st) is a fixed fiery sign ruled by the sun. Unlike the sensitive, complicated Cancerian, the Leonian is straightforward, uncomplicated, and outgoing. The sun gives him a strong, attractive personality and makes it easy for him to command loyalty from others. These qualities make him a natural leader, and the sign has long been associated with kings and potentates. The faults that sometimes afflict the Leonian are vanity, pomposity, and greed for power. At his best he is the ideal head of a large company or enterprise. Many-sided himself, he understands and appreciates the qualities of all the other types of human beings and never wastes his energies by asking anyone to do what he already knows cannot be done. Therefore, he is particularly successful in organizing activities and relegating duties. His faith and trust in humanity are, like the sun, radiated to all who know him.

# 1.

HERMAN MELVILLE, b. New York City, 1819. Critics have long observed the basic theme of male love that runs through the works of this important American writer, from the amusing and sensuous scenes between Ishmael and Queequeg sharing the same bed in *Moby Dick* to the sinister fate of Billy Budd, the "Beautiful Sailor." Only recently, however, has any scholar dared to examine Melville's life in relation to his works and suggest not only that Melville was most certainly a latent homosexual, but that the great love of his life was the lamentably heterosexual, and completely unattainable, novelist Nathaniel Hawthorne. In his biography of Melville, Edwin Haviland Miller cites example after example of the younger writer's love for the older novelist, but none as astonishing as Melville's review of Hawthorne's *Mosses from an Old Manse* (1850). Melville, who had only recently met Hawthorne and was in a state of exhilaration from their meeting, did not want his new friend to know that he was to review his book in *The Literary World*. He therefore disguised his identity by signing the review, "By a Virginian Spending July in Vermont." His infatuation with the famous writer is reflected in an extended metaphor of insemination, in which Hawthorne is clearly penetrating the love-sick Melville: "Already I feel that this Hawthorne has dropped germinous seeds into my soul. He expands and deepens down, the more I contemplate him; and further and further, shoots his strong New England roots into the hot soil in my Southern soul." Incredible!

YVES ST. LAURENT, b. Oran, Algeria, 1936. In the bad old days,

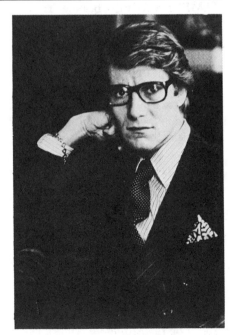

Yves St. Laurent: The March of Time.

before journalists simply said what was on their minds, *Time* magazine was the master of innuendo, taking particular delight in announcing to the world that someone was a fag without ever saying so directly. About twenty years ago, for example, when a flamboyant New York conductor reported that his car was stolen, *Time* maliciously reported that the A.W.O.L. marine caught driving it was suddenly identified by the conductor as his, er, secretary, who had merely borrowed the automobile. The *haute couturier* Yves St. Laurent's turn came when *Time* remarked that "his life with Pierre Berg, his . . . intimate of 15 years, has probably been as harmonious as most marriages." Well, it *might* have been harmonious. Right after the article appeared, the two friends suddenly split up.

# 2.

**JAMES BALDWIN, b. New York City, 1924.** One cannot underestimate the importance of *Giovanni's Room,* Baldwin's 1956 novel about homosexual love. The title has come to symbolize the confining space in which most gays were closeted in the past, and it is hardly surprising that one of the best gay bookstores in the United States has taken it as its name. Yet to limit Baldwin's contribution by referring to him as a "gay" writer is somehow to miss what he is all about. For Baldwin is not only one of the best black writers in America, but one of America's best writers period. His novels and essays about the black experience have affected two generations of readers. His first novel, *Go Tell It on the Mountain* (1953), has not lost any of its power, nor have his collected essays, *Notes of a Native Son* (1955) and *Nobody Knows My Name* (1961). But it is his *The Fire Next Time* ("God gave Noah the rainbow sign, No more

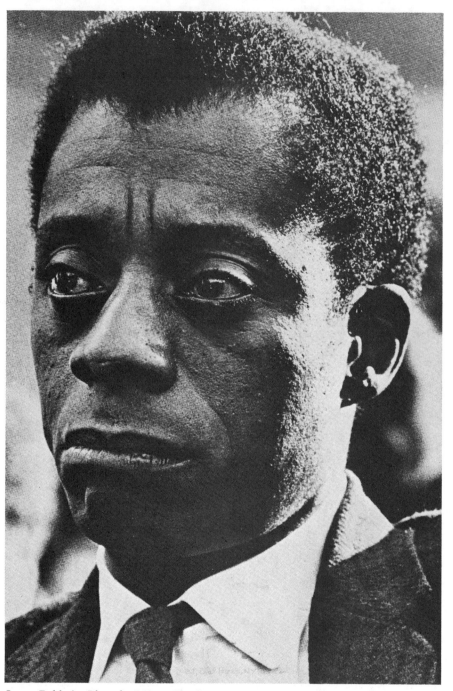

**James Baldwin:** Blues for Mister Charlie.

water, the fire next time") that grows more immediate with each passing year. In this 1963 work, Baldwin warns of the self-destruction white America is heading for if it does not rapidly, and with all its strength, undertake racial reform. The prophecy seemed to have come true in 1968, but it is apparent that Armageddon has yet to come.

# 3.

**RUPERT BROOKE, b. Rugby,**

England, 1887. Rupert Brooke was twenty-seven when he died, a poet of some promise, and very beautiful, so beautiful in fact that Lytton Strachey and John Maynard Keynes had fought each other for the privilege of wooing him when they were all students at Cambridge. As a young dandy, Brooke was present at the first performance of the Ballets Russes in London and was overwhelmed by what he saw: "They, if anything can, justify our civilization. I'd give anything to be a ballet-designer." What he became, three years later, was a soldier, and when he died in 1915 in Greece (of an illness, not in battle), he became a national symbol of fallen valor, not unlike the Greek legends of beautiful warriors cut down in battle at the height of their youthful vigor. The tone of exultation in his war poetry, the excitement with impending death (used, incidentally, by Winston Churchill and the British press for every propagandistic purpose) made Brooke a romantic hero in the popular mind. "I really think," he wrote in one of his last letters, "that large numbers of people don't want to die . . . which is odd . . . I've never been quite so happy in my life." In the years following his death, a period in which he was canonized by the public, his poetry was published in a slender volume, and a memoir by Edward Marsh appeared. One suspects that both were carefully laundered, although the poetry remains homoerotic in even a cursory reading. As Paul Fussell points out in *The Great War and Modern Memory,* there was a flowering of homosexual activity behind British lines. It was sung in the poetry of Brooke and Wilfred Owen. War, after all, was an instance in which two illegal activities—murder and loving men—were sanctioned. Both combine in the work of Brooke, even though it is doubtful, his legend having been carefully protected by his family and Edward Marsh, that we will ever really learn anything about his private life that they did not want known. It is interesting to note that in the 1920s, when that legend was still quite young, Tallulah Bankhead claimed to have read Rupert Brooke's love letters to another man.

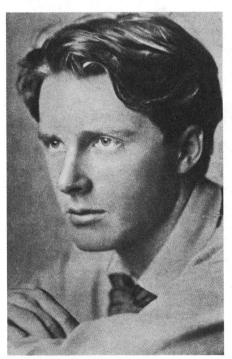

**Rupert Brooke:** The truth may never be known.

# 4.

WALTER PATER, b. London, 1839. Pater was once considered one of the greatest prose stylists in English literature, although almost no one reads him any longer. Tradition has it that he sought for the right word as laboriously as Flaubert did for *le mot juste.* The result, to modern taste at any rate, is a prose so overpolished that it is hardly the art that conceals art. Pater's eyes were focused entirely on the past, and his critical essays on aesthetic subjects—particularly on ancient Rome and on the Renaissance—have been called "reconstructions of the past toward which he turned his eyes away from the present." His greatest follower, among many, was Oscar Wilde, who has been called an unleashed version of Pater's repressed self. Wilde's favorite work by Pater was *Studies in the History of the Renaissance:* "It is my golden book; I never travel anywhere without it; but it is the very flower of decadence: the last trumpet should have sounded the moment it was written." Wilde used to tell a story (quoted in *The Oxford Book of Literary Anecdotes*) in which he delineated both Pater's repressed character and his fondness for picturesque words. One morning, before beginning his lecture, Pater asked a young man named Sanctuary to remain behind at the end. The student felt uncomfortable, but when they were left alone together, it was the professor who looked nervous. After a period of embarrassment, the young man said: "You asked me to stay behind, sir, did you not?" Pater pulled himself together: "Oh yes, Mr. Sanctuary. I . . . I wanted to say to you . . . what a very beautiful name you have got."

# 5.

AGATHON, b. Athens, Greece, c. 450 B.C. Until someone writes the definitive biography of a certain "creamy" movie star of the past, born today, let's give the day to the playwright Agathon, who was the very first dramatist to write on subjects and characters of his own invention, rather than drawing on mythology. The picture of Agathon that has survived the centuries is of an exceptionally effeminate man with plucked eyebrows, made-up face, mincing walk, and womanish clothing. This, however, is the literary invention of Aristophanes in the *Thesmophoriazusae,* a play that has been freely translated as "Ladies' Day" because it is, in part, about a particular Athenian festival sacred to women only and to which men were not admitted. In the play Agathon is asked to crash the event because he is the only man in Athens who could be admitted without having to wear a disguise. For his grand entrance, Agathon is rolled out in his bed, looking very much like a tarted-up old queen. That his audience laughed suggests that Aristophanes might have been merely exaggerating an accepted truth.

# 6.

**GOLDSWORTHY LOWES DICKINSON, b. 1862.** Dickinson, known as "Goldie" to his friends and admirers, was a professor of classics at Cambridge, where he was the hub of the so-called Cambridge Apostles, which in his time included students E. M. Forster, Bertrand Russell, Alfred North Whitehead, Lytton Strachey, Desmond MacCarthy, and Leonard Woolf. Goldie's impact on all is recorded in Forster's biography of his great teacher. Dickinson was a political writer as well as a classicist. His views were instrumental in the founding of the League of Nations, even though his own popularity declined because of his pacifism during World War I. He was revered for his wit, which even managed to creep into such somber works as the *Dictionary of National Biography.* Dickinson's write-up of the notorious educator Oscar Browning, who had been forced to leave both Eton and Cambridge for his "familiarity with young men," includes the wonderfully ambiguous line: "He assisted young Italians, as he had done young

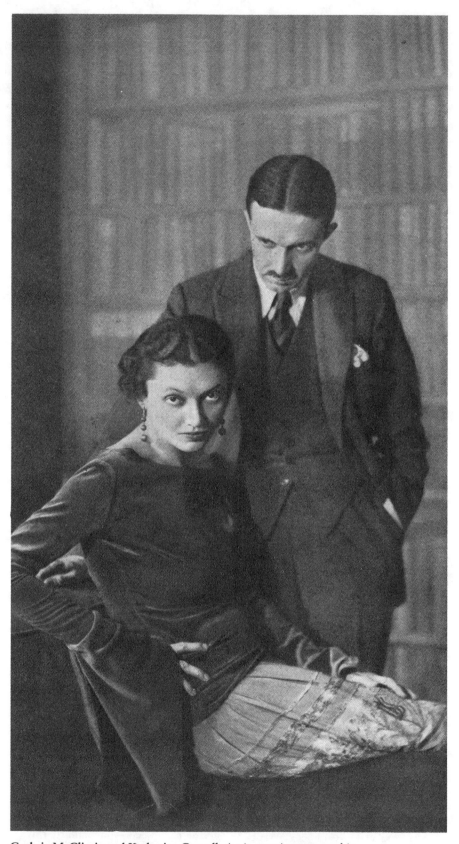

**Guthrie McClintic and Katharine Cornell:** An interesting partnership.

Englishmen, towards the openings they desired." Goldie himself cared less about openings than he did about heels and soles since he was a boot-fetishist whose tastes were only too gladly satisfied by his Cambridge students. As he wrote of one young man in his journal, "I liked him to stand upon me when we met."

**GUTHRIE McCLINTIC, b. Seattle, Washington, 1893.** *See February 16.*

# 7.

**CHARLES WARREN STODDARD, b. Rochester, New York, 1843.** Only the stout of heart or hard of head can read Stoddard today without breaking out in spots. His lush *South-Sea Idylls* (1873) depicts a land of brown-skinned gods, all young Joel McCreas and Jon Halls untroubled in paradise by the likes of Dolores Del Rio or Dorothy Lamour, all named Kana-ana or some such vowel-filled concoction, all with "lips ripe and expressive," "lashes that sweep," "eyes perfectly glorious— regular almonds," and all dropping to their knees at a second's notice. What is authentic about Stoddard is his joy in having discovered, like Paul Gauguin and Robert Louis Stevenson, an island respite from Anglo-Saxon hypocrisy. His writings, however, are not the documents of sociology that some would make them, but rather the product of a perfervid imagination.

# 8.

**SARA TEASDALE, b. St. Louis, Missouri, 1884.** It used to be fashionable in speaking of the brevity, the simplicity, the rare musical

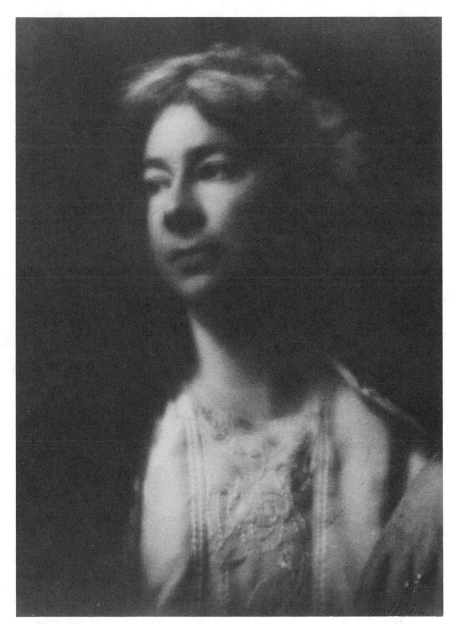

**Sara Teasdale:** A quiet at the heart of love.

quality, and the technical perfection of her poems, to imply that Sara Teasdale, something of a grown-up child, "could not adjust to the demands of maturity." What was meant by this euphemism was that a "healthy" woman was expected to yield completely to a man, and this Sara Teasdale could not do. Although she married and made a conscious attempt to "surrender herself completely" as she was ex-

pected to do, she could not succumb to an "urge" that she could not feel. The marriage endured, but it did not succeed. When the poet was forty-two she fell in love with an admiring college student named Margaret Conklin, who became the friend for whom she had been waiting all her life. The two spent summers traveling together, and Teasdale even took rooms at a nearby inn so that she could be near Conklin during her last two years in school. After the poet's divorce in 1929, they lived together until Teasdale's death at forty-nine in 1933. Of her love for Margaret Conklin, she wrote, "There is a quiet at the heart of love, / And I have pierced the pain and come to peace." As one critic has observed, the simple lyrics of Sara Teasdale are the work of "a Sappho in modest draperies."

# 9.

**REYNALDO HAHN, b. Caracas, Venezuela, 1875.** One rarely hears the music of Reynaldo Hahn today, although, as a student of Massenet, he became one of the most popular composers in turn-of-the-century Paris. Because of his popularity, Diaghilev commissioned him to create, with the young Jean Cocteau, the ballet *Le Dieu Bleu* (1912), one of the few failures of the Ballets Russes. As interest in this period of cultural history increases, Hahn is seen in more and more books (about Diaghilev, about Cocteau, about Proust) as a figure of some importance. He was a key member of the Paris homosexual set, which included, among others, Diaghilev, Lucien Daudet, Marcel Proust, and the young Jean Cocteau. He was a student and a close friend of Saint-Saëns, himself homosexual, and was Proust's first lover. It is said, in fact, that the musical battles of Hahn and Proust—Hahn championed the traditional Saint-Saëns and Proust favored the radical Debussy—led eventually to their separation. Had Hahn's musical tastes been those of his lover, the chances are that he might not have gone out of fashion so very soon.

**LÉONIDE MASSINE, b. Moscow, 1896.** As a young dancer, Massine is said to have resembled the ripening

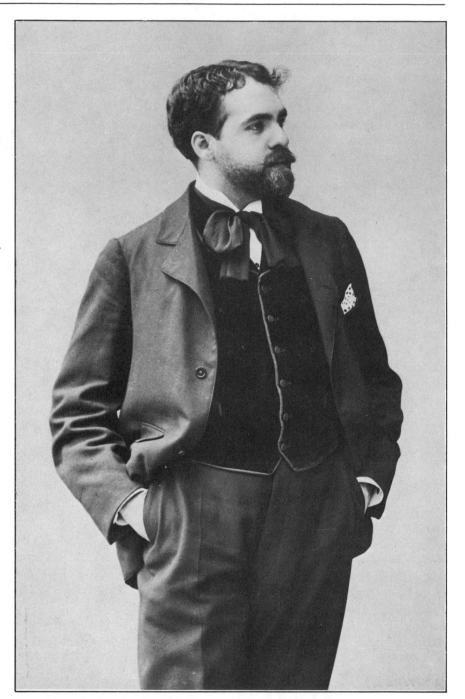

**Reynaldo Hahn:** His loyalty to the music of Saint-Saëns, and Proust's defection to Debussy, may have ended their long-lived love affair.

boys whom Baron von Gloeden photographed at Taormina. As Nijinsky's successor, both in Diaghilev's bed and as dancer and choreographer, he was, if anything, even more popular with Europe's gay set, because he was more sexually attractive than Nijinsky. Several Oxford and Cambridge dandies were known to treasure scrapbooks filled exclusively with photographs of Massine, and Harold Acton and Brian Howard, as young Eton students, are reputed to have performed behind closed blinds all the roles of their Russian idol. (They

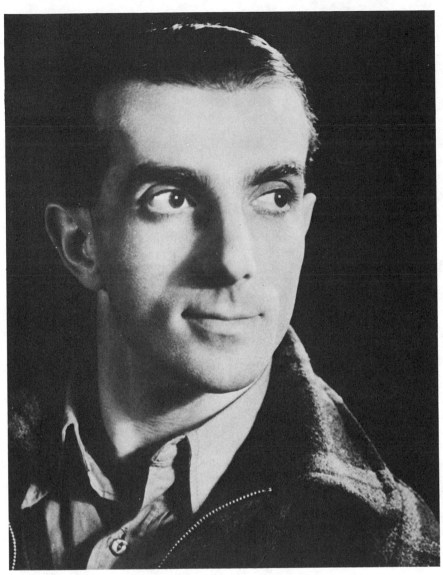

**Léonide Massine:** Undergraduates adored him.

the Théâtre Michel in Paris. Enraged at what he considered the perversion of Dada, André Breton, the spiritual leader of the Surrealists, lept upon the stage and broke Pierre de Massot's arm with the blow of a cane. Paul Eluard, another Surrealist, who took great pride in manly aggressiveness, punched two of the actors in the face. One of the actors was the playwright Tristan Tzara; the other was the writer René Crevel, among the only admitted homosexuals in the Dada movement, aside from Jean Cocteau who was Breton's *bête noir*. One of Breton's reasons for breaking with Dada was his belief that the entire movement had been polluted with homosexuals. Crevel was the founder of several short-lived literary magazines during this turbulent period. His poetry is said to be obsessed with death (his father was a suicide) and fear of castration (he vividly remembered and regretted his circumcision at age three).

were then a precocious fourteen and thirteen, respectively.) But history repeated itself. Massine fell in love with a ballerina, quarreled with his lover, and was dismissed from

Diaghilev's company. Three years later, his impetuous marriage annulled, he begged Diaghilev to take him back. Unforgiving, the impresario refused. And, by this time, he had Lifar.

# 10.

**RENÉ CREVEL, b. Paris, 1900.** How Surrealism grew out of Dada, how the Surrealists, themselves the creators of the Dada manifestoes, broke away—violently—from their former colleagues is much too complicated to attempt to explain. But the final break occurred one night in June, 1923, at a performance of the Dada spectacle *Le Coeur à Barbe* at

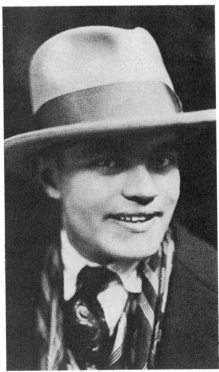

**René Crevel:** He was Charles Henri Ford's predecessor as Tchelitchew's lover.

# 11.

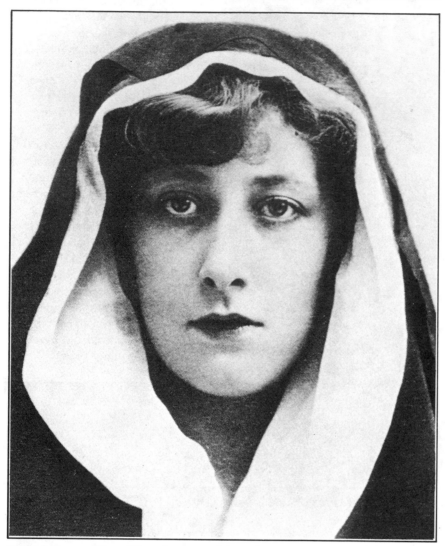

**Liane de Pougy:** After a life as the most celebrated courtesan of *la belle époque*, serving both men and women, she retired to a convent as Sister Mary Magdalene of Repentance.

**LIANE DE POUGY (née Anne-Marie de Chassaigne), b. Rennes, France, 1870.** On her first trip to Paris as a young woman, Natalie Barney walked the fashionable streets of the city studying women while her mother was at a studio studying portrait painting. One day she saw an exquisite woman in the Bois de Boulogne, and, making inquiry, learned that the fur-cloaked beauty was Liane de Pougy, the most famous courtesan in Paris. What she learned, as well, was that Liane was a lesbian, yet sold herself to men, and at a very high price. Natalie Barney resolved on the spot that she would "rescue" Liane de Pougy from her "dreadful life" and make her her own. She even went to the courtesan's house, but was turned away by the maid who informed her that Madame never rose before eleven. Just then Natalie received the news that her father wanted her to return to America, where she was to make her debut. Undaunted, she swore that she would return someday to Paris and take Liane de Pougy, whom she had only once glimpsed, as her lover. What's more, she did.

# 12.

**RADCLYFFE HALL, b. Bournemouth, Hampshire, 1880.** *The Well of Loneliness* is a badly written book, it is dated, and, God knows, it has perpetuated the myth that a lesbian is a man in a woman's body, but it is still *the* book about lesbians that everyone knows, largely because it was the first undisguised lesbian novel. The story of the book's trials, both in England and the United States, is, in a sense, more interesting to read about than the novel itself, and it attests to the remarkable courage of Radclyffe Hall to have attempted publication in the first place. What very few people know is why *The Well of Loneliness,* as well as *all* of Radclyffe Hall's other books, are dedicated "To the three of us." Radclyffe Hall's first lover was Veronica Batten, a woman more than twenty years her senior. Known

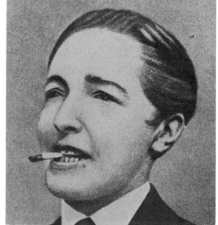

**Radclyffe Hall:** Fast cars, loose women, and "the three of us."

to her friends as "John," Radclyffe Hall, throughout her life, in fact, was remarkably promiscuous. Enormously wealthy, she had the means to pursue whatever she wanted, whether fast cars or beautiful women. Although Veronica Batten knew of her lover's adventures, she was undisturbed so long as none of these affairs developed into meaningful friendships. Her worst fears were realized when Radclyffe Hall met Lady Una Troubridge. Their friendship, it seemed, was going beyond mere sexual pleasure, and Veronica Batten determined that Una Troubridge would have to go. She quarreled with her lover and then dropped dead from a heart attack. To assuage her guilt, Radclyffe Hall took up spiritualism in a vain attempt to contact Veronica and beg forgiveness. Failing this, she forever after dedicated all her books "To the three of us."

# 13.

**MARIA CAROLINA, Queen of Naples and the Two Sicilies, b. Vienna, 1768.** *See May 12.*

# 14.

**DEMOSTHENES, b. Athens, Greece, 383 B.C.** His father, a rich manufacturer of swords and other arms, died when Demosthenes was seven. The guardians of his father's estate handled it dishonestly, and at eighteen Demosthenes demanded his rightful inheritance. After studying with Isaeus, an orator and specialist in law, Demosthenes brought charges against his guardians and finally won his case, but actually received little of what was due him. To earn a living, Demosthenes became a professional

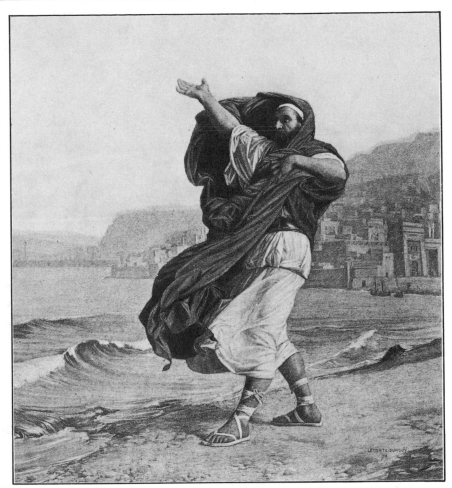

**Demosthenes:** His mother never told him that it was impolite to speak with a full mouth.

writer of speeches. According to tradition, his failure as an orator when speaking before the Assembly for the first time only stimulated him to intense study and practice, which included speaking with pebbles in his mouth and other extremely difficult exercises. Demosthenes' great talent and extraordinary self-discipline eventually made him the greatest and most famous Athenian orator.

Although it is only legend, the story about the pebbles has always been a bit troubling. How on earth could speaking with a full mouth—full of pebbles, no less—help one to speak more clearly? It doesn't make much sense. Considering Demosthenes' love affairs with the youths Cnosion and Epicrates, perhaps two myths got crossed in transmission, the pebbles actually having been rocks.

# 15.

**NAPOLEON BONAPARTE, b. Ajaccio, Corsica, 1769.** Believe what you will, but stories to the effect that the emperor of France was not the

man he was cracked up to be have circulated for more than a century and a half. The basis for these stories seems to have been the post-mortem

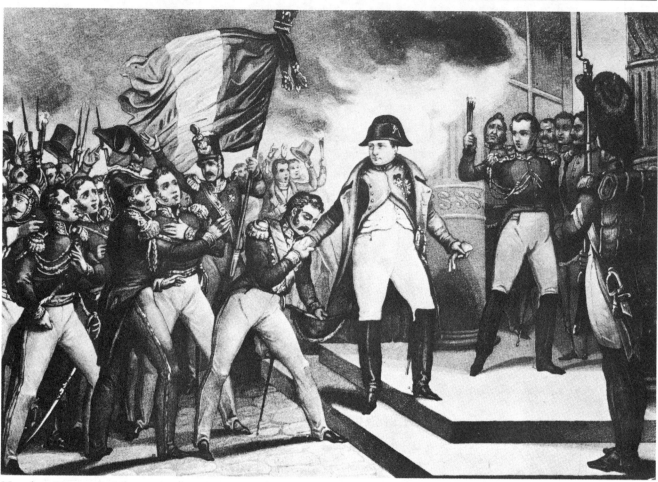

**Napoleon Bonaparte:** Hmmm. Look at them hips.

report of one Dr. Henry, revealing the "progressive feminization" that Napoleon's body had undergone through the years: "The whole surface of the body was deeply covered with fat. Over the sternum, where generally the bone is very superficial, the fat was upwards of an inch deep and an inch and a half or two inches on the abdomen. There was scarcely any hair on the body, and that of the head was thin, fine, and silky. The whole genital system (very small) seemed to exhibit a physical cause for the absence of sexual desire, and the chastity which had been stated to have characterized the deceased [Napoleon had been kept prisoner on St. Helena for seven years]. The skin was noticed to be very white and delicate, as were the hands and arms.

Indeed the whole body was slender and effeminate. The pubis much resembled the *mons veneris* in women. The muscles of the chest were small, the shoulders narrow, and the hips wide." So much for 19th-century science. It would seem as if the emperor had merely put on some weight while in captivity. And if, in fact, he *was* hung like a hangnail, why all those pictures of him with his hand inside his coat?

**T. E. LAWRENCE, b. Tremadoc, Wales, 1888.** The mere mention of T. E. (for Thomas Edward) Lawrence as a homosexual has always been controversial. Lowell Thomas, who publicized the derring-do of this great adventurer in America, just as Winston Churchill

was his chief publicist in Great Britain, was outraged at the very suggestion, calling such an "accusation" a "libel" on the good man's name. Yet, libel or no, we know that Lawrence was in love with an Arab boy, Salim Ahmed, whom he called Dahoum, and to whom he dedicated his masterpiece, *Seven Pillars of Wisdom* ("To S.A."). And we know, too, that in his retirement Lawrence hired the services of a boy named Bruce who flogged him regularly. Still, the popular film version of his life, *Lawrence of Arabia*, though falling short of providing him with a girlfriend, hardly even hints that he was gay, the famous rape scene providing only proof of what can happen to a normal Anglo-Saxon heterosexual in the heathen Middle

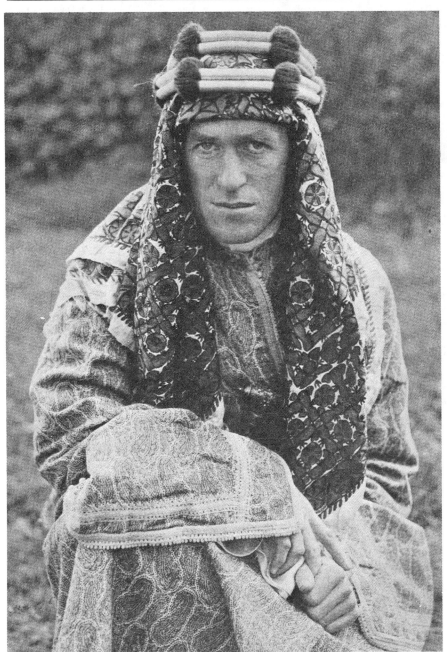

**T. E. Lawrence:** El-Orens, Destroyer of Engines.

East. There are even some readers, who, finding *Seven Pillars of Wisdom* too romantic for their blood, doubt that such a rape ever even occurred. The real question, it would seem, is not whether Lawrence was in fact raped by a Turkish officer, but to what extent El-Orens, the Destroyer of Engines, might have actually enjoyed it.

# 16.

**MONTY WOOLLEY** (né Edgar Montillion Woolley), **b. New York City, 1888.** The bearded actor is best remembered as he was in late middle age, when he became known to moviegoers in such films as *The Man*

*Who Came to Dinner, The Pied Piper,* and *Since You Went Away.* His great ambition, to play George Bernard Shaw, was never realized, and one can only wonder what the old curmudgeon would have thought of an American bugger impersonating him in films. Woolley was a lifelong friend of Cole Porter, the two having met as students at Yale. Although Porter's Hollywood biopic would make one think that Woolley, who consented to play himself opposite Cary Grant's Porter, was about half a century older than his friend, they were in fact contemporaries. And they were also "fuck buddies" (their term) together. If Porter's special interest was rough trade of any type, white or black, Woolley's preference was for black men, generally supplied him by an assortment of New York pimps. His taste, as a matter of fact, led to his ultimate estrangement from Porter late in life. Woolley fell in love with one of his employees, a black manservant, and the two lived together as lovers. Porter, whose snobbism was legendary—after all, he was from the *crème de la crème* of Peru, Indiana—liked black men well enough to pay for their stud service, but there was no way that he would ever accept one as an equal.

# 17.

**ROGER PEYREFITTE, b. Costres, Tarn, France, 1907.** For a time Roger Peyrefitte was very much the best-selling *enfant-terrible* of the contemporary French literary world, a specialist in scandal. He has been attacked as a pornographer, a scandal-monger, and a mischief-maker, all of which are true, but he is essentially a very funny satirist of French manners and hypocrisy. One of his more recent books, *Les Juifs* (The Jews)

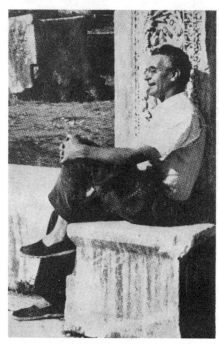

**Roger Peyrefitte:** An uncanny eye for the controversial.

caused a sensation because it "proved" that virtually everyone of any importance at all—from the Pope to Winston Churchill to John F. Kennedy—is Jewish. He was, needless to say, attacked for his "anti-Semitism," when in fact his entire point was to skewer anti-Semitism. Its critics notwithstanding, the book sold 200,000 copies in France alone. A few years back, he caused a minor scandal by accusing Pope Paul VI of being homosexual. Since he was never prosecuted, one can assume either Christian charity or no contest on the part of Rome. His gay novels, *Special Friendships* (1945) and *The Exile of Capri* (1961), the latter a fictionalized biography of Adelsward Fersen, are particularly recommended.

# 18.

**SIR FRANCES ROSE, b. 1908.** The English artist was the last, and probably the most infamous, though the least known, of Gertrude Stein's many protégés. Several of Francis Rose's drunken escapades are wonderfully recollected in Samuel M. Steward's *Dear Sammy.* One story, peculiarly or not-so-peculiarly omitted from the artist's autobiography, *Saving Life* (1961), is about Luis, his *valet de chambre.* In 1952 Alice B. Toklas wrote Sam Steward to tell him that Francis Rose "was in a good deal of trouble with Luis his *valet de chambre* boyfriend." A casual encounter betwen the artist and a Spanish gypsy boy in front of a bistro called La Reine Blanche in Paris had resulted in not only an evening pickup, but in the young man being hired for the entire summer, as both valet and bedmate. As Sam Steward tells it, "It was only after Luis got into some trouble with the *gendarmérie* over a stolen bicycle that Francis—called to help him out of his difficulty—examined his papers and discovered the boy was his illegitimate son. This episode titillated both France and England for some time." It certainly titillated Alice B. "Francis," she wrote, "is saying that he is going to recognize Luis so that he will inherit his title!! As yet this tale has not been confided to any English friends—who would put him straight about bastards inheriting titles. . . ."

# 19.

**GABRIELLE "COCO" CHANEL, b. near Issoire, France, 1883.** She designed the most simple, the most elegant, the most beautiful clothing of the 20th century and became rich from her good taste. She was the saint who paid for the funeral of poet Raymond Radiguet, "Monsieur Bébé," Cocteau's boy lover. She designed the costumes for most of Cocteau's productions. She sheltered Cocteau when he was down and out, loaned him money, paid his bills. Her life was, in many ways, indistinguishable from his. And yet she still lacks a biographer with the stature of a Francis Steegmuller, who could capture her word portrait on paper, fearlessly. Whatever she was, she was not the sanitized shell designed for Katharine Hepburn to portray on Broadway. One would like to know everything possible about this woman whom Noel Coward recalled meeting in a Paris bomb shelter at the beginning of World War II. She had entered the shelter, followed, a few discreet steps behind, by her maid who carried Madame's gas mask on a satin pillow.

# 20.

**PAUL TILLICH, b. Starzeddel, Kreis Guben, Prussia, 1886.** What? The famous theologian? The one who preached that every Yes must have its corresponding No, and that no human truth is ultimate? Yes, and if you doubt it, read his wife's autobiography, which, in its own beautifully-written way, is far more racy than some contemporary fiction. It appears that Hannah Tillich liked it with Paulus, with other men, and with other women; Paulus liked it with Hannah, with Hannah and other women, with other women, and with Hannah and other men. In fact the Harvard theologian liked it in almost every configuration. Given the limited number of human permutations and combinations, one would think it inevitable that snake eyes would have had to be rolled. But not necessarily. Tillich called his homosexuality "latent."

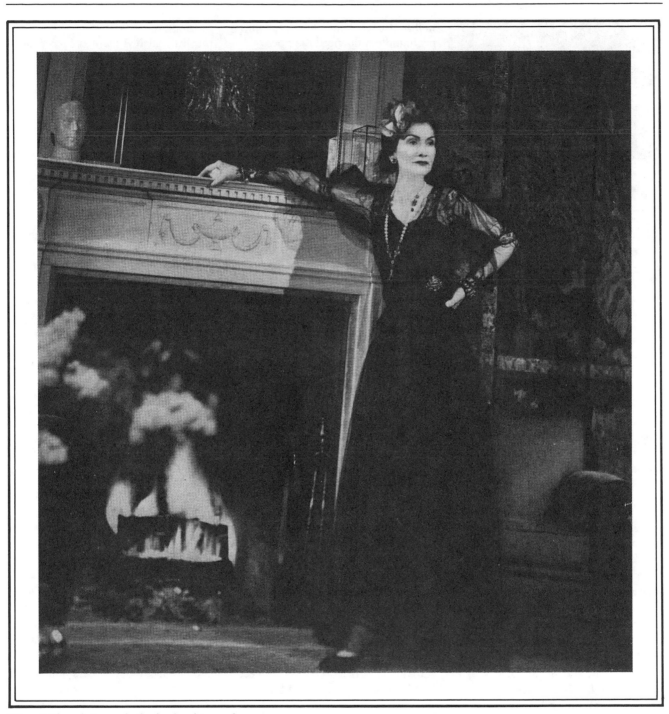

"Coco" Chanel: In need of a fearless biographer.

# 21.

**AUBREY BEARDSLEY, b. Brighton, England, 1872.** Beardsley epitomized to a greater degree than any other English artist of his time the *fin de siècle* style embodied in the Art Nouveau style, and yet his influence was far greater in France than it was in his native country. His work was worshipped by Bakst,

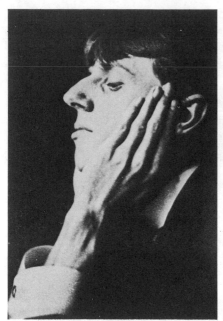

Aubrey Beardsley: "If I am not grotesque, I am nothing."

Iribe, and other artists who collaborated with Diaghilev to create the Ballets Russes. Beardsley's drawings profoundly influenced the poet Maurice Rostand, the gay son of Edmond Rostand, author of *Cyrano de Bergerac.* Rostand *fils,* an early friend of Cocteau, modeled the images in his poetry on Beardsley drawings, as he did his own appearance. Maurice Rostand and his dear mother, whose side he rarely left, used to promenade hand-in-hand down Parisian boulevards, the son's make-up far more colorful than his mother's, his hair bleached, and his eyebrows plucked. Beardsley's professional affiliation with Oscar Wilde, as everyone knows, ruined him, and he died from tuberculosis less than three years after Wilde's famous trial and imprisonment. Ironically, it has long been believed that Beardsley was not himself gay and that his ruin was largely a case of "guilt by association."

# 22.

**JAMES KIRKWOOD, b. Los Angeles, 1927.** Some time ago, an editor at a major book club in New York had just gone through a perfectly lousy series of business meetings. Feeling generally rotten, and using a manuscript that had just arrived from a publisher as an excuse, he locked himself in his office, told his secretary that he was not to be disturbed, and started to read. By the time he finished page one, he was already laughing; by the end of chapter one he was still laughing; by the end of the manuscript he was feeling terrific and had decided to buy book club rights to the book. Calling the publisher's representative, he made an offer for the rights, on condition that the publisher would set up a luncheon date with the author. As the book club editor explained, "If the guy is so funny on paper, what must he be like in real life?" Besides, he said, he'd treat since working authors are not always particularly well-heeled. The lunch was set up. The book was *P.S. Your Cat Is Dead;* the author, James Kirkwood. And he *was* as funny in real life. The book club editor learned that he was the son of pioneer film stars James Kirkwood and Lila Lee, that he had spent his entire life in show business, first as a movie brat, then as an actor-singer-dancer, and had had a moderate success as an author with two novels to his credit, *There Must Be a Pony* and *Good Times/Bad Times,* both particularly popular with gay males because of their gay sub-themes. What the book club editor didn't know was that his lunch partner was then putting the finishing touches on the book for a musical called *A Chorus Line.* Had he known that, and had he been clairvoyant, he would have asked Kirkwood to pay for his own goddam lunch and for his, too.

# 23.

**HERBERT POLLITT, b. 1871.** Herbert Who, you're asking, right? Well, we've already met Liane de Pougy (August 11), and we've been introduced to Aubrey Beardsley (August 21). Herbert Pollitt was an English transvestite actor who used the stage name "Diane de Rougy" (derived from the name of Liane de Pougy, who was a Folies-Bergère dancer as well as a courtesan) and was a close friend of Aubrey Beardsley, who, as we've already learned, some believe to have been straight, despite his odd-duck friends. Herbert Pollett, Folies-drag and all, was an early lover of Aleister Crowley, whom we'll meet on October 12.

# 24.

**THE ERUPTION OF MT. VESUVIUS, 79 A.D.** The catastrophic eruption of Vesuvius that buried Pompeii, Herculaneum, and Stabiae under cinders and ashes had one salutary effect. It preserved the ruins of Pompeii with magnificent completeness—down to the fresh colors of the wall paintings. Much of what we know about ancient Roman culture has been learned from excavating the ruins of Pompeii. Among the treasures preserved are aspects of that civilization that would surely have been destroyed by the followers of St. Paul had not the lava of Vesuvius preserved them. These are the famous homosexual graffiti scrawled on walls around town. Some of the more choice examples are (in Latin, naturally), "On this spot Auctus fucked Quintius," "I want to fuck a humpy number," and, even more remarkable, a series of comments (written by different hands) on the talents of one particularly well-hung stud, e.g., "Phoebus the perfume maker fucks real good." There are no phone numbers, of course.

# 25.

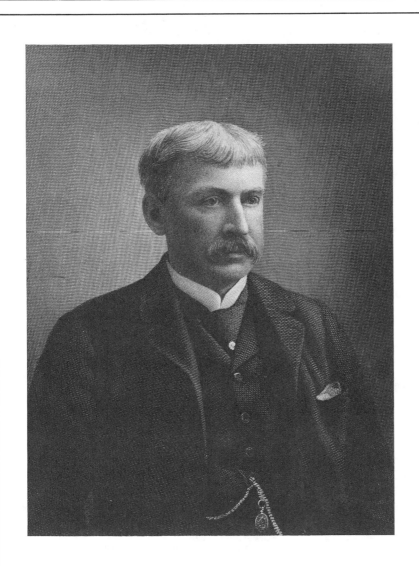

Bret Harte: The fastest gun in the West?

**BRET HARTE (né Francis Bret Harte), b. Albany, New York, 1839.** The author of "The Outcasts of Poker Flat" and "The Luck of Roaring Camp" was one of America's first commercially-successful writers. Lionized back East as the epitome of the Western man, the transplanted Californian toured the cities of the East, complete with Western gear, and cashed in on his popularity by living up to his readers' expectations. When European newspapers picked up on his success, he was invited to tour abroad, since the English and the Germans in particular were completely mad (as the Germans still are) for cowboys. So Harte continued to live the part, becoming more and more extravagant in his tastes as he became more and more famous. The pen-and-ink cowboy has always been thought of as gay, even though the evidence is largely superficial. As his obituaries put it, "He never married."

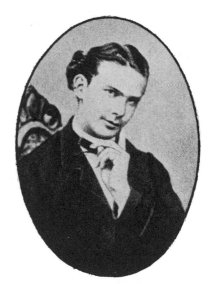

Ludwig II: Bonkers.

**LUDWIG II, King of Bavaria, b. Nymphenburg, Bavaria, 1845.** Poor Ludwig was so batty that it hardly pays to dwell on him. That wretch of a genius Richard Wagner played up to the king's fondness for handsome men by spinning fantasies of his own about brawny blond heroes of the Aryan past, but the result, to say the least, was some of the greatest music ever written. The king's indulgences, including the expense of building a series of fairy-tale castles and supporting Wagner's elaborate productions, nearly depleted the Bavarian treasury. Here, too, the present has benefited from the past. If you've not visited Ludwig's castles, particularly Neuschwanstein, you have no idea of what the gay temperament really is. (Perhaps a doctoral candidate will someday write a thesis comparing Ludwig's gay decor with that of William Randolph Hearst's San Simeon, which surely defines straight kitsch.) Sad to say, Ludwig was raised in such ignorance of sex that he was already a grown man when he learned the bare rudiments from his handsome equerry, Richard Hornig. Yes, that is a final "g."

herited his gayness from a celebrated ancestor, a bishop who had been caught in bed with a soldier in 1822. Noel was one of Whitman's earliest admirers in England and wrote a letter to the poet whom he had only "met" in *Leaves of Grass* itself: "The proclamation of comradeship seems to me the grandest and most tremendous fact in your work and I heartily thank you for it."

# 26.

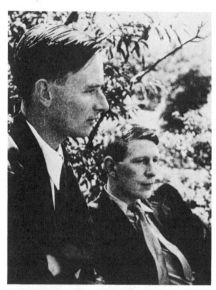

**Christopher Isherwood and W. H. Auden:** When the world was young and gay.

**CHRISTOPHER ISHERWOOD, b. High Lane, near Stockport, Cheshire, 1904.** There is very little that can be said about this important writer that he has not already said about himself. For the past decade, his published writings have been retellings, the third and fourth time around, of material that already appears, perhaps more imaginatively, in his fiction. *Christopher and His Kind,* for example, is less an autobiography than it is a context for the infinitely more rewarding *Berlin Stories.* Isherwood is really the little girl with the little curl. When he is good, he is very, very good; and when he is bad, . . . well, you know the rest of the rhyme. Among the good—in fact, the best— is *A Single Man,* still the most perfect novel ever written about a gay male. It is one of those works of art—like the last fifteen minutes of *Der Rosenkavalier,* or the last five minutes of Chaplin's *City Lights*—that could make even a stone weep.

# 28.

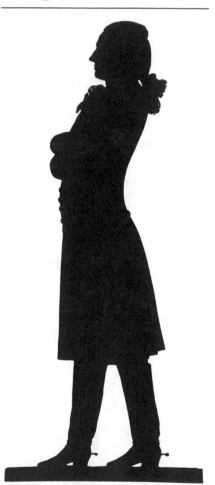

**Johann Wolfgang von Goethe:** Details obscured by shadows.

**JOHANN WOLFGANG VON GOETHE, b. Frankfurt am Main, 1749.** Attempting to show why some thinkers over the centuries have suspected the German genius of being

# 27.

**RODEN NOEL (né Roden Berkeley Wriothesley Noel), b. 1834.** Noel was an English poet and critic from a distinguished family, related on one side to Lord Byron, about whom he later wrote a book. He was also the first person ever taken to bed by the very timid John Addington Symonds (*see October 5*). Noel, who married and raised a family to carry on his line, had a rare sense of humor about his "condition," claiming that he in-gay is about as loaded a proposition as suggesting that Jesus and his twelve Disciples were members of the international homintern. Dare to lay a finger on Goethe and there are people out there gunning for you. Various commentators, nonetheless, have suggested that the "evidence" exists in Goethe's own works for those who care to look. Start with the master's *Diwan* lyrics, progress to *Wilhelm Meister,* move on to the essay on Winckelmann. Above all, read Edward Carpenter's passages on Goethe in *The Intermediate Sex* (1912) and the poet Edgar Lee Masters' biography of Whitman (1937), in which he suggests that Goethe, Whitman, Shakespeare, Marlowe, Michelangelo, and, yes, Jesus were all "Uranians."

**COUNT LEO TOLSTOY, b. Tula, Russia, 1828.** The great Russian novelist's marriage was so stormy, so emotionally volatile, that it deserves a place in military history. Tolstoy spent his last years either separated from his countess or playing Socrates to her Xanthippe. So embattled was their life together that she became increasingly jealous of her famous husband's closeness to the manager of their landed estates and tried to prove that the relationship of the two men was homosexual. Tolstoy died before his wife could confirm or dismiss her suspicions.

# 29.

**EDWARD CARPENTER, b. Brighton, Sussex, 1844.** In recent years, the great English "sexual emancipator" has been rediscovered, principally by gay activists and scholars investigating the social history of homosexuality. Although much has been written about him, and

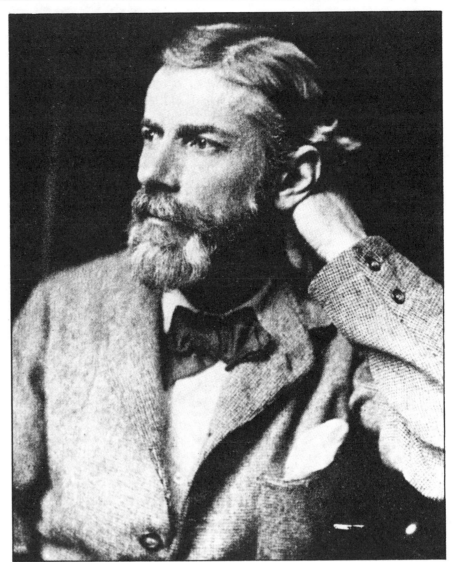

**Edward Carpenter:** The English Whitman.

although readers are seeking out his many books, a modern biography is still badly needed. He was inspired, in part, by Whitman's poetry, eventually came to America to meet Whitman, and spread the gospel according to St. Walt throughout England. Believing the effeminacy of "Uranians" a myth, he affected a form of macho dress, as did his working-class lover George Merrill, that make them both look, almost a century later, oddly contemporary. Any number of stories could be told about Carpenter, but, against the hope that the reader will at least

become acquainted with him in Jonathan Katz's *Gay American History,* one story will have to suffice: Carpenter's boyfriend, George Merrill—a rough, tough "working-class bloke from the slums," was so ignorant that, when he heard that Gethsemane was the place where Jesus had slept on his last night, he asked in all innocence, "Who with?" E. M. Forster, who was a disciple of Carpenter, visited Carpenter and Merrill one day, when Merrill stroked Forster's rear end "gently and just above the buttocks." As Forster described it, "The sensation was unusual and I still remember it. . . It seemed to go straight through the small of my back into my ideas, without involving my thoughts. If it really did this, it would have acted in strict accordance with Carpenter's yogified mysticism, and would prove that at that precise moment I had conceived." What Forster had conceived, in fact, was his gay novel *Maurice,* which he began to write as soon as he left Carpenter's house.

# 30.

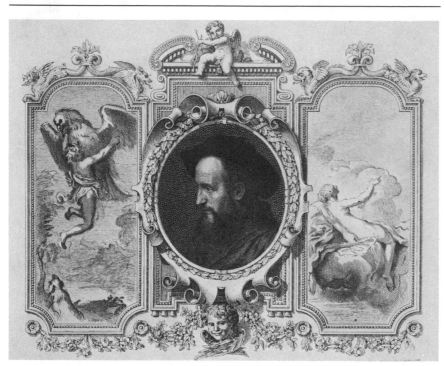

**Correggio:** What do his paintings tell us about him?

**CORREGGIO (né Antonio Allegri), b. Correggio, Italy, 1494.** In the century and a half since apologists began compiling lists of famous practitioners to justify homosexuality, the name of the Italian painter Correggio has always enjoyed a prominent place on most lists. Many of his paintings are noted for the almost unearthly beauty of their male nudes, and have certainly been admired by gays through the centuries, but the paintings themselves appear to be the only "evidence" that Correggio was himself homosexual. Nothing of what is known of his biography would seem to support explicitly what appears implicit in his works.

# 31.

**CALIGULA (Gaius Caesar Germanicus), b. Anzio, Italy, 12 A.D.** Back in the dim '50s, the epidemic of biblical and classical extravaganzas from Hollywood reached a new height, or low, depending on one's point of view. One learned all sorts of interesting things about the past from these flicks. All women in classical Rome, for example, whether freeborn or slave, wore the same type of kiss-proof lipstick; were sentenced to death if their two-piece dancing-girl togas were not sufficiently high to cover any hint of a navel; were tortured if caught on the streets of Rome without sandals that were laced provocatively to the thigh. During this time actor Jay Robinson offered two scenery-chewing performances as the mad emperor Caligula in two 20th-Century Fox epics, *The Robe* and its sequel, *Demetrius and the Gladiators.* So effective was Robinson in his epicene camping, his evil vamping, his insane torture of innocent Christian Hollywood extras, that by the time he threw his eighty-fifth Christian to a couple of toothless lions, one small child, biting his fingernails, leapt to his feet in a crowded theater and exclaimed, "Boy, am I glad I'm Jewish!" Actually, Robinson's performance was not too different from the behavior of the real Caligula. Only Heliogabalus seems to have outdone him in licentiousness. If it moved, Caligula wanted it, male or female. His taste in women was certainly catholic, since it included his sisters. His taste in men was equally far-ranging and included a priest whom he enjoyed screwing in public during religious ceremonies, an actor with whom he enjoyed smooching during meetings of state, a stud with whom he maintained a friendly contest as to who would outlast the other in a friendly orgy, and an officer in his guards whose buns he particularly admired. It was the latter, the guard named Chaerea, with whom he came a cropper. Part of Caligula's fun with his guard consisted in taunting him in front of his peers for having played bottom to his top The lovely emperor would regularly force his guard to kiss his middle finger in public. To repay Caligula for his kindness, Chaerea hacked him to death with his sword and finished off what was left of him with his dagger. Caligula was twenty-nine.

## Other Personalities Born in August

1. **Claudius,** Roman emperor, 10 B.C.
   **Stuart Merrill,** American poet, 1863
   **Walter Griffin,** American poet, 1937

2. **Adolf Hausrath,** German theologian and novelist, 1837
   **Roy Dean,** American photographer, 1925

3. **H. C. Brunner,** American writer, 1855
   **Gordon Merrick,** American novelist, 1916

4. **Edward Irving,** English theologian, 1792
   **Percy Bysshe Shelley,** English poet, 1792

6. **Alfred Lord Tennyson,** English poet, 1809
   **Andy Warhol,** American artist and professional celebrity, 1927
   **Martin Duberman,** American historian and playwright, 1930

7. **Alice James,** Henry's sister, 1848

9. **Dolores Klaich,** American writer, 1936

12. **Edith Hamilton,** American classicist, 1867

13. **Lucy Stone,** American abolitionist and feminist, 1818

14. **William Flanagan,** American composer, 1926

16. **Abbé de Choisy,** French cleric and transvestite, 1644
    **Giovanni Bosco,** Italian saint, 1815
    **Dennis Altman,** Australian writer and activist, 1943

17. **Kurt Hiller,** German activist, 1885
    **Wallace Hamilton,** American writer, 1919
    **Larry Rivers,** American artist, 1923

19. **Nicola Porpora,** Italian composer, 1686

**David Rothenberg,** American writer and activist, 1933

21. **Jules Michelet,** French historian, 1798
    **Edith Simcox,** English writer, 1844
    **Lili Boulanger,** French composer, 1893
    **Mort Crowley,** American playwright, 1935

22. **Claude Debussy,** French composer, 1862

23. **Newton Arvin,** American literary critic, 1862

24. **Theodor Neuhof,** German adventurer, 1694

26. **Guillaume Apollinaire,** French poet, 1880

28. **Karl Heinrich Ulrichs,** German sexologist and activist, 1825

29. **Harry Conover,** model agent, 1911
    **Thom Gunn,** English-born American poet, 1929

31. **Commodus,** Roman emperor, 161
    **Warren Miller,** American writer, 1921

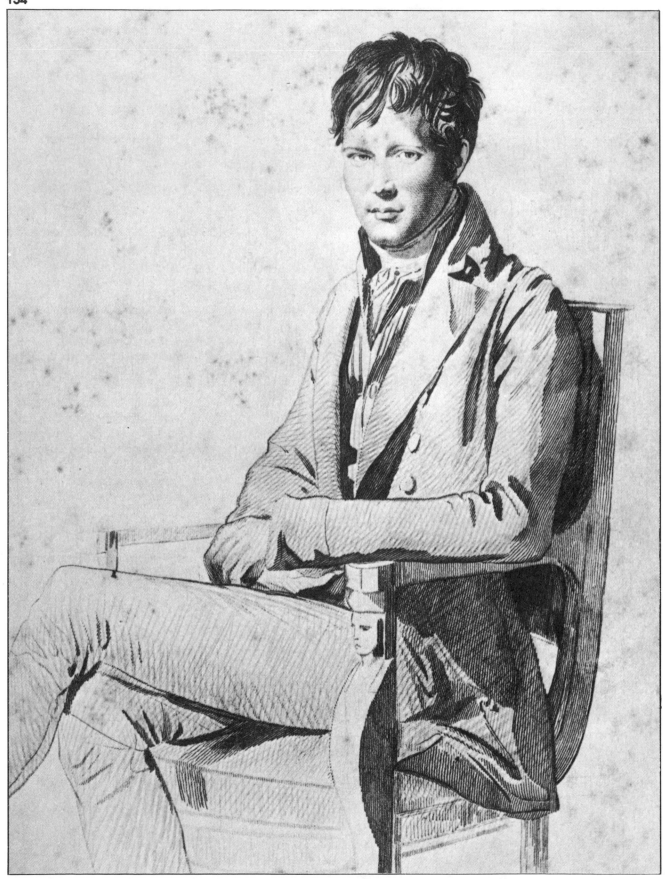

**Alexander von Humboldt:** Although his father and Napoleon mocked his interests as unmanly, he was one of the true geniuses of the 19th century.

# SEPTEMBER

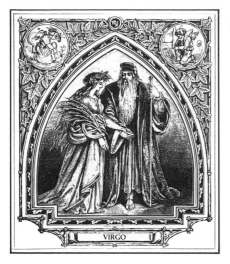

VIRGO

**Virgo** (August 22nd to September 21st) is a mutable earthly sign. Like Gemini, Virgo is ruled by Mercury and is mental in character. But the Virgoan tends to supply his mental talents to more practical activities than does the Geminian. Virgoans are down-to-earth, methodical, conscientious, and skilful with their hands. They are fond of things to do with the country and the soil. They are aloof by nature and do not as a rule make many friends. The chief characteristic of a Virgoan at his best is his wonderful power of discrimination. He brings a clear vision to whatever work is entrusted to him and sees at a glance all the practical possibilities and opportunities for usefulness involved. At his worst, however, the Virgoan sees only the impossibilities and the flaws—and finds them, by preference, in work done or schemes drawn up by others. Virgoans can be very, very picky.

# 1.

**SIR ROGER CASEMENT, b. Kingstown, County Dublin, Ireland, 1864.** Roger Casement was a good man. In the course of British consular service, he exposed the atrocious conditions imposed on gatherers of wild rubber in the Congo. His report served as grounds for the extinction of the Congo Free State in 1908. He exposed similar conditions in South America and was knighted for his services. Obviously, anyone this decent must have had enemies, and Casement had them by the carload. Though an Ulster Protestant, Casement became an ardent Irish nationalist. He went to Germany to seek aid for the Irish Revolution of 1916, and, England being at war with Germany, found himself upon his return arrested, tried, and convicted for high treason. What sealed

Casement's doom was the admission as evidence of his diaries. Meticulously kept, they recorded all of Casement's sexual encounters, itemizing both the amount of the transaction (if the stud was for hire) and the size of his equipment. It made for sensational evidence in 1916: "Stanley Weeks, 20, stripped, huge one, circumsized; swelled and hung quite." "Huge tram inspector . . . stiff as sword and thick and long." "Mario: Biggest since Lisbon July, 1904 and as big." "Beautiful muchacho . . . black and stiff as poker." "Enormous 19 about 7" and 4 thick; into me." "I to meet enormous 9; will suck and take too." Casement was done for. That he was on trial for treason and not for buggery did not matter. His homosexuality simply tightened the noose. When he was found guilty, protest was world-wide. But when the British government leaked word of the contents of the "black diaries," all

protest suddenly stopped. Roger Casement was hanged on August 6, 1916, a martyr for more than Ireland alone.

# 2.

**BRYHER, (neé Annie Winifred Ellerman), b. Margate, Kent, England, 1894.** Now, the relationships that follow are complicated, so pay attention; they won't be repeated. Ellerman, who called herself 'Bryher," was a New Woman, an Edwardian in search of the avantgarde. She traveled abroad and sought out as many of the remarkable people of her time as she could find and thus became an intimate of Havelock Ellis, Freud, Norman Douglas, Joyce, Gide, Stein, Hemingway, and others. During much of this period between the

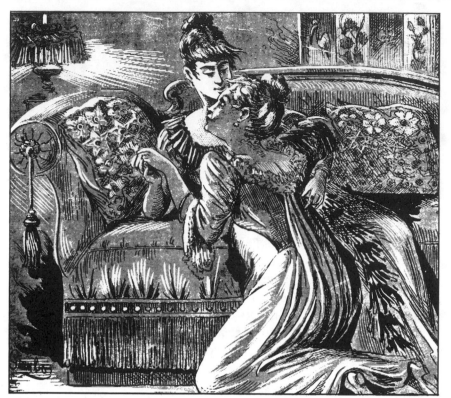

**Lesbians on the cover of The Police Gazette, 1893:** The headline screamed, "Good God! The Crimes of Sodom and Gomorrah Discounted."

wars, Bryher's traveling companion was the American poet, Hilda Doolittle, who called herself "H.D." and was the founder of Imagism. Bryher and H.D. were lovers. H.D.'s husband was the English poet Richard Aldington, among whose works was a volume of verse about two lesbian lovers, *The Love of Myrrhine and Konallis.* Although H.D. was in the process of shedding her husband, Bryher was in the process of acquiring one, the gay American writer Robert McAlmon. Their marriage, quite unlike that of H.D. and Aldington, which had produced a child, was a *mariage de convenance.* Bryher wanted to be free of her family and McAlmon was in need of the money that the wealthy Bryher could provide. But this marriage, convenient as it might have been, eventually ended in divorce. Bryher, undaunted, took another husband, this time Kenneth MacPherson, who had written a

novel about male homosexuality. Together with her second husband, Bryher established *Close Up,* perhaps the finest magazine devoted to the art of the silent film. Meanwhile, H.D. and Bryher had set up house together in Switzerland, H.D. was writing poems, Bryher historical novels, McAlmon was in Paris publishing avant-garde literature at the Contact Press, and Richard Aldington was writing poetry and novels and finding himself a new wife. McAlmon, Aldington, and Bryher all wrote autobiographies. Reading them is like watching *Rashomon.*

# 3.

**CHARLES VICTOR DE BONSTETTEN, b. Berne, Switzerland, 1745.** As a young man, the handsome Swiss writer was one

of those consciously unconscious charmers who could entice the birds from the trees, especially if the birds were unmarried middle-aged men. In maturity, Bonstetten's best known work was a study of the influence of climate on different nations, the north being exalted at the expense of the south. In his youth, Bonstetten's most famous work was the job he did on poet Thomas Gray. (*See December 26.*)

# 4.

**HANS AXEL, COUNT VON FERSEN, b. Stockholm, Sweden, 1755.** Descended from the Scottish McPhersons, Count Fersen was general, statesman, and lover of three different Swedish kings. So handsome that he was known as *le beau Ferson,* he turned the heads of Gustavus III, Marie Antoinette, Gustavus IV, and, possibly, Charles XIII before the latter ascended to the Swedish throne. Although the reason for his horrible death has never been satisfactorily explained, it may possibly have been the result of rumors about his involvement in the death of Christian of Augustenberg or about his sexual hold over the Gustavian dynasty. Whatever the reason, a savage mob tore him to pieces in the streets of Stockholm as police looked on and did nothing. He had been beaten with canes and umbrellas and then kicked to death.

# 5.

**TITUS (Titus Flavius Sabinus Vespasianus), b. Rome, 39 A.D.** There's nothing sensational or lurid here, so we can hurry through the life of Titus and on to something more interesting. Titus was a good emperor.

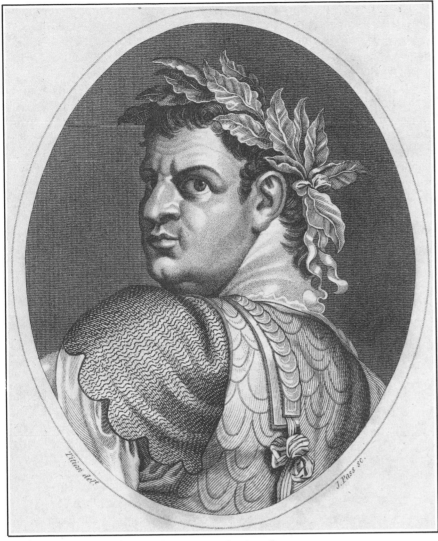

**The Emperor Titus:** Was he a Roman Goody Two-shoes?

Having served for eight years as co-ruler with his father, the emperor Vespasian, Titus, on his ascension to the throne, was a benevolent ruler who stopped persecutions for treason and was lavish with gifts to his subjects. He completed the Colosseum and built a luxurious bath. During his reign occurred the eruption of Mt. Vesuvius, and Titus was active in aiding the injured and homeless. So good was Titus that he is said to have given up the licentiousness of his youth, when his preferences ran particularly to handsome dancers. He is supposed to have given up cavorting with other men out of respect for his high office. *What do you mean you're disappointed in this write-up and that Titus had to be more than just a Roman Goody Two-shoes?* O.K. O.K. There *are* some ancient sources that imply that Titus did with his palace eunuchs what he no longer did in public with his dancers, the hypocrite.

**JOHN POWELL, b. Richmond, Virginia, 1882,** When anyone's entry in a standard reference work begins with a sentence like, "His mother was a descendant of Nicholas Lanier, a court musician to Charles I," then you know that there's a shortage of important information to follow. John Powell was both a pianist and composer. As a pianist he concertized throughout the world, but, as anyone who has ever visited Dubrovnik or Liverpool or Altoona, Pennsylvania, knows, it's possible to perform 'round the world and still not be a pianist of the first order. As a composer Powell's interests turned to American folk music, which has more or less placed his compositions in cold storage against the day when audiences are again interested in pieces with such names as *Negro Elegy, In Old Virginia,* and *At the Fair.* His lover was composer Daniel Gregory Mason, whose father was one of the founders of the Mason & Hamlin Piano Company, but not under Charles I.

# 7.

**ALBIUS TIBULLUS, b. Pedum, near Rome, c. 48 B.C.** Tibullus is chiefly known as a love elegist. His graceful poems convey genuine tenderness for the two women he calls Delia and Nemesis, and the personality of the poet that emerges from his elegies is gentle and sometimes melancholy. Like Catullus, Tibullus writes about his love for women and his love for boys, and his poems about his lusting after the handsome youth Marathus are simultaneously bitter-sweet and funny. The poems to the street-wise Marathus outline, first of all, the poet's stratagems for bedding him. The one thing he will not do in order to have Marathus is bribe him. Money corrupts, Tibullus tells us, not without irony. In a second poem, the poet's strategies have obviously not worked. Marathus couldn't care less. But the poet has a new plan. He will give the young man his slave girl, Pholoe, if only Marathus will sleep with him. As Tibullus tells the girl about how handsome the youth is, both poet and slave girl grow more and more desperate to have Marathus. In the final poem, none of Tibullus's strategies, including the bait of Pholoe, have worked in luring the young man to his bed. In the end, he is finally aware of Marathus's game. A rival of the poet, who has obviously been making it with the boy, has told him not to put out except for cold cash. Money corrupts, all right. But Tibullus never tells us whether or not he told the little pricktease where to go or simply reached in his toga for his wallet.

# 8.

**RICHARD LION HEART, b. Oxford, England, 1157.** Richard I saw little of England and was concerned with it chiefly as a source of revenue, but his military career and his personal qualities have made him a central figure in English romance and an English symbol of chivalry. Richard's chivalrous reputation is known to all English-speaking schoolboys through Sir Walter Scott's *Ivanhoe.* What Scott doesn't tell them, however, is that as a young man Richard fell in love with the king of France. As a chronicle of Henry II records (in John Boswell's translation): "Richard [then] duke of Aquitaine, son of the king of England, remained with Philip, the king of France, who so honored him for so long that they ate every day at the same table and from the same dish, and at night their beds did not separate them. And the king of France loved him as his own soul; and they loved each other so much that the king of England was absolutely astonished at the passionate love between them and marveled at

it." Richard, who was sincerely devout, was several times warned to "repent," but never completely abstained from his interest in men. Once, when he ignored the warning of a religious hermit to "be mindful of the destruction of Sodom" and to "abstain from what is unlawful," he took seriously ill and resolved to do something special as penance. He married shortly thereafter. Life, however, was apparently lonely for his wife, for Richard continued to pursue his battles and his men, never produced an heir, and, so far as we know, may never have consummated his marriage. After Richard's death, his wife had to sue the pope for recognition as Richard's widow. Apparently, the repentant sinner had not bothered to advertise his marriage hither and yon.

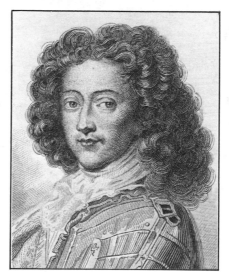

**Louis II de Bourbon,** Prince de Condé: One whore knew all there was to know about the other.

**LOUIS II DE BOURBON, PRINCE DE CONDÉ, b. Paris, 1621.** Known as "the Great Condé," this greatest of French generals was an intimate of Molière, Racine, Boileau, Boussuet, and La Bruyère. He also had the misfortune to be acquainted with "Madame"—whom we have already met—the gossipy wife of Philip, duc d'Orléans, who spread the word

about Condé's amours with his own sex. Condé, a clever gent, went to great pains to establish a reputation for himself as a great womanizer, but between the sharp tongue of Madame and the word of the well-known courtesan, Ninon de Lenclos, who was in a position to know, Condé fooled no one with his boasts.

# 9.

**CAPTAIN WILLIAM BLIGH, b. 1754.** Yes, Virginia, there really was a Captain Bligh, and, aside from his temper, he did not resemble Charles Laughton. Nicknamed "Breadfruit Bligh," not because of his stomach but because he had discovered breadfruit on one of Captain Cook's voyages, and because the famous journey of *H.M.S. Bounty* was in quest of breadfruit for transplanting in the West Indies, Bligh not only survived the mutiny and his 4,000-mile voyage in an open boat (all but one of the mutineers perished on Pitcairn Island), but he resumed his career, eventually becoming governor of New South Wales. The story of the mutiny suggests that Bligh might very well have had the hots for Fletcher Christian, a thought not lost on Byron when he came to write his version of the *Bounty* story, *The Island,* and one that would certainly have been explored (as in *Billy Budd*) if Melville had written the potboiler that eventually became the 1935 film. The theme never develops in the movie, possibly because, as Pauline Kael points out in an entirely different context, Clark Gable looks oddly tubby in tight white pants.

# 10.

**HILDA DOOLITTLE, b. Bethlehem, Pennsylvania, 1886.** *See September 2.*

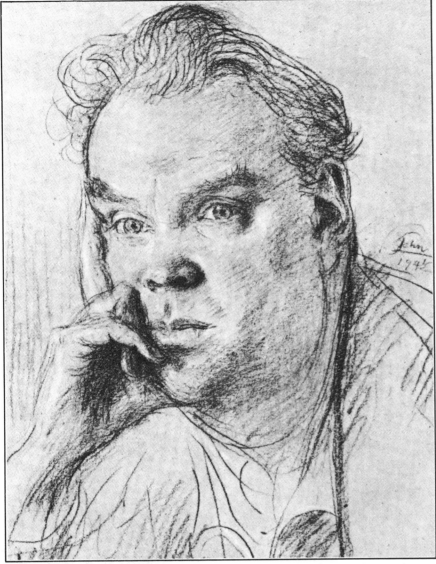

**Cyril Connolly:** He it was who wrote, "Imprisoned in every fat man a thin man is wildly signaling to be let out."

**CYRIL CONNOLLY, b. Coventry, England, 1903.** Connolly, one of the "bright young men" of the 1920s and one of the dandies featured in Martin Green's *Children of the Sun,* is one of the few modern critics who is fun to read, not merely because his prose style is so clear, so seemingly effortless, but because what he says is frequently unexpected and is original and fresh even when one disagrees. Though polite, he is fearless, is willing to back his own literary taste, to tilt at established reputations, to make fun of the pompous and pretentious. He gets under people's skin, in other words, because he frequently says what most do not want to hear. He is also capable of writing on virtually any subject, and in fact does, with the result that his enemies point out gleefully that no Connolly piece is ever without digressions that interfere with his argument. Edmund Wilson, no slouch himself as a critic, once defended Connolly's digressions as an extension of his *jeux d'esprit* and predicted that Connolly's critical pieces would remain classics of the language. It is impossible even to suggest the range of subjects covered by this fine writer, but no one has ever written more trenchantly than Connolly on the effects of the British public school system. No one else has ever said in print what is obvious to many foreigners who visit England. Where else on earth, he asks, can one find grown men who are completely hung up on the love affairs they had when they were thirteen?

# 11.

**D. H. LAWRENCE, b. Eastwood, Nottinghamshire, 1885.** What is one to make of this powerful but uneven writer, a man who has come to be seen as the high-priest of heterosexual love? Basic to David Herbert Lawrence's writing are characters struggling to resolve their fundamental needs with the demands and restrictions of a repressive society, and one senses this struggle within Lawrence himself. No one who has ever read Lawrence can deny a strain of homoeroticism that runs throughout his work, intensely in such works as "The Prussian Officer" and *Women in Love* (particularly the suppressed Prologue) and unconsciously in even *Lady Chatterley's Lover.* As to the latter, it may never have occurred to Lawrence, but the idea of the lower-class gamekeeper providing the aristocratic Constance with orgasm after orgasm is precisely the English homosexual fantasy that accounts for the fact of so many famous English upper-class men shacked up with lorry drivers, steam fitters, and construction workers. It is the fantasy-reality not only of E. M. Forster's *Maurice,* a Lady Chatterley in reverse, but of Forster himself. Lawrence's own struggle may very well have been the containment of what he himself saw as a homosexuality he could not accept. Katherine Mansfield's biographer

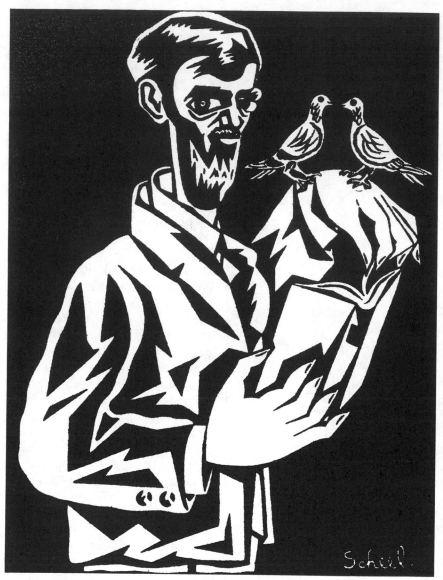

**D. H. Lawrence:** The author of *Aaron's Rod* was infatuated with another writer's husband.

suggests that Lawrence was physically attracted to the writer's husband, Middleton Murry, and it is known that at one time Lawrence had become so friendly with a handsome farm boy named William Henry that his wife Frieda adamantly refused ever to allow the young man to enter the Lawrences' house. Since Frieda's hackles were raised whenever anyone attempted to threaten her hold on Lawrence, one can only suspect that she probably realized what the writer himself did not.

# 12.

**MAURICE CHEVALIER, b. Paris, 1889.** Maurice Chevalier was an institution. In America, at least, the response was positively Pavlovian. Just to hear an "oo-la-la" or a "gay Par-ee" and Maurice of the curled-lip sprang to mind immediately. So much did he ooze exported Frenchiness that one began to suspect that the accent itself was fake and that he

had probably been born in Cedar Rapids. There was something of the runny cheese about him even in his youth, and he perfected a rakish wink, which was calculated to entice moviegoing matrons out of their step-ins, but which was only slightly to the right of Liberace's. And he could do the cutest things with a straw hat and cane that made one want to shake him. But the ladies loved Maurice and that's all that mattered. His career was clouded when he was accused of having "col-

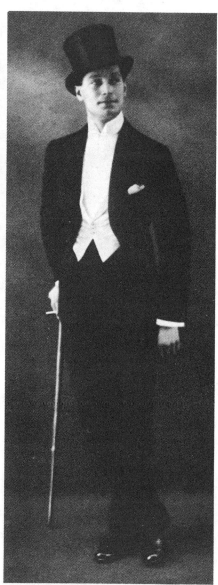

**Maurice Chevalier:** Every little breeze seems to whisper. . . .

laborated" with the Vichy government, and, for a while, every little breeze seemed to whisper that there was something between him and his valet, Felix Paquet. Recently, and posthumously, his politics during the war were declared pure. No one has said anything one way or the other about M. Paquet.

# 13.

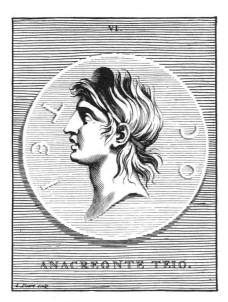

**Anacreon:** Oh say, can you see . . . ?

**ANACREON, Teos, Ionia, c. 570 B.C.** Why celebrate the Greek lyric poet's birthday today, when it is impossible to know his exact date of birth? Because Francis Scott Key wrote "The Star-Spangled Banner" today in 1814, that's why. And what does one have to do with the other? Simply this: Anacreon's poems were largely about boys he diddled, such youths as Smerdis, Leukaspis, Simalus, Euryalus, and Bathyllus, to name but a few. The structure of these poems was so popular in its own time that other poets imitated the so-called *Anacreontics*. Anacreon was rediscovered by English poets who delighted in imitating his style.

The vogue for *Anacreontics* in English culminated in the popular song "Anacreon in Heaven," and, as every schoolboy knows, the music to the song eventually became the tune for the American national anthem. Francis Scott Key's words may have been inspiring in the past, but they're impossible to memorize because archaic. If you doubt this, listen to the mumbles that pass for words when the song is sung at your next high-school graduation. And watch the people shifting uneasily from one foot to the other while staring at their shoes. And the tune itself is positively unsingable. There have been several attempts to convince Congress to seek a new national anthem, but no such luck thus far. If you want to accelerate this movement, just let the Moral Majority know that the anthem has everything to do with some foreign fag who used to dip his dork in little boys *just like theirs.* That oughta do the job.

# 14.

**ALEXANDER HUMBOLDT (Friedrich Heinrich Alexander, Freiherr von Humboldt), b. Berlin, Germany, 1769.** The great German naturalist and traveler, one of the geniuses of the 19th century, lived such a full life and made so many contributions to science that there is no way to do justice to him in a brief space. From 1799 to 1804 he made his renowned expedition with A. J. A. Bonpland to Central and South America and Cuba, a journey which in effect laid the broad foundations for the sciences of physical geography and meteorology. Humboldt explored the course of the Orinoco and the sources of the Amazon, establishing the connecting systems of the two. He ascended peaks in the Peruvian Andes to study the relation

of temperature and altitude, made observations leading to the discovery of the periodicity of meteor showers, and investigated the fertilizing properties of guano. In 1808 he settled in Paris and published his findings in some twenty-three volumes. During this period he also established the use of isotherms; studied the origin and course of tropical storms, the increase in magnetic intensity from the equator toward the poles, and volcanology; and made pioneer investigations on the relationship between geographical environment and plant distribution. All this was undertaken before middle age. In his sixties he was exploring Russia and Siberia, and he was working without stop until he died at ninety. Humboldt was an extraordinarily handsome man, and pictures of him rendered throughout his long life reveal good looks undimmed by age and a lean, trim body, apparently kept in good shape because of the physical requirements of his explorations. He has always been thought of as homosexual, with the first rumors having begun with the suspicion that he and Bonpland were lovers. What was suspected seemed confirmed to his contemporaries when he named his valet Seifert his sole heir.

**KATE MILLETT, b. St. Paul, Minnesota, 1934.** This deeply unconventional woman is not the victim of her own honesty, as the spiritually blind maintain, but was steamrolled by the hypocrisy of her own liberal readers, alas. When *Sexual Politics* was published in 1971, it created a storm not felt in the women's liberation movement since Betty Friedan's book had set postwar women's lib in motion. For a time, Millett was the darling of the movement—bright, articulate, gutsy. Then she published *Sita,* an autobiographical work that reinforced in print what some already knew—that Millett was bisexual. In an instant, she was discarded as a

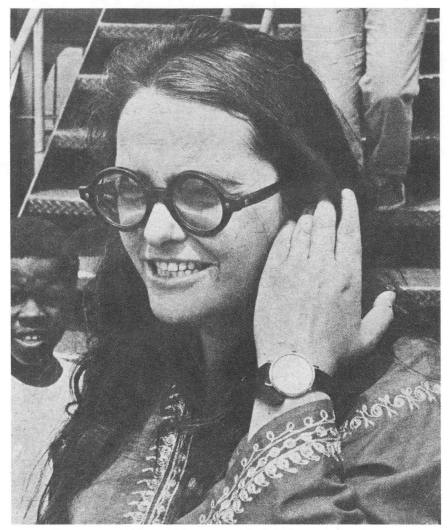

**Kate Millett:** A victim of her own honesty or of others' hypocrisy?

sexuality candidly, differing only in the stories used to illustrate his sexual preferences. According to Spartianus, Trajan was the proud possessor of a *paedogogium,* a road-show harem of boys that he took along with him on campaigns, apparently for his and his officers' pleasure. He also profited from the change of Roman mores that permitted him to receive without censure what he was so freely giving to his eunuchs. Rome's highly appropriate tribute to this good emperor—the Column of Trajan—is indeed a monumental erection.

# 16.

**WILHEIM VON GLOEDEN, b. Wismar, Germany, 1856.** At the turn of the 19th century and well into the opening years of the 20th, photographs by this German artist were circulating all over Europe—and for many different reasons. People who collected and mounted picture postcards in albums wanted the art postcards from the little Sicilian town of Taormina. They wanted them for the section of their albums that featured exotic and remote areas of the globe, or they wanted them for the section devoted to classical civilization or tableaux of historic scenes. Most people who wanted von Gloeden postcards, however, wanted them for one reason only—for the naked Sicilian boys that were featured on them. Von Gloeden photographs almost always show a boy, or a group of boys, in poses that are like classical sculpture come to life. The boys are clad in togas, or wearing wreaths of laurel, or illustrating scenes that are right out of classical poetry: an older man placing a hand on the buttocks of an adolescent boy, a boy looking longingly at another youth. To our eyes these photographs look faintly absurd,

leader, since it was deemed inappropriate that one of *them* should be leading *us.* Perhaps it's in the stars that women born on this day should be abused for their forthrightness. Millett shares a birthday with

Margaret Sanger (b. 1883), who dared campaign for birth control when polite Americans were busily pretending that they didn't even know how babies were made, no less prevented.

# 15.

**TRAJAN (Marcus Ulpius Trajanus), b. Santiponce, Spain, 53 A.D.** Trajan was the first non-Italian to serve as Roman emperor. An exceptionally efficient man, he was one of Rome's "good" emperors. His accomplishments were many, not only in battle,

but in the construction of public works, including aqueducts, theaters, the restoration of the Appian Way, the draining of the Pontine Marshes, and the building of the massive Forum of Trajan. All the ancient sources discuss Trajan's homo-

even naive. Yet they exist in a context that is very much of a piece with their origins. If Oscar Wilde's "bible" was Walter Pater's book on the Renaissance, Wilde was not alone in his appreciation of the historic period that had rediscovered the glories of Greece and Rome. The architecture, art, and writing of von Gloeden's era all reflect a new enthusiasm for the Renaissance. Von Gloeden's photographs are therefore very much of their period. But despite his obvious pederasty, the pictures themselves are not erotic for what seems a simple reason. Not one boy in any of the photos seems happy to be there, not one is happy in his nakedness. They are desperately poor and joyless and are posing because the Baron is paying them to. Ultimately that is what makes most erotic photography fail.

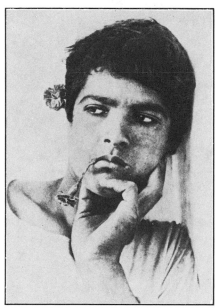

**"Jealousy":** The astonishing popularity of this photograph by Wilhelm von Gloeden tells us volumes about our ancestors, the proper Victorians.

# 17.

## BARON FRIEDRICH VON STEUBEN, b. Magdeburg, Prussia,

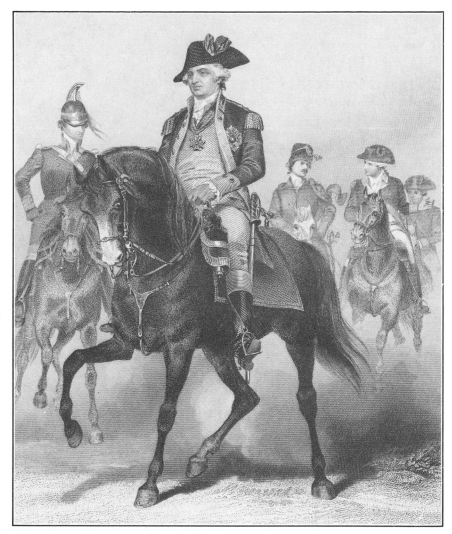

**Major General Baron von Steuben:** Daddy to two boys not his own.

1730. Steuben was an aide to Frederick the Great and instituted important reforms and training in the Prussian army before he lost royal favor, supposedly because he had taken "indecent liberties" with young men. His troubles at home were instrumental in his offer to instruct the Continental army in America, where Congress accepted his services and made him inspector general. At Valley Forge in the winter of 1777-78 he shared the sufferings of the ill-fed and ill-tended men as he organized and disciplined them into a powerful striking force. The effect was seen at the battle of Monmouth (1778), when he rallied his men after the retreat was begun by Charles Lee. He also commanded in the trenches at Yorktown. Steuben spent his fortune in the service of the young United States and was finally repaid by a pension voted by Congress, as well as by large tracts of land granted by various states. To help him share his retirement, he legally adopted two American patriots, Ben Walker and William North, and made them his sole heirs. The two handsome young men were not part of the government pension. Steuben, an honest man, paid for their maintenance himself.

# 18.

**GRETA GARBO** (né Greta Gustafsson), b. Stockholm, Sweden, 1905. Only a cad would suggest that you dig up a copy of the forgotten *Here Lies the Heart* by Mercedes de Acosta and read the silly section on Garbo. Dig up a copy of the forgotten *Here Lies the Heart* by Mercedes de Acosta and read the silly section on Garbo.

# 19.

**HENRI III, Fontainebleu, France, 1551.** In the final years of his reign (he died at thirty-seven), convinced that France was in the hands of scheming ministers and clergy, Henri abandoned himself completely to his homosexuality by attempting to rival the excesses of the most licentious Roman emperors. He surrounded himself with handsome young men, his *mignons,* whose fancy dress set the fashion for 16th-century Europe, but who nonetheless offended bourgeois mentality because they were "*frisés, fraisés, poudrés, perfumés*" (curled, ruffled, powdered, scented). Henry's passions included throwing orgies only slightly less wild than those of Heliogabalus, dressing up in drag, playing with teeny lap dogs, and indulging in a touch of sado-masochistic sex, where, surprisingly, he was S, not M. (On days of penitence, the Catholic Henri took great delight in flagellating his Confraternity of Penitents. As the penitents marched in the holy procession before him, the sight of rivulets of blood slowly staining their white linen robes made him wield his whip even harder.) The same blood-hungry Henri was known to be so effeminate that he would run, shriek-

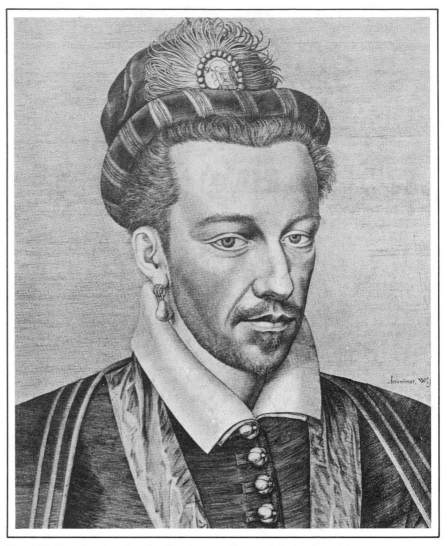

**Henri III:** Powdered, painted, effeminate, and, surprisingly, S not M.

ing, to hide in cellars during thunderstorms. Of his *mignons,* the best known was Saint-Mégrin, of whom it was said: "When he died, he gave his soul to God, his body to the ground, and his arse to the Devil."

# 20.

**TIPPU SAHIB, b. Mysore, India, 1753.** Tippu, last maharajah of Mysore, spent his entire life resisting British designs on India. It was, of course, a losing battle, but one that was fierce and bloody nonetheless. Long before Mahatma Gandhi conceived the idea of passive resistance as a means of toppling British rule, Tippu had his own way of dealing with Imperialism. The fierce warrior, known as the Tiger of Mysore, used to supervise the gang rape of captured British soldiers. It is not known whether a well-known oil company had Tippu in mind when it came up with an ad campaign featuring a cuddly tiger holding the nozzle of a gas pump. "Put a tiger in your tank," the ad said. And some did.

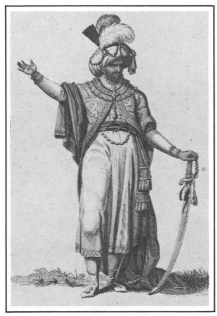

**Tippu Sahib:** A tiger in their tanks?

# 21.

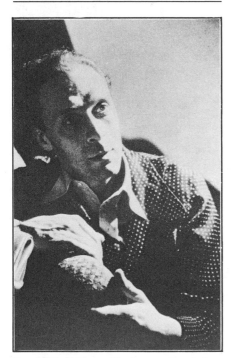

**Pavel Tchelitchew:** His lovers played the field because he spent himself in painting, not in sex.

**PAVEL TCHELITCHEW, b. Moscow, 1898.** The paintings of Tchelitchew, like those of any other artist, progressed through several different stages. Two of these are immediately recognizable as uniquely Tchelitchew's to anyone even casually interested in modern art. In the mid-1930s, the Russian-born American artist became increasingly preoccupied with the problems of perspective and metamorphosis. In *Portrait of My Father* (1939), for instance, a winter landscape becomes a Bengal tiger holding a black snake in its mouth; and the children in his famous symbolic canvas *Hide-and-Seek* (1941) become a gnarled tree. In 1943 he began his series of "interior landscapes" or anatomical paintings in which he depicted figures whose skeleton or veins showed through their skin. Before these two well-known periods of his career, Tchelitchew worked both in Berlin and Paris, where he intermixed realistic subjects and Cubism (*Figures,* for example, depicts a sexual assault featuring three male nudes). Much of Tchelitchew's work is decidedly erotic, and these very beautiful works not originally designed for public display should be collected and published. His lovers included the Surrealist René Crevel and the American writer Charles Henri Ford. Ford has recently said that since Tchelitchew poured so much of himself into his work, sex was not of paramount importance to him in his friendships. Tchelitchew was once a favored protégé of Gertrude Stein, but they parted company after the artist was taken up by Edith Sitwell, Stein's chief rival as a discoverer of bright young men. When Tchelitchew was banned from Stein's salon, he began to spread the funny, but savage, rumor that the disfiguring hump on Alice B. Toklas's forehead was in reality "Gertrude's baby."

# 22.

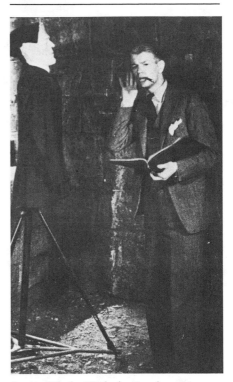

**James Whale:** With the Frankenstein Monster before there was any possibility of mating it with Elsa Lanchester.

**JAMES WHALE, b. 1889.** In 1930 the British stage director went to Hollywood to film his stage production of *Journey's End* and stayed to make other movies, including four classics of the macabre: *Frankenstein* (1931), *The Old Dark House* (1932), *The Invisible Man* (1933), and, perhaps best of all, the witty *Bride of Frankenstein* (1935). Among his many other films is the best of the three Hollywood depictions of *Showboat,* the 1936 black-and-white version with Irene Dunne. Whale, who was very much his own man and who did not think that anyone would much care anyway, lived openly as a homosexual in discreetly closeted Hollywood. His lover was the producer David Lewis. But there was no way that he could run counter to America's, and

Hollywood's, growing conservatism as the Depression waned. By 1940 no studio would risk hiring him, and he never worked again.

with a tambourine, '*Videsne ut Cinaedus orbem digito temperet?*' translatable as both 'Do you see that queer's finger beating the orb?' and 'Do you see how this queer's finger

governs the world?' " The audience immediately took this as a reference to Augustus and broke into wild applause while staring at the imperial box.

# 23.

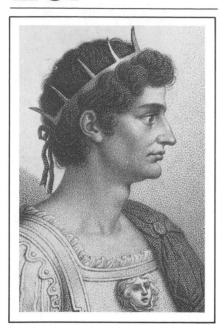

**Augustus Caesar:** Uncle Julius's peg-boy.

**AUGUSTUS CAESAR (Caius Octavius), b. Rome 63 B.C.** Octavius, as he would have been called before he became the first Roman emperor, was a young opportunist who literally rose on his hands and knees. It's a wise child who knows his uncle, and Octavius regularly put out for his uncle, Julius Caesar, an investment that paid off in the end. He also lured the powerful Roman statesman Hirtius to his bed and received 3,000 pieces of gold for his pains, a favor he returned when he became emperor by having Hirtius murdered to prevent him from ever telling the tale. But he could not effectively stifle what was already popularly known. In *Jonathan to Gide,* Noel Garde tells how secret the emperor's secret really was. Once, when Augustus was attending a play, "an actor spoke a line about an effeminate eunuch priest

# 24.

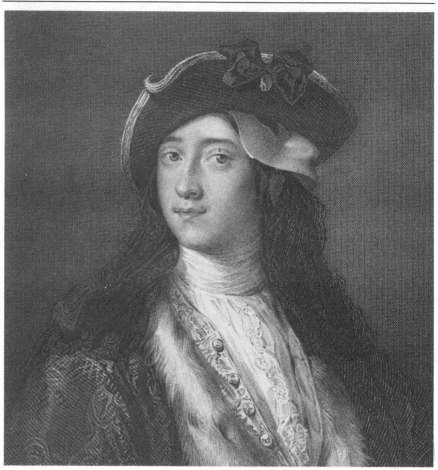

**Horace Walpole:** Locked in a closet at Strawberry Hill.

**HORACE WALPOLE, b. London, 1717.** Like his famous father, Robert Walpole, Horace Walpole spent much of his life in the service of his government, but his primary concern was with the arts. He was a master at finding ways to spend his extraordinary fortune and devoted twenty years to altering his villa in the Gothic style, a style that he almost single-handedly revived. Strawberry Hill, his Gothic castle, was decorated by the very gay John Chute, the

spiritual father of two centuries of gay interior designers. Walpole, whose novel *The Castle of Otranto* (1764) created the vogue for Gothic novels, is one of the most famous closet cases in recorded history. Although surrounded by homosexual friends—some flamboyant like Chute, some repressed like the poet Thomas Gray—Walpole spent most of his life hopelessly in love with his heterosexual friend Henry Seymour Conway, to whom he addressed very beautiful love letters. Ironically, when Walpole died he left Strawberry Hill to Conway's daughter, Mrs. Damer, without ever having known that she was one of the most celebrated lesbians of the 18th century.

# 25.

**JEAN HENRI DUNANT, b. Geneva, Switzerland, 1828.** In 1862, Dunant, a Swiss philanthropist published his *Un souvenir de Solférino,* a description of the sufferings of the wounded at the battle of Solférino and a plea for organizations to care for the war wounded. There was an immediate response, out of which eventually grew the Red Cross. In 1901 Dunant shared the first Nobel Peace Prize. It has long been suspected that after his death Dunant's family not only bowdlerized the philanthropist's memoirs, but falsified them through additions not written by Dunant himself. He is thought to have been homosexual, but there is no way to know for certain.

# 26.

**T. S. ELIOT, b. St. Louis, Missouri, 1888.** Here are the facts. When Thomas Stearns Eliot was living in Paris before World War I he met a French medical student named Jean Verdenal in the Luxembourg Gardens. Verdenal was waving a branch of lilac at the time. Verdenal died in the Dardanelles in 1915. Eliot dedicated to him his first published book, *Prufrock and Other Observations,* adding an epigraph from Dante's *Purgatory*: "Now can you understand the quantity of love that warms me towards you, so that I

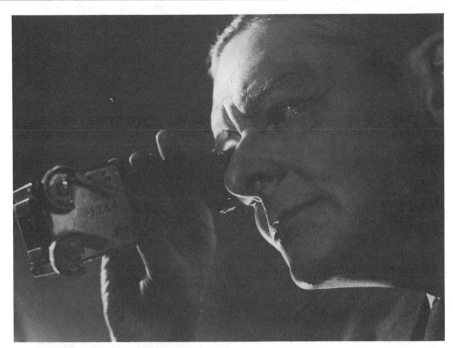

**T. S. Eliot:** The poet's adolescent lines on masturbation: "Then he knew that he had been a fish/With slippery white belly held tight in his own fingers,/Writhing in his own clutch, his ancient beauty/Caught fast in the pink tips of his new beauty."

forget our vanity, and treat the shadows like the solid thing." That is all we know about his friendship with the young medical student, and all that we are likely ever to know. Here are other facts. Eliot had a horror of the female body, he feared it and thought it "smelled." He had an abhorrence of sex in general, although, as a boy, he masturbated guiltily (and once wrote a magnificently sensuous poem about it). He was obsessed with the thought that *every* man wanted to kill a

woman, and without irony extended *his* fantasy to include all men. His first marriage was miserable in that his wife laughed in his face at the very idea of sleeping with him. These are the general facts, and various interpretations will be offered by biographers as long as people read Eliot's poetry. Thus far, interpretations have run in two obvious directions. Of course he was completely asexual. Of course he was a latent homosexual. Both seen unfair. He was simply T. S. Eliot.

# 27.

**ROBERT PATRICK (né Robert Patrick O'Connor), b. Kilgore, Texas, 1937.** This is how the playwright Lanford Wilson begins his introduction to *Robert Patrick's Cheep Theatricks* (yes, the author's name is part of the title): "Bob told me this introduction should begin,

'Bob Patrick's plays are stars shooting across the cobalt night sky—snowflakes that for a second enhance the eyelashes of the blushing Muse!' or some such. But I really can't capture the preposterous pop jargon that Bob nearly invented. If I did begin this introduction that way, I couldn't finish

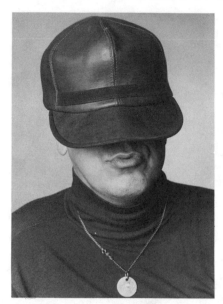

**Robert Patrick:** Antic, brilliant, one of a kind.

it—not the way he would." There's a lot in that small paragraph, even though Wilson goes his own way after dropping it, telling us about Bob's life in the theater—how he's done everything from act and sing and direct to tend the door, run the lights, mop the floors, and, for all we know, wash the clothes of indigent actors appearing in his plays. These are facts, but the real Bob Patrick is in that first paragraph. For Bob is right. His plays *are* shooting stars. They burn bright, brilliant, but only for a moment, retained in memory. And they are snowflakes, as many and as dazzling as the stars, no two the same. And Wilson is right to find Bob's language impervious to imitation. Bob invents the right sentence for the right occasion, and if there's only one that's right, he'll find it, quickly (for Bob is very, very fast), efficiently (for Bob is very, very intelligent), and humorously (for Bob is very, very funny). Bob is also always telling you what to do (notice Wilson's first sentence). You're rarely aware of his bossiness in his plays because his messages are subliminally told. Ask anyone who has just

emerged from a Patrick play what he has ordered them to do and they'll know. New York's most frequently produced playwright wants us simply to be good to one another, and has found a thousand star-and-snowflake ways to tell us how.

# 28.

CARAVAGGIO (Michelangelo Merisi da Caravaggio), b. Caravaggio, Lombardy, 1573. Caravaggio was in every way a rebel. A profound realist, he was accused of imitating nature at the expense of ideal beauty. In religious scenes his use of models from the streets was considered irreverent. He worked directly on the canvas, unheard of in his time. He was a brawler, a drinker, a fornicator, a fugitive who had killed a man. Because he knew the underside of life and painted it, because he associated freely with the underclass, because he died degraded and forlorn, he is thought by some to have been classically gay. We have no proof, nor will we ever.

# 29.

WILLIAM II RUFUS, b. Normandy, 1056. The second surviving son of William the Conquerer was nicknamed Rufus for his full red beard and fiery complexion. Almost every ancient source agrees that he was "effeminate," "vain," "wicked," and a "sodomite," and long passages spun from these chronicles have concluded that he was extravagant in dress and talk, "a feudal Oscar Wilde" one modern writer calls him. If the man is so wicked, so potentially intriguing, why is this daily entry so brief

when others, with far less interesting subjects, are so much longer? Because John Boswell in his *Christianity, Social Tolerance,* and *Homosexuality* uses the legendary reputation of King William to show just how unreliable the ancient chronicles can be. Only a ninny would believe everything he reads in print. Let the brilliant Dr. Boswell show you why William II Rufus was not necessarily gay in his magnificent book.

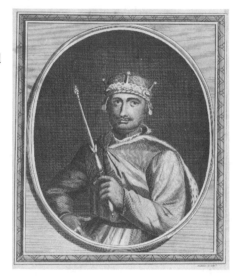

**William II Rufus:** Don't believe everything you read in the papers.

# 30.

TRUMAN CAPOTE, b. New Orleans, Louisiana, 1924. "I was a beautiful little boy," Truman Capote says, and the talk-show viewer blinks his eyes in disbelief. Knowing only the name, the puffy face, and the voice that the Smithsonian should display as a national treasure, the wide-eyed viewer does not know that Capote is correct. "I was a beautiful little boy," he says, "and everyone had me—men, women, dogs, and fire hydrants." Sad, sad, oh sad, to think what fame and wealth and for-

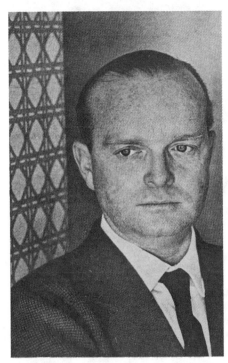

**Truman Capote:** Gore Vidal boasts that his work has been studied by a Professor Dick while Capote's has been analyzed by a Professor Nance.

ty years can do to a man. Write us an autobiography, Mr. Capote, or something beautiful like so many of your early books. But give us something lest we think that of the women, men, and dogs you had, you were left with only the fire hydrant.

## Other Personalities Born in September

1. **Emma Stebbins,** American sculptor, 1815

2. **Rev. John M. McNeill,** Jesuit scholar, psychotherapist, and writer, 1925

3. **Sarah Orne Jewett,** American writer, 1849
   **James Nolan,** American poet, 1947

6. **Guillaume Cardinal Dubois,** French statesman, 1656
   **Julian Green,** French writer of American parentage, 1900

7. **Valerie Taylor,** American writer, 1913

8. **Marie Thérèse Louise, the Princess de Lamballe,** aristocratic lover of Marie Antoinette, 1749

9. **Paul Goodman,** American poet-reformer, 1911

10. **Pope Julius III,** 1487
    **Mary Oliver,** American poet, 1935

12. **Grace Greenwood** (née Sara Jane Clarke), American writer, 1840

13. **J. D. Beazley,** English classical scholar, 1840

14. **Eric Bentley,** English-born American translator, critic, director, 1916

15. **Titus Oates,** English conspirator, 1649
    **Karl Philipp Moritz,** German novelist, 1757

    **Umberto II,** exiled king of Italy, 1904

16. **Mikhail I. Kutuzov,** Russian general, 1745

17. **Charles Tomlinson Griffes,** American composer, 1884

18. **Gerald Tyrwhitt-Wilson, Lord Berners,** English composer and artist, 1883
    **Francis Grierson** (né Jesse Shepard), English-born Amercian writer and singer, 1848

21. **Philippe, duc d'Orleans,** French nobleman and transvestite, 1640
    **Sir Edmund Gosse,** English critic and translator, 1849

26. **Jean-Louis André Theodore Gericault,** French painter, 1791
    **Sir Anthony Blunt,** English art historian and the "Fourth Man" in the Burgess-Maclean spy case, 1907
    **Andrea Dworkin,** American writer and feminist, 1946

27. **Louis XIII,** French king, 1601
    **Vincent Youmans,** American song writer, 1898

28. **Johann Mattheson,** German organist, singer, and composer, 1681

30. **Rumi,** Persian poet, 1207
    **Johnny Mathis,** American popular singer, 1935

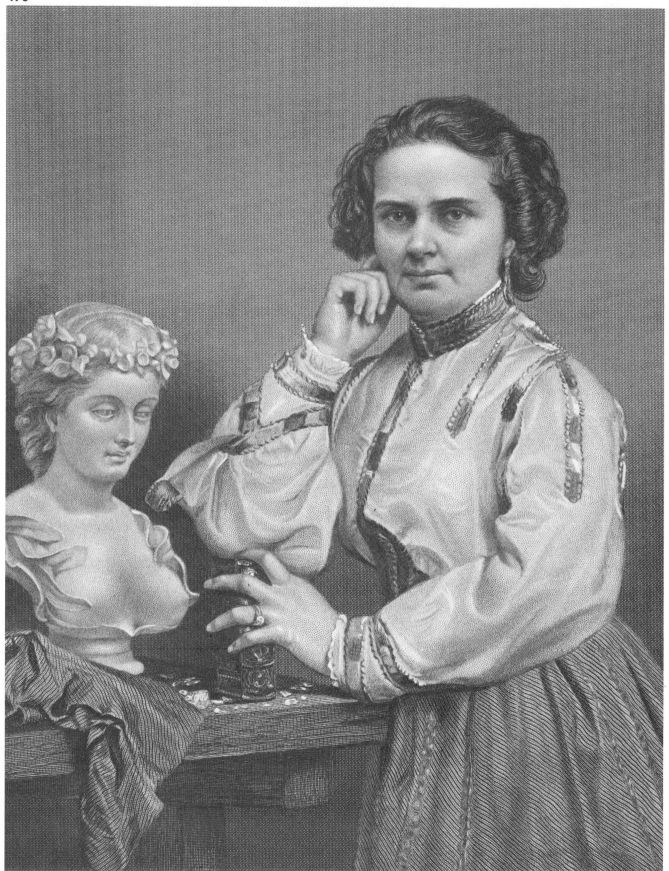

**Harriet Hosmer:** Of Charlotte Cushman's female "Jolly Bachelors," she alone was a "buddy" of the famous actress and not a lover.

# OCTOBER

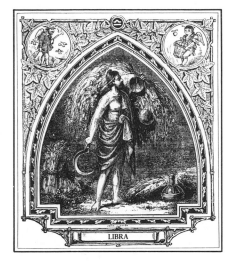

LIBRA

**Libra** (September 22nd to October 22nd) is a cardinal airy sign ruled by Venus. This is one of the most easy-going and gentle of all the signs of the Zodiac. The scales symbolize a love of harmony and balance and a distrust of unpleasantness and conflict of any kind. Unlike the Virgoan, the Libran is sociable and outgoing, and generally makes many friends. Like the Taurean, who is also ruled by Venus, the Libran is fond of the opposite sex, and generally successful in his affairs. His balanced outlook and dislike of extremes make him a good diplomat, but they can also lead to weakness and an inability to commit himself. Librans hate injustice and unfairness and everything ill-proportioned and ugly in life, and also dislike exaggeration and all feelings that are morbid, depressing, or strained. Librans are seldom introspective and self-analytical and tend to live a good deal in the present by leaving the past to the concern of others.

# 1.

**WILLIAM BECKFORD, b. Font-hill Gifford, Wiltshire, England, 1760.** The rich have all the fun. When he was eleven years old, William Beckford inherited his father's vast fortune. The rest of his life was devoted to spending it. Along the way he also wrote several highly imaginative books, the most famous of which is the oriental romance *Vathek*, a bizzare but enormously entertaining book that anticipates the epicene lushness of Oscar Wilde's *Salome* by a century. Well educated and courtly, he was the quintessential dandy. Even in his teens he was the especial favorite of aristocratic dowagers. When Beckford was nineteen, he became obsessed with ten-year-old William Courtenay, a provocative upper-class nymphet naturally skilled in the art of seducing "older"

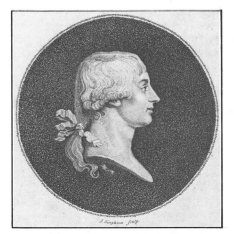

**William Beckford:** A mistake in gender.

men. When, five years later, "Kitty" Courtenay and Beckford were caught *in flagrante delicto* (the newspapers called the affair "a grammatical mistake in regard to the genders"), Beckford was obliged to flee to Switzerland, where he spent the next ten years in exile. With his young wife conveniently dead, and having fulfilled his obli-

gation to his class by reproducing his kind, Beckford, at twenty-six, was now free to pursue a life lived entirely for his own pleasure. Travels throughout Europe and a steady stream of conquests followed, including the famous castrato Pacchierotti, who was in turn thrown over for a young Venetian nobleman whom Beckford called his "pagan idol," and, somewhere along the way, seventeen-year-old Gregorio Franchi, who remained with Beckford for forty years. Beckford returned to England in 1794 and immediately began work on Fonthill Abbey, the Gothic castle that dwarfed Walpole's more modest Strawberry Hill. Called "Beckford's Folly" by neighboring squires who watched its construction, it cost the equivalent of about $10 million. Its size can be imagined by the wall—12 feet high and 7 miles long—that surrounded it. Within this castle was one of the most extraordinary art collections in Europe, the library of Edward Gibbon, purchased at his death, and a fleet of male servants with names, selected by Beckford, right out of *La Cage aux Folles*—Miss Long, the Doll, Bijou, Miss Butterfly, Countess Fox, and Madame Bion. As the years passed, this young, rich, talented, happy queen developed into an old, rich, talented, happy queen. The moral would seem to be that money can, and does, buy happiness no matter what the spoilsports say.

# 2.

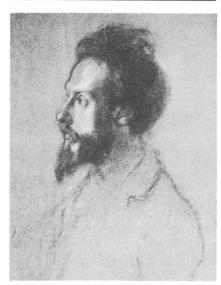

**Charles Ricketts:** Gay stability in Victorian England.

**CHARLES RICKETTS, b. Geneva, Switzerland, 1866.** There have almost always been homosexual couples, living discreet and not entirely secret lives together, that have managed to enjoy happy partnerships free of scandal and sensation. Such a marriage—and a marriage it was—was enjoyed by Charles Ricketts and Charles Shannon, two English artists of note. Although both pursued independent careers as painters (Ricketts was also a

stage designer whose work anticipated that of Bakst), they served as joint editors of the *Dial* before Ricketts founded the Vale Press in 1896 and designed some of the most beautiful collectors' books ever printed. Their friendship was an open secret and they moved undisturbed within London's gay circle throughout the Oscar Wilde years and after. Both, in fact, were present at the gay twenty-first birthday party for Vyvyan Holland, Oscar Wilde's son. (Other stalwarts present at this gala coming of age included Henry James, Ronald Firbank, Robbie Ross, and Reggie Turner.) Ricketts and Shannon lived together for more than fifty years. Their greatest problem seems to have been what to do if the telephone rang and someone asked for "Charlie."

# 3.

**CAMILLE SAINT-SAËNS b. Paris, 1835.** Saint-Saëns began his musical career as a child prodigy and pursued a life in music until he died at eighty-six. He was an exceptional pianist and organist, who composed works, as he put it, "as an apple-tree produces apples." He brought forth prodigious quantities of musical apples, and if some, to modern ears, are a little green or even rotten, they are more than made up for by the large number of perfect, polished fruit. It costs a great deal of money to be a full-time composer, and Saint-Saëns was no struggling artist in a rooftop garret. He was supported by a large behest from an older friend, Henri Libon, and the nature of their friendship has always been open to interpretation. There's no question, however, about Saint-Saëns' own homosexuality. Al-

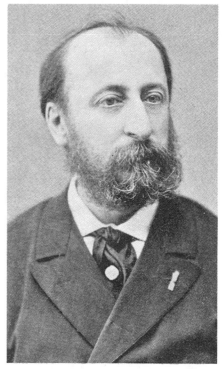

**Camille Saint-Saëns:** In old age pissoirs were for peeking.

though he is reported to have had a marked preference for Algerian boys, he was a devotee of Parisian pissoirs even in old age. In an amusing memoir, the composer Henri Busser (1872-1937) records coaxing his ancient colleague, now reduced to merely peeking, from the local pissoirs. Saint-Saëns was certain in his tastes. Once, when asked whether he were homosexual, the composer replied, "No, no, my dear, I am a pederast." Not everyone, after all, acknowledges that the two are not synonymous.

**GORE VIDAL, b. West Point, New York, 1925.** Gore Vidal is America's foremost essayist, one of America's best novelists (and one capable of distinguishing between a "serious" work and an entertainment), a political thinker to reckon with, a mortal enemy of Truman Capote ("I can't read him; I'm diabetic"), and a savage wit (when asked whether the first person he slept with was a man or a woman, he replied, "I don't know, I was too polite to ask"). He is sharp, outspoken, and not afraid of no one, no way, no how. It's nice to have him on *our* side.

# 4.

**MARIE CORELLI (Mary Mackay), b. England, 1864.** No precise date of birth is known for this English novelist since she was adopted in infancy by the poet Charles Mackay. If Hall Caine *(see May 13)* was the Harold Robbins of the Victorian era, then Marie Corelli was its Jacqueline Susann. Corelli was a master at tickling the Victorian libido while remaining primly moral. Instead of multiple orgasms there was a great deal of nostril-flaring in her books. The Prince of Wales, who preferred flaring his own nostrils to reading about it, was nonetheless one of Corelli's biggest fans, as was his mama Victoria, who was not particularly known for her literary taste. Is it any wonder that Marie Corelli, like Hall Caine, became enormously rich? Available to help her spend her fortune was her lifelong lover Bertha Vyver, whom Corelli called "Mamasita" and "Darling Ber." In return, Big Bertha called Corelli "Little Girl." All but one of Corelli's biographers agree that besides hugging each other a lot and combing each other's hair, which was permissible in a Victorian "romantic friendship," they most certainly flared nostrils together, which was not. The story goes that while in Reading Gaol, Oscar Wilde was constantly bothered by a prison guard who fancied himself a literary connoisseur. Day after day he would ask Wilde remarkably obtuse questions about authors and their

books. One day the guard asked Wilde if he considered Marie Corelli a "great writer." Said Wilde when he recovered from his shock: "Now don't think I have anything against her *moral* character, but from the way she writes, *she ought to be here.*"

# 5.

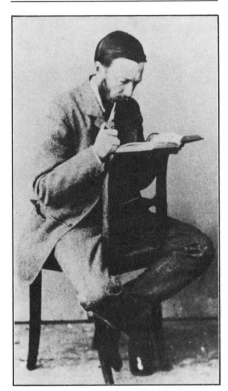

**John Addington Symonds:** A fearless pioneer.

**JOHN ADDINGTON SYMONDS, b. Bristol, England, 1840.** To be a homosexual in Victorian England meant membership, if one dared, in an underground fraternity. For to speak candidly of one's tastes was to open oneself to criminal prosecution, if scandal, or one's enemies felt inclined to claim a pound of flesh. One of the few Englishmen of the day who came closest to crusading for public acceptance of "inversion," as he called it, was

John Addington Symonds. Homosexuality was his obsession. It was the "problem" in modern ethics that most deeply touched on his life, and he refused to hold back both questions and intelligently-considered answers. In 1877 he lost his chair of poetry at Oxford because he was openly "familiar" with boys and left England for Italy, dedicating the rest of his life to exploring the problem. The result of his labors was *A Problem in Greek Ethics* (1833) and *A Problem in Modern Ethics* (1891), pioneering works of sexual apology. Symonds was a painfully honest man. Walt Whitman, who for reasons of his own was not, was hounded for twenty years by Symonds who wanted to know whether the author of "Calamus" was gay. The poet, to his eternal shame, said no. Had Whitman not died shortly after his response, Symonds would undoubtedly have asked again. He was not the kind to take no for an answer.

# 6.

**KAROL SZYMANOWSKI, b. Timoshovka, Ukraine, 1883.** In his autobiography, *My Life and Loves,* pianist Arthur Rubinstein speaks of his friendship with the important Polish composer Karol Szymanowski, who was gay. Rubinstein speaks of a wealthy friend and admirer who had invited the composer several times to visit Italy. "After his return," the pianist writes, "he raved about Sicily, especially Taormina. 'There,' he said, 'I saw a few young men bathing who could be models for Antinous. I couldn't take my eyes off them.'" Rubinstein does not mention that Szymanowski had been visiting the isle of Wilhelm von Gloeden, and one wonders, in fact,

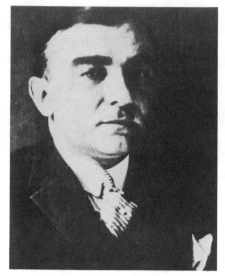

**Karol Szymanowski:** In love with von Gloeden's Taormina and its boys.

whether the German photographer was Szymanowski's wealthy friend. New recordings have marked a recent reawakening of interest in Szymanowski's music, which is all to the good. How many recordings of Beethoven's Fifth do the record companies think we need?

# 7.

**CHEVALIER D'ÉON (Charles Gemeviéve Louise Auguste André Timothée d'Éon de Beaumont), b. Burgundy, France, 1728.** If you look up *eonism* in your dictionary, you may or may not find it. It's a pseudo-scientific word for transvestism that has the quaint ring of Stekel or other *Herr-Doktors* who were writing in turn-of-the-century Vienna when people seem to have been having love affairs with their piccolos or putting clown hats on their penises. The Chevalier d'Éon, a century before, loved to dress in drag. Supposedly, the French adventurer originally had been sent on various spying missions disguised as a woman and so liked the feel of silk and satin

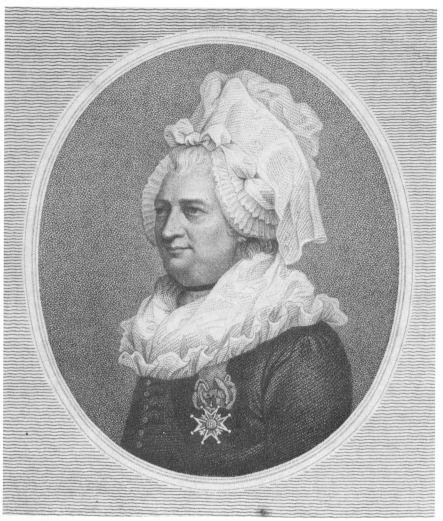

**The Chevalier D'Éon:** Bets were laid on whether he was male or female.

that he decided to stay in costume for the rest of his life. Not that he had much choice. When word got out that he really liked taking four hours to dress each morning, King Louis XV decreed that the chevalier *had* to wear women's clothing forever after. For years people laid bets on d'Éon's sex, but a post-mortem examination of his body conclusively established the fact that he was very much a man.

**JAMES WHITCOMB RILEY, b. Greenfield, Indiana, 1849.** In the days when schoolmarms were intent on seeing to it that schoolboys

would grow up hating poetry, they force-fed liberal doses of James Whitcomb Riley, who had gained immense popularity with his series of poems in the Hoosier dialect written under the pseudonym "Benjamin F. Johnson of Boone." His verses were collected under the title *"The Old Swimmin'-Hole" and 'Leven More Poems."* Well, shucks, land's sake alive, it turns out that old Jimmy Riley act'lly liked lovin' li'l boys 'bout 'lebenty-'leben times more than writin' poetry. Or, that's at least what Charles Warren Stoddard, who knew him, claims in his letters and journals.

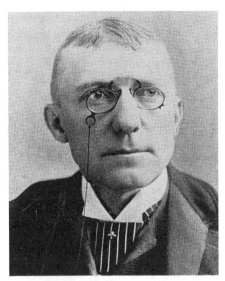

James Whitcomb Riley: Hours spent down by the old swimmin'-hole.

# 8.

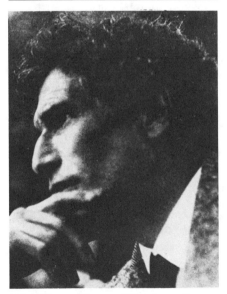

John Cowper Powys: Ripe for rediscovery.

**JOHN COWPER POWYS, b. Shirley, Derbyshire, England, 1872.** Here's a subject for a college term paper, and it's free for anyone who wants to take it up. John Cowper Powys's best-known novel is *A Glastonbury Romance* (1933), a modern adaptation of the myth that Joseph of Arimathea possessed the Holy Grail. Powys has written that the hero of this novel is autobiographical. Since the novel is about a young man who loves a male friend better than his lady love, what exactly does Powys mean by "autobiographical"?

# 9.

**SIMEON SOLOMON, b. London, 1840.** The last time we met this English artist *(see April 5)* he and Algernon Swinburne were chasing each other naked through the house of Dante Gabriel Rossetti. But that friendship was soon to end. In 1873, Solomon, one of along line of artists in his family, was arrested in a London public urinal. In his hour of need, Solomon learned that his fair-weather friend Swinburne would no longer deign to be seen in his company, no less run naked with him through the houses of their mutual friends. For a time, Solomon was the lover of Oscar Browning, the Eton master and Cambridge tutor who was forced to leave both schools because of homosexual scandals. His paintings and drawings, many of which are erotic and explicitly gay, have never been collected in a published volume, much as the artist's name is rarely found in any but the most complete reference books. More's the pity, since his work may be said in many ways to virtually define Victorian art.

# 10.

**HARRIET HOSMER, b. Watertown, Massachusetts, 1830.** In 1908 newspapers reported that Miss Harriet Goodhue Hosmer, the famous sculptor, had died. If obituaries reserved the phrase "he never married" for male homosexuals, there was no need to do so for females. The title "Miss" announced to the world that the deceased was unmarried, and that was sufficient. Since almost no one believed that lesbianism was even possible, there was no need to report, even in polite code, what didn't exist. Harriet Hosmer's widowed father raised her as a boy, encouraged her to become a physician, and did not deny her his blessing when she decided to become a sculptor instead. When she was about twenty she fell under the spell of Charlotte Cushman, who convinced her to study sculpting in Italy, where she presided over a colony of lesbians who called themselves the "Jolly Bachelors." What was unusual about this friendship, given the mesmeric power that the actress seemed to have over fluttering, feminine types, was that Hosmer, herself masculine in demeanor, seems to have been accepted as an equal from the beginning. If ever two women can have been called "buddies" it was Cushman and Hosmer. They were particularly fond of shocking the Roman gentry by riding astride their horses, instead of the proper side-saddle, and by riding in male attire. Hosmer went on to become one of the most successful sculptors of her day, her most famous work, "Puck," perhaps the most frequently reproduced sculpture of the late 19th century. For the remainder of Cushman's life, the two friends lived either under the same roof or in close proximity to one another, buddies to the end.

# 11.

**ELEANOR ROOSEVELT, b. New**

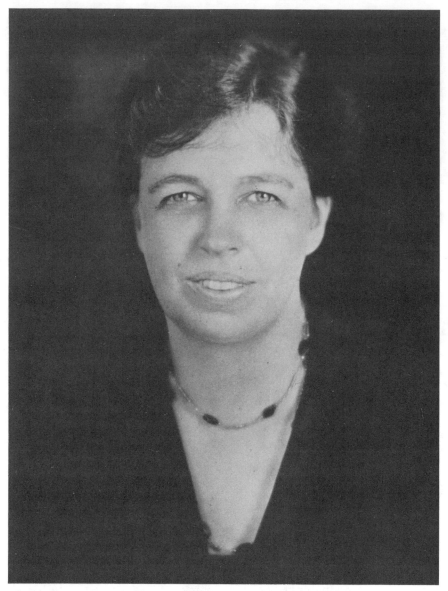

**Eleanor Roosevelt: A "romantic friendship" or a real romance?**

"Hick darling . . . Oh I want to put my arms around you . . . I want to hold you close. . . ."

# 12.

ALEISTER CROWLEY (né Edward Alexander Crowley), b. Leamington, Warwickshire, England, 1875. There can be no fence-straddling with Crowley. Either you consider him nuts, bonkers, loony, albeit brilliant, fascinating, and maybe even a bit of a con-man—or you're completely in his thrall, agreeing with the English Satanist that he is what he said he was: "He Who Is Above the Gods." Much depends, however, on how you feel about his central message. That is, once you strip away all the trappings of this extraordinary character—the magic rings, the incantations, the orotund language which is very much like W. C. Fields crossed with Mandrake the Magician—his motto is simplicity itself: Do whatever you wish. And that exactly is what Crowley did throughout his life, although having a pocketful of inherited money helped, not to mention a couple of pounds here and there from ardent disciples. Is it any wonder that this hashish-smoking, yoga-practicing, occult-preaching self-described religious prophet was immensely popular in our own 1960s and '70s? In his own time, he was called "The Beast" and "The Wickedest Man in the World." His shaved head, powerful glance, and magnetic personality enabled him, like Rasputin, to sleep with scores of female disciples, but his background was strongly pederastic. His writings reveal this side of his nature, especially *White Stains, The Scented Garden of Abdullah the Satirist of Shiraz,* and a

York City, 1884. The controversy over Eleanor Roosevelt's friendship with the journalist Lorena Hickok will probably be with us for the next century or until all parties with a vested interest in the outcome are long dead and gone. And that, perhaps, is as it should be. When Mrs. Roosevelt discovered that her husband was sleeping with her social secretary, she found solace where she could. That her family and official biographer explain her closeness to Lorena Hickok as "a romantic friendship right out of the 19th century" is hardly incorrect. She was of the period, and, as her son says, she grew up at a time when women spoke about their love for other women in florid language. But, as we know, the term "romantic friendship" by no means precludes a physical relationship. For the moment, all we know is that Eleanor Roosevelt found herself in need of a friend; that Lorena Hickok was, in fact, a lesbian; and that Eleanor Roosevelt wrote her friend some very moving, if provocative letters:

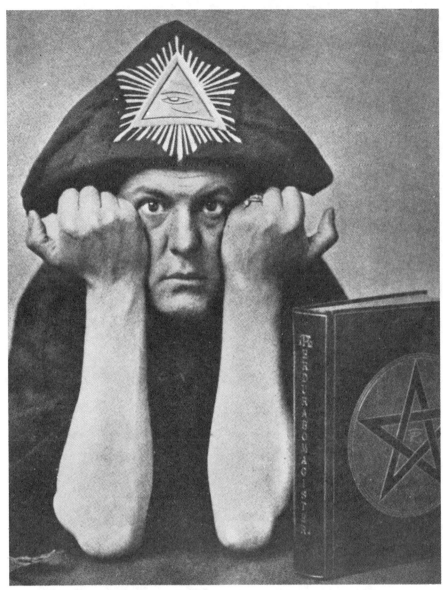

Aleister Crowley: Did he make the hat himself? Were there stores where they could be bought ready-made? If so, can I buy one?

poem that begins "I was bumming a boy in the black-out. . . ." Crowley changed his name from Edward Alexander to Aleister because of his belief that "to become famous it is necessary to bear a name with the metrical value of a dactyl followed by a spondee." He was known, even in old age, for his quick wit. Once, when a woman asked him which American woman's college would be most suitable for her daughter, he replied, "Radclyffe Hall."

# 13.

RICHARD HOWARD, b. Cleveland, Ohio, 1929. *The Advocate* has summarized this important poet's career: "Richard Howard has written seven books of poetry (the third, *Untitled Subjects,* secured him a Pulitzer Prize in 1970) and two books of criticism: *Alone with America* and *Preferences.* He has translated more than 150 books from the French; he is poetry editor [for several publications]; he teaches at three universities and has been president of P.E.N.—American Center. In 1980 Howard was given an Award of Merit from the American Academy of Arts and Letters and was made a Chevalier de l'Ordre National du Merite by the French government." He is also gay and up-front about it. Why outline his credentials here? For a simple reason. When someone comes to write a *Gay Book of Days* a century from now, it will be filled with hundreds of Richard Howards of the present—brilliant, hardworking, accomplished contributors to their fields, all of whom "happen to be gay."

# 14.

VERNON LEE (née Violet Paget), b. Boulogne-sur-Mer, France, 1856. Vernon Lee, as Violet Paget signed her many books on Italy (where she spent most of her life), was a Victorian down to the final snap on her corset, and that was her problem. She fell in love with three women in succession, fully expected to live out her life with each, and fell swooning to her bed each time the friendship ended. She was aristocratic, a snob, and the pleasure in reading her on Italian art and culture is very much like reading Edith Wharton's prescriptions for upper-class American taste. What happened to Lee's first love no one knows. To the end of her days she kept a faded picture of her over her bed. Her second love announced her marriage to (horrors!) a Jew, which required a double dose of smelling salts. Her third just drifted away. A three-time loser, she never tried again and lived in dejected loneliness for almost forty years. Dame Ethel

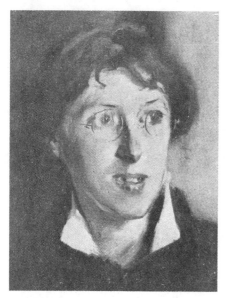

**Vernon Lee:** Imprisoned by Victorian propriety.

Smyth, who had been around, believed that Lee, alas, "was the chastest of beings and refused to face the fact or indulge in the most innocent demonstrations of affection, preferring to create a fiction that those friends were merely intellectual necessities."

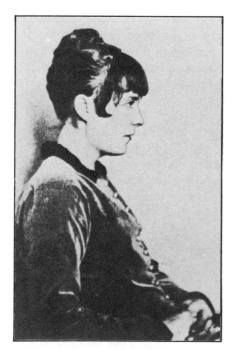

**Katherine Mansfield:** Her "slave" was a woman named Ida Baker.

**KATHERINE MANSFIELD, b. Wellington, New Zealand, 1888.** Time has been good to this exquisite writer who died of tuberculosis when she was only thirty-four. With each passing year, as the reputations of men who surrounded her begin to slip, she is seen as the major writer that she was. In many ways, she is the British Chekhov, and her quiet stories are frequently painful commentaries on the inadequacy of human relationships. Although she had many affairs with men and was married to John Middleton Murry, her diaries and letters reveal her to have been a lesbian, and a troubled one at that.

# 15.

**JOHN HERVEY, BARON HERVEY OF ICKWORTH, b. 1696.** History has given Lord Hervey a raw deal. Or rather, the undiminished fame of Alexander Pope has. In the 1730s erupted one of the most famous and venomous literary feuds in history. Pope, supposedly jealous that his friend Lady Mary Wortley Montagu had taken up with Hervey, began satirizing Hervey's effeminacy in his poetry, most notably as "Lord Fanny" in *Imitations of Horace* and as "Sporus" in the *Epistle to Dr. Arbuthnot.* If Pope's picture of the mincing Lord Fanny had not set London laughing, the reference to Sporus had literate London holding its sides, since Sporus was the boy "bride" of Nero who would bare his rear for the emperor to attack in public. (At the same time, Nero's "husband" was Doryphorus, who would return the favor in kind—also in public.) Hervey, understandably upset by these jibes, responded with verses of his own that ridiculed the crippled poet's hideous hump and his less than no-

ble birth. London found this hilarious, too. Eventually, the feud died down and was forgotten. Unfortunately for Hervey, however, he has remained Lord Fanny and Sporus for the past two centuries and probably forever. The trouble is that in school everyone reads Pope, and no one Hervey. (Incidentally, it has long been rumored that Alexander Pope himself had more to hide than his hump.)

# 16.

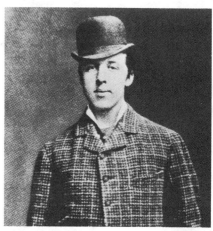

**Oscar Wilde:** "I have never admitted that I am more than twenty-nine, or thirty at the most. Twenty-nine when there are pink shades, thirty when there are not."

**OSCAR WILDE (Oscar Fingal O'Flahertie Wills Wilde), b. Dublin, Ireland, 1856.** There is no way to do justice to Oscar Wilde in this short space. Above all, one wants to avoid the controversy that will circle about his head till the end of time: Was he truly a martyr to a noble cause, or, in fact, a fool whose arrogance in initiating his famous trials caused not only his ruin, but untold misery for both his colleagues and the next three generations of British homosexuals. He was a great writer and an even greater wit, so let's leave the matter at that.

# 17.

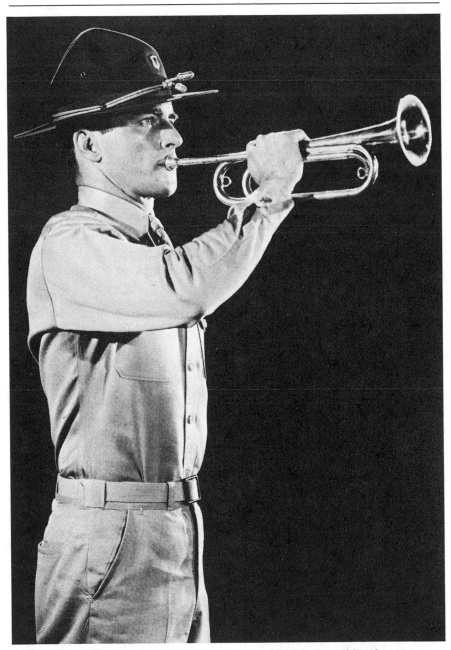

**Montgomery Clift:** That's odd. Tallulah Bankhead said he never blew *her*.

**MONTGOMERY CLIFT, b. Omaha, Nebraska, 1920.** It's often claimed that Clift, even earlier than Brando, introduced an intense naturalness to the screen, thus influencing an entire generation of postwar actors, Brando included. That Clift was an actor's actor, that he was much studied and even imitated, is undoubtedly true, although one approaches "firsts" in any area with a certain amount of caution. (Where do film theorists put John Garfield, for example? He was completely different from any other screen actor as early as 1938, and certainly as "natural," whatever that means anyway.) As two biographers have already shown, Clift gradually burned himself out and was dead at forty-five from long abuse of drugs and drink. To what extent his homosexuality, a secret carefully guarded from his ticket-buying female fans, was responsible for his brooding unhappiness is difficult to say, although the strain of having to live two lives must have been enormous. If Clift's Hollywood career came to an end, it was because he was growing older and because he was a troublesome drunk, not because he was homosexual. The question, of course, is whether he would have been a drunk had he not been gay. Probably, but who can say for certain?

# 18.

**JEAN JACQUES RÉGIS DE CAMBACÉRÉS, b. Montpellier, France, 1753.** Throughout the career of this revolutionist and legislator, his chief interest was in developing the principles of revolutionary jurisprudence. Although it is generally believed that he was solely responsible for legalizing in France homosexual relations between consenting adults in private, that is an oversimplification based on the irony that he himself was gay. He was of course one of the principal framers of the Code Napoléon. Cambacérès's homosexuality was well known, and he was commonly called "Tante Urlurette." The triumverate of Napoleon, Cambacérès, and Lebrun, in fact, was popularly known as *Hic, Haec,* and *Hoc,* Latin for "this one" in male, female, and neuter genders respectively. Cambacérès, the story goes, was once late for an appointment with Napoleon and offered the excuse of having "been with a woman" to the annoyed emperor. "Been with a *woman?*" Napoleon sniffed. "Next time tell her this: 'Take your hat and cane and leave me.' "

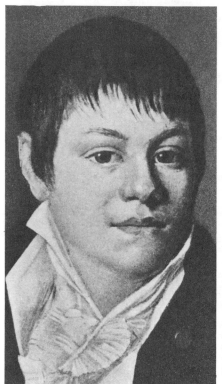

Heinrich von Kleist: Death was the only way out.

**HEINRICH VON KLEIST, b. Frankfurt-an-der-Oder, Germany, 1777.** This Romantic novelist-poet-playwright achieved in death what he could not accomplish in life: His works were finally taken seriously. None of his literary efforts had any real success during his short lifetime. Poverty-stricken and despondent, he killed himself and a friend, a Frau Vogel, in a joint suicide pact when he was thirty-four. Although he was older than the budding English poet, Kleist in death became the German Chatterton, revered by his contemporararies. His letters reveal him to have been homosexual, the letters to his friend Ernst von Pfuel particularly passionate in their out-

pouring of love: "You are my Greek god, dear youth. I want to sleep with you, embrace you. When you bathe in Lake Thun, I stare at your magnificent body with the longing of a girl." Kleist was of a distinguished Prussian military family. The way out was clear.

# 19.

**DIVINE (né Glenn _____?_____), b. Baltimore, Maryland, 1946.** Since it's a woman's prerogative to lie about her age, we don't care that the date is really much closer to 1938. For what different does it make? The star of *Pink Flamingos, Female Trouble,* and other films is The Most Beautiful Woman in the World, and when you're The Most Beautiful Woman in the World, what difference does anything make? Having come a long way from the days when Glenn's grandma, outraged at finding the boy in drag, chased him across their lawn while he was wearing only a slip and outsized hat, Divine now lives in a penthouse off Fifth Avenue with a longtime male friend. Divine claims that being a sex symbol has its advantages—like getting through security at airports. "They open my bags and see two tits staring up at them and they slam it closed. You could smuggle heroin in them."

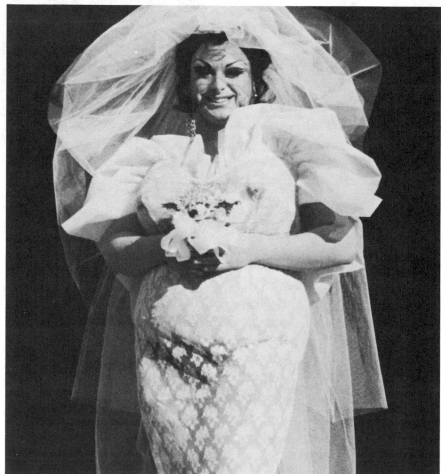

Divine: White for the blushing virgin bride.

And he's intelligent, too, and has a clear understanding of just why he is so popular: "When you think of a bombshell, you think of Monroe or Mansfield, you don't think of a three-hundred pound man. People like to be shocked." And if there's anyone on earth who can shock people, it's Divine—with a little help from his director, John Waters, of course. So let's all wash a couple of Once-A-Month Wormers down with a double scotch in honor of Divine, who, John Waters tells us, really *did* eat dog doo at the end of *Pink Flamingos.*

# 20.

**ARTHUR RIMBAUD, b. Charleville, France, 1854.** Like Emma Bovary, who was bored with middle-class respectability, Arthur Rimbaud was from Charleville. When he was seventeen, he came upon the twenty-seven-year-old Paul Verlaine and his pregnant wife. Spying Mme. Verlaine's swollen belly and sniffing the air of respectable poverty, he determined that he would lead Verlaine out of this bourgeois trap. That he succeeded all too admirably is a matter of history. So is the story of their wretched life together, blessedly brief. And, of course, the shooting, Verlaine's imprisonment, and Rimbaud's renunciation of his poetry. He was nineteen when he abandoned literature, but he did not give up men. Almost immediately after his disastrous affair with Verlaine, he fell in love with nineteen-year-old Lucien Letinois. Eventually he wandered around the world, finally becoming a trader in Abyssinia. He died at thirty-seven with the name of his faithful native boy Djani on his lips.

# 21.

**TED SHAWN, b. 1891.** As John Paul Hudson writes, "This world-renowned choreographer and dancer—though somewhat overshadowed by his wife Ruth St. Denis's towering talent—helped liberate our dance" from its classical past. "Developing part of the famous 'Denishawn Creed,' which held that the body ought to be freed from the bonds of tradition and allowed to respond to the natural rhythms of the breath and the pulse," Shawn helped to gain acceptance of male dancers in America, as Nijinsky and the Ballets Russes had done in Europe. To prove that the dance could be "masculine," Shawn formed an all-male troupe in the 1930s. Its serious intent notwithstanding, its appeal to novelty was little different from that of Evelyn and Her All Girl Orchestra during the same decade. Shawn is said to have been fond of sending friends nude pictures of himself and did so well into his seventies.

# 22.

**LORD ALFRED DOUGLAS, b. 1870.** That his life was ruined by the celebrated trials of Oscar Wilde is hardly debatable. Forever after he would be known as "Bosie" to the world, the boy lover of Oscar Wilde, the son of the 8th Marquis of Queensberry, who was so enraged by his son's cavorting with the notorious dandy that he couldn't even spell the word properly when he labeled Wilde a "Somdomite." Still, he was as thoroughly unpleasant as a grown man as he was when young. A snob, an anti-Semite, and a bit of a liar, too,

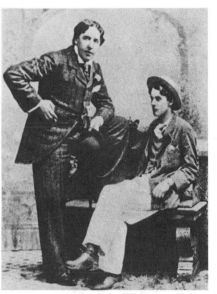

Oscar Wilde and Lord Alfred Douglas: The twerp on the right is "Bosie."

Douglas, who never had to worry about money as do lesser mortals, published tolerably good poetry, cranked out reminiscences that vilified almost everyone from the Wilde circle, eventually married, and declared to the world that he had long ago thrown off his childhood vices. That the latter was a lie may be seen in Sam Steward's indelible portrait of him in *Chapters from an Autobiography.*

**JOHN REED, b. Portland, Oregon, 1887.** Isn't it odd? In Warren Beatty's film biography of the co-founder of the American Communist Party, *The Exclusively Heterosexual Adventures of Warren and Diane,* there's no mention of John Reed's gay poems. Fancy that. But then, Mabel Dodge Luhan, who published them, did know him a little better.

# 23.

**NED ROREM, b. Richmond, Indiana, 1923.** When he was born into a humble Quaker household in

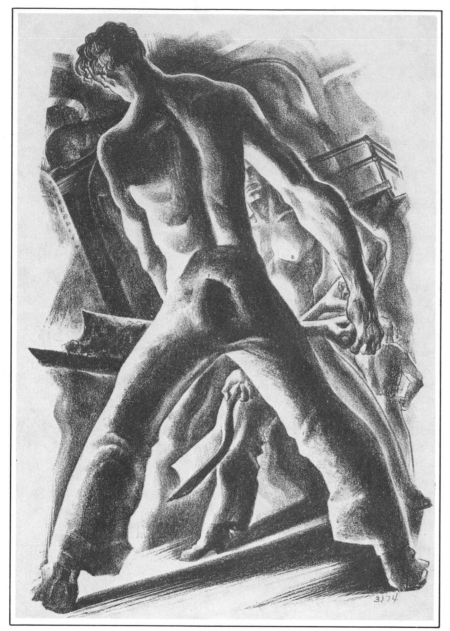

**John Reed:** As a stoker on a Scandinavian ship to Russia.

literally and figuratively on both sides of the Atlantic. *The Paris Diary,* which, in its highly literate style, was nonetheless a kiss-and-tell memoir of a devastatingly handsome homosexual making the rounds of the French cultural circles of the 1940s and '50s, was a smash success. And it didn't exactly hurt Rorem's popularity in the concert hall. Somewhere along the way from Indiana to Paris he must have come across Mae West's famous line: "Keep a diary and someday it'll keep you."

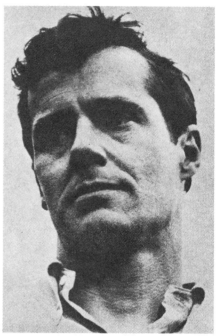

**Ned Rorem:** Four-times blessed.

# 24.

pancake-flat Indiana, Ned Rorem was four-times blessed. He is a prolific composer of rare talent, certainly the American heir to the great tradition of the French art song. He is a writer and critic of note, incisive and witty by turns. He is the closest thing to Apollo that the Hoosier State has yet produced (although it acquitted itself admirably in turning out James

Dean). He is a Scorpionian and, hence, has spent a fair share of his life in the sack, which, considering the time devoted to turning out his prolific compositions and essays, must have meant many, many twenty-hour days. Put these four gifts together and they spell Ned Rorem's *Paris Diary,* the first of his published diaries to scandalize the musical world and titillate laymen

**AUGUST VON PLATEN** (**August, Graf von Platen-Hallermünde**), **b. Ansbach, Germany, 1796.** There must be something in the air under the sign of Scorpio. Like Ned Rorem, the German poet and dramatist August von Platen wrote it all down. His detailed, explicit diaries, published in unexpurgated form at the turn of the century, long after his death, are remarkable for their homosexual revelations, documenting gay life in German universities of the early 19th century. His intense crushes, idealizations, and subsequent disenchantments are not at all dissimilar from those of, say, Emerson or Thoreau in the United States, and his lamentable habit of fixing his desires on the unattainable are typical of youthful homosexual experience in any age in any culture. The diaries are psychologically authentic, far more convincing than Platen's appended prologue in which, anticipating publication, he bewails the cruel Providence that made him different. "Why is it impossible for me to love women?" he cries. "Weep with me, that I should have suffered so unspeakably."

wore an Izod shirt, or carried a tennis racquet to the Hamptons.

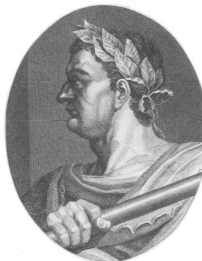

Domitian: He never wore an alligator on his toga.

and in earning the anachronistic title that some historians accord him, "the Voltaire of the Renaissance." A more important image, apt but oversimplified, is the belief that "Erasmus laid the egg and Luther hatched it." The "egg" of course is the Reformation, in which, Erasmus's ideas notwitstanding, he did not participate, choosing instead to work for reform within the Church itself. As to what else Erasmus might have laid, no one knows. He was a priest, after all, but in the 15th century that hardly meant obedience to the oath of chastity. All that is known is that he had no particular interest in women and that he wrote letters to other priests that may be read as homoerotic.

# 25.

DOMITIAN (Titus Flavius Domitianus), b. Rome, 51 A.D. Why all the fuss about the film *Making Love?* What was so special about the bland, perfect doctor leaving his bland, perfect wife for that bland, perfect writer, eventually to wind up in the arms of that bland, perfect lawyer? Domitian, emperor of Rome, left his wife for another man, and none of them were bland or perfect. Domitian, who was every bit as much of a tyrant as his father Titus was a pussycat, fell in love with the mime Paris and ditched his wife, Domitia, to be with his new lover. All Rome was shocked, but not quite so shocked as when the emperor remarried his discarded wife and ultimately dispatched Paris for cuckolding him via his cuckolded wife. Domitia, who had had quite enough, saw to it that her husband, who was not very popular anyway, was murdered by a freeman named Stephanus. And not one of them had his teeth capped,

# 26.

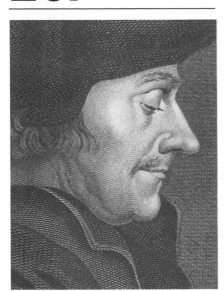

Desiderius Erasmus: One historian (with a straight face, no less) said that Erasmus laid an egg and Luther hatched it.

DESIDERIUS ERASMUS, b. Rotterdam, The Netherlands, c. 1466. The great Dutch humanist spent much of his life seeking reforms within the Roman Catholic Church, in editing classical texts,

# 27.

KATHERINE HARRIS BRADLEY, b. Birmingham, England, 1848. The other half of "Michael Field." *See January 12.*

# 28.

EVELYN WAUGH, b. London, 1903. After gallantly protecting T. S. Eliot from "the specious assumption that he was homosexual," T. S. Matthews in *Great Tom,* suddenly became viciously ungallant: "It is peppery, glaring little men like Evelyn Waugh who are sexually suspect—as his diaries bear witness." Aside from the psychologically interesting oppositon of "great" Tom and "little" Evelyn, it's perfectly clear that the former editor of *Time* magazine has no particular liking for either homosexuality or for Evelyn Waugh. The very word "suspect" is suspect. Many people disliked

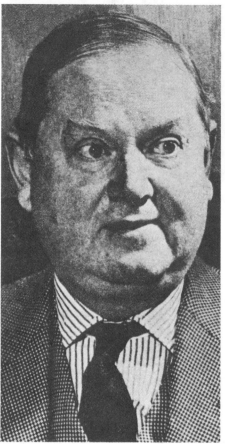

**Evelyn Waugh:** How much of Charles Ryder is based on young Evelyn Waugh?

Evelyn Waugh personally. He could be unkind, ungenerous, ornery. But he was one of the greatest English prose stylists of the 20th century, if not the greatest, and the idea of thinking of this giant as "little" is odd. Yes, his diaries do clearly reveal his homosexuality. But then, so do his novels, particularly the quasi-autobiographical *Brideshead Revisited*, in which the friendship of Charles and Sebastian, despite the limitations of what Waugh was permitted to write in the early 1940s, is magnificently drawn. It is obvious that as a young man Waugh passed through the same "extreme homosexual phase" that he describes in Charles. But, like Charles, he too married and passed on to another stage of his life. Doubters should realize that for centuries this was the upper-class English way. What's more, to a certain extent, it still is.

# 29.

**SIR WALTER RALEIGH, d. London, 1618.** Was Sir Walter Raleigh Marlowe's lover? Don't laugh. Anything is possible, especially when so little is known about both. For many years this provocative possibility has been suggested, even though it is based entirely on speculation. As everyone knows, Marlowe is supposed to have written "The Passionate Shepherd to His Love," which begins with the charming invitation, "Come live with me and be my love." A twin poem, "The Nymph's Reply," appeared shortly thereafter, and some advance the romantic notion that it was written by Raleigh out of love for Marlowe. The response, of course, is typically coy (Well, no, what do you think I am, but of course you know I mean yes when I say no, and you aren't really thinking of taking my virginity with that big thing, are you, you beast, but if you don't you know I'll die, etc.). It's probably the best of the many no-but-I-mean-yes poems in the language, at least until it was answered by Marvell in "To His Coy Mistress": Look, if you don't screw now, when are you going to do it? In the grave? So shut up and let's get it on. Good for Marvell!

# 30.

**PISISTRATUS, b. Athens, Greece, c. 605 B.C.** The first tyrant of Athens was Pisistratus, a temperate ruler who enforced the liberal laws of Solon and did much to improve the economic lot of the Athenian common man at the expense of the aristocrats. He also encouraged poets and artists, welcoming them to his court. During his reign many magnificent temples were built, and he may possibly have ordered that the first edited texts of the *Iliad* and the *Odyssey* be made from the oral tradition. His favorite boy was the youth Charmus, whom he guarded jealously. His son Hippias, who coveted the boy, kept his distance until his turn to squeeze the Charmus came upon his father's death.

# 31.

**NATALIE CLIFFORD BARNEY, b. Dayton, Ohio, 1876.** For over sixty years, Natalie Barney was the doyenne of Parisian lesbians. A good poet in her own right, and enormously wealthy, she was in many ways a female adventurer, a seducer ("Seductress," as in the title of one of her biographies, would probably have amused her) who knew whom she wanted and usually got her. We've already met her through the painter Romaine Brooks (*see May 1*) and the courtesan Liane de Pougy (*see August 11*). Perhaps this is the moment to tell the perhaps apocryphal story of the dissolution of her love affair with Dolly Wilde, Oscar Wilde's niece. At sixty, and very much resembling Benjamin Franklin, Natalie dispatched Dolly by buying her a one-way ticket to London and showing her out the door. Feeling guilty, she is said to have devoured an entire chocolate cake in one sitting in order to console herself. She was the very milk of human kindness.

**MARIE LAURENCIN, b. Paris, 1885.** Although she was described by her lover Apollinaire as a Cubist, Marie Laurencin belonged

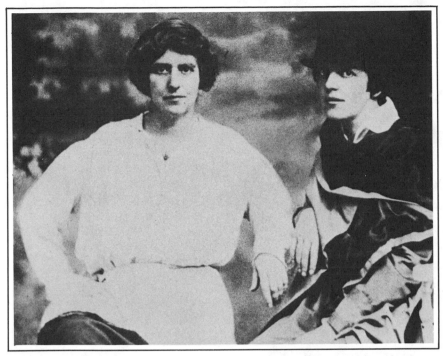

**Natalie Barney and Romaine Brooks:** "Indiscretion," Barney wrote, "has always seemed to me one of the privileges of tact."

to no school of painting. She painted portraits of some of the best-known people of her time (including W. Somerset Maugham and Jean Cocteau), created fashion designs for Paul Poiret, designed sets for both the Ballets Russes and the Comédie Française, illustrated books (her illustrations for the poetry of Sappho are particularly relevant here). She is, however, best known for her paintings of young girls. As she herself put it, "Why should I paint dead fish, onions, and beer glasses? Girls are so much prettier." After a succession of male lovers, she settled down with Suzanne Morand, at first her maid, whom she legally adopted so that the young woman could inherit her estate.

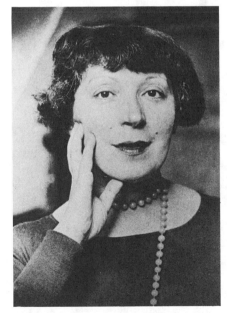

**Marie Laurencin:** Thank heaven for little girls.

## Other Personalities Born in October

1. **Paul I,** Russian czar, 1754

4. **C. A. Tripp,** American sociologist and writer, 1919

6. **John Gambril Nicholson,** English poet, 1866
   **Gerald Heard,** English writer, 1889

7. **John Horne Burns,** American novelist, 1916

8. **Edgar Saltus,** American novelist, 1855

9. **Jim Owles,** American activist, 1946

11. **Stark Young,** American writer and educator, 1881

12. **Henry More,** English philosopher, 1614

14. **Sumner Welles,** American statesman, 1892

15. **Virgil,** Roman poet, 70 B.C.

16. **Laud Humphreys,** American sociologist and writer, 1930

18. **Sarah Jennings Churchill, Duchess of Marlborough,** intimate of Queen Anne, 1660
    **Prince Eugene of Savoy,** Franco-Italian Austrian general, 1663

19. **Umberto Boccioni,** Italian painter and sculptor, 1882

20. **Robert Peters,** poet and literary scholar, 1924

26. **Donn Teal,** American writer and activist, 1932

28. **Anna Dickinson,** American feminist, 1842

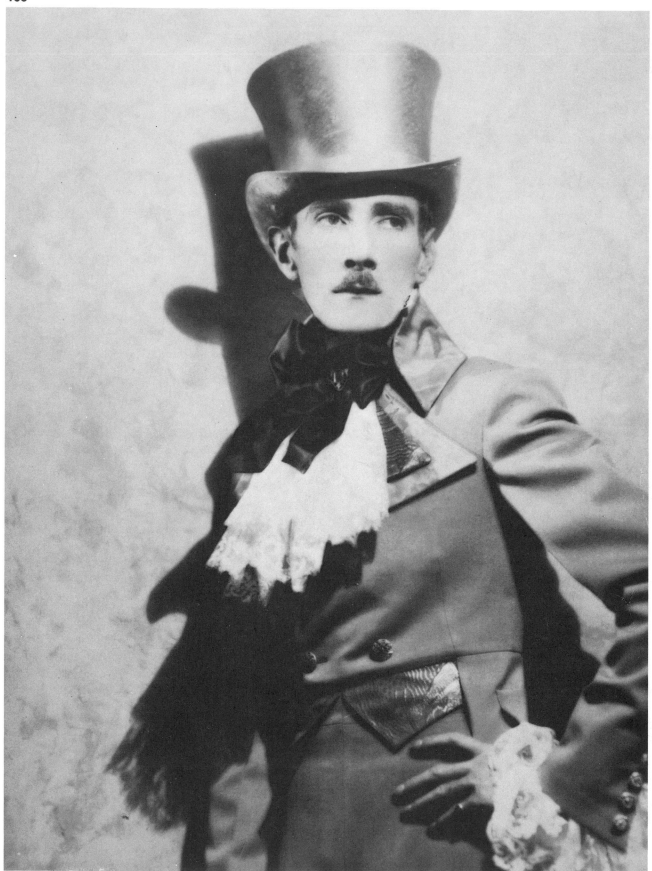

**Clifton Webb:** A battle to the finish with Tallulah Bankhead over the affections of a handsome Austrian army officer.

# NOVEMBER

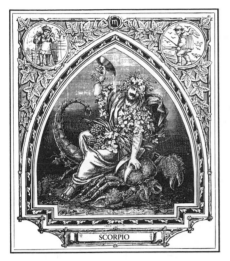

SCORPIO

Scorpio (October 23rd to November 21st), a fixed watery sign ruled by Mars and Pluto, has all the energy and forcefulness of Mars, combined with the emotional intensity associated with its watery nature. The Scorpionic type is extreme in his feelings towards others, sensitive to injury, quick to anger. He is ambitious and dislikes playing second fiddle. He can be vindictive and cruel. More than any other sign, Scorpio is associated with sexual energy. Writers as different as Manilius and Alberuni agree in attributing rulership of the genitals to Scorpio. A son of Scorpio essentially seeks power. At his best, therefore, he seeks absolute self-mastery first. The destruction of egotism is his chief goal. At his worst, he can be not merely wicked, but fiendish, and will seek mastery over others. The ideal Scorpionic type has a magnificent physique and phenomenal powers of endurance. The weak son of Scorpio will abuse his body with excesses of alcohol and drugs.

## 1.

**STEPHEN CRANE, b. Newark, New Jersey, 1871.** Had he lived beyond the mere twenty-eight years allowed him, Crane would undoubtedly have become the greatest American novelist of his day. As it is, he produced two fine books well in advance of his years, *Maggie: A Girl of the Streets* (1893) and *The Red Badge of Courage* (1895). Obsessed by urban street life, Crane left behind an unpublished novel, *Flowers of Asphalt,* a realistic portrayal of a gay male prostitute at the turn of the century. No one knows what became of the manuscript or who destroyed it. The reason why it disappeared, however, is much more certain. The trial of Oscar Wilde, only five years before Crane's death, drove the subject underground for more than a generation.

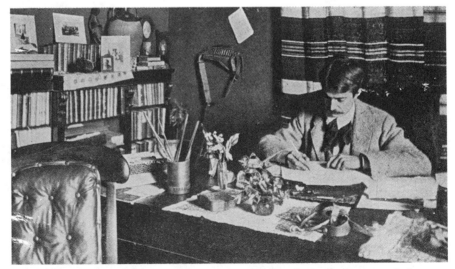

**Stephen Crane:** Hamlin Garland tried to dissuade him from writing a novel about a male prostitute, but he persisted.

## 2.

**VASSILY SAPELNIKOV, b. Odessa, Russia, 1868.** Sapelnikov, who became one of the foremost Russian pianists of his day, knew a good thing when he saw it. His teacher was the renowned composer Peter Ilyich Tchaikovsky, twenty-eight years his senior, who was known to enjoy performing duets with his students. Natural talent notwitstanding, young Sapelnikov made his way to the composer's bed and to instant patronage. Nothing new here. The music Mafia to this day is said to use the casting couch as frequently as Hollywood.

**CASEY DONOVAN (né Calvin Culver), b. New York State, 1943.** Like the Biograph Girl, Casey Donovan was probably the first male porno star to have his name above the title. Audiences were so taken with his winning personality, not to mention his other charms, that letters started pouring in to the theatres showing his films demanding to know the identity of the incredible blond with the amazing buns. And so, taking the name of one of the characters he played in a film, Calvin Culver, a stage actor and former teacher in a private school, became Casey Donovan. If Casey became a star, it was not merely because of his good looks and riveting personality. The persona he developed had a basis in common fantasy. He revolutionized skinflicks by making the merely prurient psychologically probable by suggesting that the boy next door had all the stuff that erotic dreams are made of. His screen persona radiates warmth and intelligence, attributes that are his off-screen. In real life, in fact, he is something of a Clark Kent, attractive but unprepossessing. But once his clothes are off, it's not Clark Kent; it's not the boy next door. My God, it's Superman!

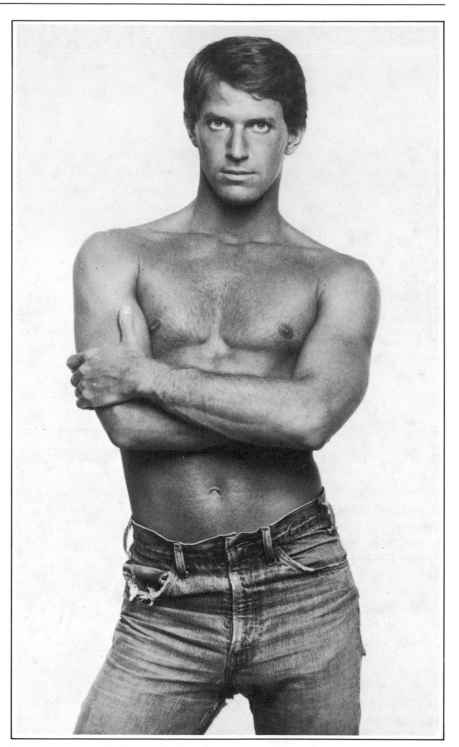

Casey Donovan: Oh, how I adore the boy next door . . . .

**TERENCE McNALLY, b. 1939.** In 1965 a play opened on Broadway that received what were probably the worst reviews in history. So outraged were most critics with a play called *And Things That Go Bump in the Night,* by a young playwright named Terence McNally, that almost to a man they spewed out a torrent of abuse and venom that was unprecedented. Many people reading the news-

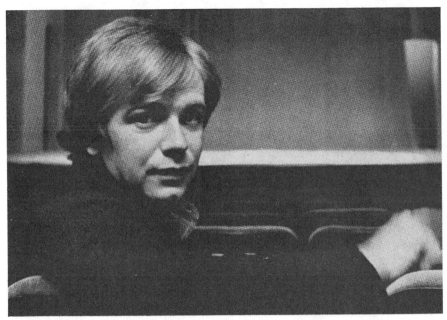

Terence McNally: An unfailing gift of wild comedy.

papers that day were able to read between the lines. If the play was that "bad," then it either had to be so bad that it was hilarious—or perhaps the critics, who can be pretty stupid when you come down to it, had actually missed the point. A good number of people resolved to see this "atrocious" play, a resolution easy to keep because the acting company vowed to keep it running at only $1.00 a ticket. The line for tickets stretched around the block for days, and, of course, the play *was* hilarious, but not because it was bad, but because it was authentically funny, outrageous, in bad taste, everything that made it fun and even meaningful. McNally went on to write many other plays, including *The Ritz*, which, when it was filmed, introduced millions of obviously startled movie goers to the world of gay baths, not to mention their comic possibilities.

# 4.

**J. R. ACKERLEY, b. Herne Hill, England, 1896.** By all accounts, Joe Ackerley was a "writer's writer" because, remarkably selfless, he devoted a good portion of his creative years to helping young writers working on their manuscripts, and assisting them to get published. His own published works are few in number, but each of them is perfect, a polished gem, including at least two minor masterpieces of English prose, the unforgettable *My Dog Tulip*, perhaps the most perceptive and moving book ever written about the mutual dependence of man and dog, and *My Father and Myself,* an autobiographical work that is almost indescribable because of the many layers of truth that it explores, from the inability of human beings ever to understand one another fully, no matter how closely related, to a profound understanding of the nature of one's own homosexuality. Ackerley's life was intertwined with that of his friend E. M. Forster, and a greater study in contrasts cannot be imagined. Joe Ackerley was a remarkably handsome, well-built man. Forster, of course, had been described by Virginia Woolf as "timid as a mouse." Despite his many years at the B.B.C. and as editor of *The Listener,* Ackerley made no bones about his homosexuality, his masculinity insulating him from gibes or insults. Any sniggering was immediately met with a string of epithets, ending with "bloody pack of arse-holes." Ackerley spent his life in quest of "the Perfect Friend," and, there being no such critter, never found him. He settled, however, for second best. Since one of his best friends was a local constable, he serviced two generations of the police force. Needless to say, it was he who introduced Forster to his future lover Bob Buckingham. It was also Ackerley who waged a long battle to convince Forster to "come out" publicly. "Look at Gide," Ackerley would say. "But Gide has no mother," Forster whined. Ackerley is a wonderful, wonderful writer. Read him.

# 5.

**JAMES ELROY FLECKER, b. Levisham, London, England, 1884.** Publicity helps. Flecker was the contemporary of Rupert Brooke. Both died young during World War I. Brooke, because of his jingoistic attitude toward war (useful to the government) and his good looks became an instant legend. Flecker, who lacked both utility and looks, did not. Brooke continues to be read. Flecker, who was the superior poet, is known to few readers. Flecker's *Collected Poems* (1916) were published the year after he died at thirty. His poetry shares one trait in common with Brooke's: the sexuality is ambiguous. There is no question, however, that Flecker was gay. His lover was the classicist J. D. Beazley, one of the world's great authorities on Greek vases.

# 6.

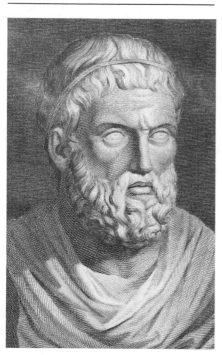

**Sophocles:** If Freud was so smart, how come Oedipus and Electra are not gay?

SOPHOCLES, b. Colonus, near Athens, Greece, c. 495 B.C. Sophocles, of course, has come down to us as the author of tragedies, two of which, *Oedipus Rex* and *Electra,* have been ill-used by Freud and his followers to beat up on mommies and daddies of gay men and women. No one seems ever to have questioned why, if Oedipus was so hung-up on his mother and hated his father, *he* didn't grow up to be a faggot. What's more, Electra, who hated her mother and loved her father, doesn't show the slightest sign of dykiness. Sophocles' greatness as a

dramatist notwithstanding, he is remembered as the comic butt of Euripides' ridicule because his clothing had been stolen by a male hustler when he wasn't looking. His own two favorite butts belonged to the boys Smicrines and Demophon.

# 7.

RUTH PITTER, b. Ilford, Essex, England, 1897. Since making a living from poetry is virtually impossible, most poets, unless they are independently wealthy or kept, work at whatever it is that will keep them alive while they devote their lives to the Muse. Ruth Pitter was a clerk in the War Office during World War I, after which she took up pottery painting, eventually becoming a partner in a furniture and gift store. Her many volumes of poetry—from *First Poems* (1920) to *Still by Choice* (1965)—contain some of the best lyrics in modern English. When the critics tell you that "her poetry is not profound," that really means that it is accessible, a serious flaw as we all know, since in our time "difficult" has come to mean "good" for some peculiar reason. If you like Edna St. Vincent Millay, you'll like Ruth Pitter. And for the same reasons.

# 8.

NERVA (Marcus Cocceius Nerva), b. Narnia, near Rome, c. 30 A.D. Nerva was the first of the so-called "Good Emperors" of Rome, but, like almost all the others, he slept with women and with boys. Contemporary gossip records that his most celebrated liaison was with his imperial predecessor, Domitian. It appears that Domitian, while a student, had the same problem that

most modern students have—a shortage of funds. So he did what a minority of young scholars continue to do today. He turned a few tricks, one of whom was the Roman senator Nerva, later the emperor.

# 9.

JAMES RENNELL RODD, b. 1858. Rodd is a not particularly important minor English poet and is included here not only out of desperation for someone of interest born today, but because he may possibly have had a disastrous love affair with Oscar Wilde. No one seems to know what exactly caused his bitter estrangement from the one and only Oscar, but in 1881 he sent Wilde a chilling prophecy—"At thy martyrdom the greedy and cruel crowd to which thou speakest will assemble; all will come to see thee on thy cross, and not one will have pity on thee!" Methinks, James Rennell Rodd, thou wast possibly a witch.

# 10.

VACHEL LINDSAY, b. Springfield, Illinois, 1879. The poetry of Vachel Lindsay is no longer fashionable, and that's too bad since it contains a rhythmic vitality that has all but gone out of contemporary poetry once it became so damnably cerebral. Lindsay is perhaps best known for his poetic apostrophe to the Salvation Army in "General William Booth Enters Heaven," although it is questionable whether he ever made it past the Pearly Gates himself since he not only liked the boys too much, but ended his days as a suicide, both offenses that would

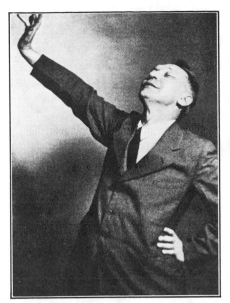

**Vachel Lindsay:** Boomlay, boomlay, boomlay, boom.

remove his verses from today's suburban libraries if the PTAs only knew. When he was in his forties, Lindsay lost his heart to the dazzlingly good-looking Australian composer and pianist Percy Grainger, as had the Norwegian composer Edvard Grieg before him. Lindsay killed himself in 1931, a year before Hart Crane leaped into the sea; his only biography was published during the Eisenhower years, a decade before homosexuality was officially invented. If it took biographers almost a century to acknowledge Whitman's gayness, Lindsay should be due for a serious biography around the year 2021.

**ERTÉ (né Romain de Tirtoff), b. St. Petersburg, Russia, 1892.** The flamboyant designer has become virtually synonymous with Art Deco, which is unfortunate since Erté's work represents an extreme of the style, but not the style itself. It's perhaps not incorrect to say that Erté creations make the most outrageous clothing designed by MGM's Adrian look like nuns' habits. Erté's name can safely be

added to that small list of gay male favorites—Judy Garland, Bette Davis, Angela Lansbury, Bette Midler—that either sends one swooning with rapture or jumping for cover behind the nearest sofa.

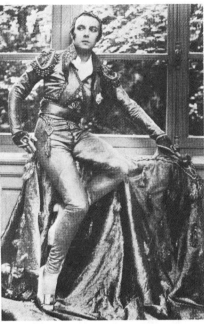

Erté: Brilliant flamboyance.

**RICHARD BURTON (né Richard Jenkins), b. Pontrhydfen, Wales, 1925.** One can only respect Burton for his candor. Given his burly masculinity and ham-hock fists, who would have dared blink an eyelash when he mentioned a bit of homosexual exploration in his youth to *People* magazine? 'Perhaps most actors are latent homosexuals and we cover it with drink. I was once a homosexual, but it didn't work."

# 11.

**DAVID IGNATIUS WALSH, b. Leoninster, Massachusetts, 1872.** Walsh was U.S. senator from Massachusetts when he became involved in a homosexual "scandal" in 1942. In *The Homosexual Matrix,* C. A. Tripp tells the sad

story of how the government raided what it called "a male brothel" (possibly a bathhouse?) near the Brooklyn Navy Yard. Arrested was the manager, Gustave Beekman, who was told that he could expect a lighter sentence if he cooperated with the government in naming clients, especially foreign agents who were suspected of blackmailing gay Navy men in an attempt to gain military secrets. Several foreign agents were in fact arrested. Also named as a regular patron of the "house on Pacific Street" was Senator Walsh, chairman of the Senate Naval Affairs Committee. Walsh, whose name was plastered across the tabloids for weeks, was cleared by his colleagues in the Senate after a favorable report from the F.B.I. Beekman, whose position was not exactly one of privilege, was tried on "sodomy" charges and was sentenced to twenty years in prison, every day of which was served.

# 12.

**ST. AUGUSTINE (Aurelius Augustinus), b. Tagaste in North Africa, 354.** Augustine, following the example of St. Paul, set the standard for the confessional literature that was to flourish in the centuries following. The pattern, of course, is a detailed listing of one's sins, followed by a narration of some event or events that made one yearn for salvation, and then an enunciation of the pains and joys of penance with the hope of future redemption. Augustine confessed not only to having fathered an illegitimate son, but to a friendship that was classically homoerotic. When he was a young man, his closest friend died and Augustine contemplated joining him in death. "I felt that his soul and mine were 'one soul in two bodies': and there-fore life was to me horrible, because I hated to live as half of a life; and therefore perhaps I feared to die, lest he should wholly die whom I loved so greatly. My long-ing eyes sought him everywhere."

Augustine, of course, cast off all sins of the flesh and went on to become one of the great founders of Christian doctrine, a doctrine that urged the rest of us sinners to follow his example.

ponents of Whitman's poetry in Bri-tain. He married a widow older than himself and eventually wrote several works jointly with his grown step-son. During the last four years of his life (he died at forty-four), he found the paradise he had yearned for in the South Seas. Is it merely coincidence that others who had yielded to the seductive islands and to the bodies of their natives were homosexual or bisexual—Gaugin, Stoddard, Maugham?

# 13.

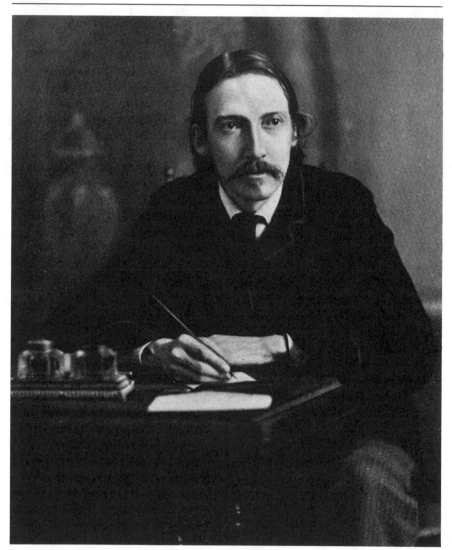

Robert Louis Stevenson: What would a modern biographer make of his life?

**ROBERT LOUIS STEVENSON, b. Edinburgh, Scotland, 1850.** There has always been an air of mystery associated with the roman-tic character of Robert Louis Stevenson. Did the author of *Dr.*

*Jekyll and Mr. Hyde* possess a dual nature himself? The question, though unanswerable, has been often raised. Was there, in fact, a homosexual side to Stevenson? He was one of the outstanding pro-

# 14.

**JOSEPH R. McCARTHY, b. near Appleton, Wisconsin, 1908.** Good Lord, no one wants to claim the Red-baiting senator from Wiscon-sin, especially when one thinks of the number of lives he destroyed, gay and straight. But there's no get-ting around the fact that Drew Pearson, who had a nose for news, recorded in his diaries the rumors that were circulating around Washington regarding McCarthy's alleged homosexual activities. C. A. Tripp in *The Homosexual Matrix* suggests that the senator was in fact gay. If this was so, then we are reminded of the sad truth that it sometimes takes one to hate one.

# 15.

**CHARLOTTE MEW, b. London, 1870.** This English poet committed suicide in 1928 after destroying almost all of her poetry. Two slim volumes remain, with a total of only fifty poems or so. It used to be believed by the credulous that Mew was a perfectionist who destroyed the poems that did not measure up to her exacting standards. But times

change, and it is now more or less accepted that Mew destroyed any evidence of her lesbianism in her works. Since what remains is very fine indeed, the destruction of the majority of her work can only be called a major loss to English letters.

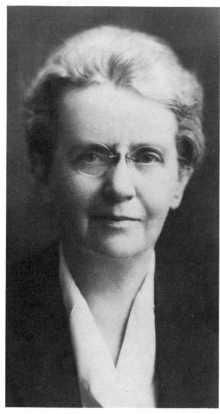

**Dr. S. Josephine Baker:** When it came time to capture Typhoid Mary, they said: "Let George do it."

**DR. S. JOSEPHINE BAKER, b. Poughkeepsie, New York, 1873.** Dr. Baker was the pioneering public-health physician known as "George" to her lover, I. A. R. Wylie. *(See March 16.)*

# 16.

**TIBERIUS (Tiberius Julius Caesar**

**Augustus), b. Rome, 42 B.C.** The emperor Tiberius was the predecessor of Caligula (*see August 31*), and he was certainly the appropriate curtain-raiser. His sexual excesses were widely known, especially when he "retired" to Capri, governing Rome via correspondence, and becoming the patron saint of that future gay mecca. Suetonius reproted that Tiberius trained young children, whom he called his "minnows,"to stay between his legs while he was swimming so that they could lick and nibble him until he came. Supposedly, he used unweaned infants for the same end on dry land. This may not have been known in New York and Hollywood night clubs of the early 1940s, but Tiberius may very well have originated the conga line. For ancient Rome's jet set he popularized the "daisy chain," or *spintriae*—a "conga line" of people joined front and back in sexual union. There is no mention in Suetonius as to whether this fad was accompanied by music with a Latin beat.

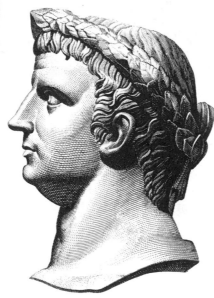

**Tiberius:** Inventor of the Roman conga line and other diversions.

# 17.

**LOUIS HUBERT GONZALVE LYAUTEY, b. Nancy, France, 1854.** Lyautey was one of the most successful imperialist rulers in history. It was he who governed Morocco for the French, developed its economy, extended its borders, and pacified native resistance. During World War I, even with diminished troops, Lyautey maintained an iron rule over the French protectorate. During his administration, inadvertently perhaps, Morocco became a place of refuge for homosexuals from all over Europe who came to sample the delights of the native population. Lyautey is one of the many real-life homosexuals who people Roger Peyrefitte's novel, *The Exile of Capri.*

# 18.

**CATHERINE TOZER COOMBES, b. Axbridge, Somersetshire, England, 1834.** One day in 1897, a little old man, penniless and disheveled, walked into an English police station and begged for admission to a county poorhouse. "I am a woman," the man said, thus opening the strange case of Kate Tozer. To escape a brutal husband, she said, she had dressed in male attire and lived as "Charlie Wilson," a house painter, for almost half a century, fearing all those years that her husband might find her if she were not so disguised. The novelist Charles Reade, fascinated by this story, investigated it on his own and discovered that it was only true in part. What had really occurred was this: Kate Tozer had indeed mar-

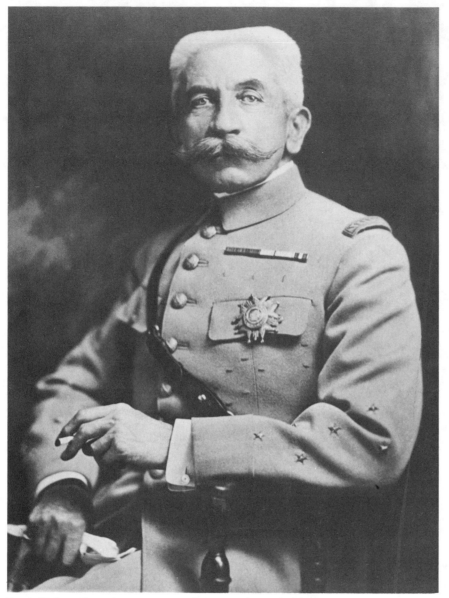

Louis Hubert Gonzalve Lyautey: Take me to the Casbah . . . .

## 19.

**CLIFTON WEBB, b. Indianapolis, Indiana, 1889.** Long before he became universally known as a movie actor in middle age, Clifton Webb was a Broadway star, dancing and singing his way through a string of musical comedies from childhood through the 1930s. By the time he first bared his viper's tongue in *Laura,* filmgoers had forgotten the silent films he had made in the 1920s. Webb's old-maidish ways, particularly in the Mr. Belvidere series, and his snobbish priggishness in such films as *The Razor's Edge,* proved a goldmine for 20th Century-Fox and kept him gainfully employed for many years. In real life, the actor was supposedly very much like the characters he played. He lived together with his mother, Maybelle, who was the scourge of Hollywood since wherever Clifton went, mamma went too. In her nineties, Maybelle was still Clifton's best girl and was very likely to stop a Hollywood party by doing her famous can-can for the umpteenth time. Humphrey Bogart once invited Webb to a party and added, "Bring your fucking mother and she can wipe up her own vomit this time." Mamma Maybelle finally kicked off, and sonny was inconsolable, weeping buckets and taking to his bed for months. As Noel Coward put it, "It must be tough to be orphaned at seventy-one." In his rare excursions away from Maybelle, Webb, especially in his youth, was irrepressible. Once both he and Tallulah Bankhead were smitten with the same handsome Austrian army officer and vied for the uniformed stud. While Tallulah did her stuff vamping him, Webb retreated for a moment, and returned with an armload of roses.

ried Tom Coombes, but he had not mistreated her. Having inherited ten pounds from an aunt, she appeared dressed as a man before her husband one day and announced, "I am no longer Kate. My name is Fred." They continued to live together as Tom and Fred, both working as house painters. Then one day "Fred" fell in love with a Nelly Smith and they eloped, together with Tom. When the police, spurred on by Nelly's parents, broke down the Coombeses' door, they found Tom smoking his pipe and reading a newspaper while "Fred" and Nelly went at it on the sofa. It's only after "Fred" got out of jail that she became "Charlie Wilson" and eventually settled down and found herself a nice bride named Anne Ridgway, about whom, alas, he tells us nothing. One would like to hear *her* story.

To Tallulah's amusement and the officer's shock, Webb danced around the man and began pelting him with flowers. Tallulah walked off with the prize.

# 20.

**DANIEL GREGORY MASON, b. Brookline, Massachusetts, 1873.** The American composer, author, lecturer, and teacher was the lover of composer-pianist John Powell. (*See September 6.*)

# 21.

**VOLTAIRE (assumed name of François Marie Arouet), b. Paris, 1694.** Voltaire blew hot and cold on the subject of homosexuality. Although he is known to have sampled the delights of same-sex sex on one occasion, he nonetheless admonished a friend who wanted to try it a second time: "Once, a philosopher," he proclaimed, "twice a sodomite!" Voltaire was locked in a love-hate relationship with Frederick the Great, with whom he spent agonizing, ecstatic years. In her biography of Frederick, Nancy Mitford writes that "nobody who studies the life of Voltaire can doubt that he had homosexual tendencies, and one wonders whether his feelings for the king were not exacerbated by unrequited passion." Whatever his personal reservations about homosexuality, the famous French writer was forthright in declaring that sodomy, "when not accompanied by violence, should not fall under the sway of criminal law, for it does not violate the rights of any man." We will probably never

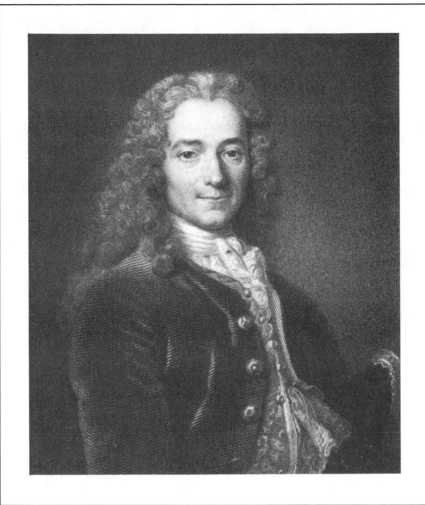

**Voltaire:** What did he mean by "I kiss your rod"?

know why Voltaire once signed a letter to a male friend, *"E vi baccio il catzo,"* which politely translated means, "I kiss your rod."

# 22.

**ANDRÉ GIDE, b. Paris, 1869.** Nobel Prize for Literature or no, Gide, like any other human being, was at his absolute worst in an argument, and the almost lifelong feud between him and Jean Cocteau was a low-point in both their careers, not unlike the spectacle of Gore Vidal and Truman Capote going at each other like Paulette Goddard and Rosalind Russell in *The Women.* Yes, a couple of bitchy one-liners emerge from the fracas, but the image of two men in a hair-pulling melee still remains. The Cocteau-Gide feud, which lasted for more than forty years, all the while aired in public, stemmed from simple jealousy. Gide was enraged that Cocteau had kept his young lover Marc Allégret out all night and had, presumably, slept

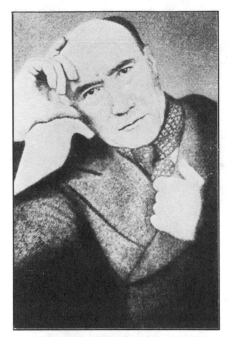

**André Gide:** Muhammed be praised . . . and praised . . . and praised. . . .

have an orgasm after a night of fucking? I'll bet he couldn't even produce an erection!" But, dear Wystan, what's sauce for the gander is not necessarily sauce for the goose.

### BENJAMIN BRITTEN, b. Lowestoft, Suffolk, England, 1913.

The composer's musical output was enormous, and it is much too soon after his death to know what will continue to be performed and what will not. For the moment, Britten is definitely an acquired taste, and the empty seats at the Met, as opposed to the standing room only at Co-vent Garden, would indicate that operas like *Peter Grimes* do not always travel well, that perhaps the musical establishment is pushing a bit too hard, as if the British sun will set if "the greatest English com-poser since Purcell" is not im-mediately embraced by the world. One imagines, too, for the sake of the living, that it may be some time

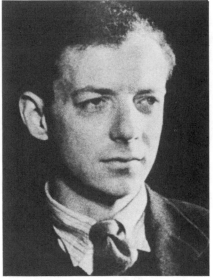

**Benjamin Britten:** His most beautiful music was composed for Peter Pears.

before a straightforward biography is published.

### BILLIE JEAN KING, b. Long Beach, California, 1943.

When Billie Jean King defeated Bobby Rigg in the sexist battle of the cen-

with him. Gide confessed years later that he wanted to kill his rival, but decided that blood drawn from words would kill more painfully than a single bullet. There is nothing to equal one writer putting another down, and Gide was a master of the art. Not that he wasn't on the receiving end at times. His famous story in *Si le grain ne meurt* about how his doubts about the gay life vanished when he came five times in a single night with Muhammed, a boy pro-cured by Oscar Wilde ("that perfect little body, so wild, so ardent, so somberly lascivious"), was seriously doubted by W. H. Auden. Auden, who thought "that dreary im-moralist" a liar, challenged the French writer's veracity in public. According to Auden's biographer, Charles Osborne, Auden could not believe that Gide could have had sex with the boy all night and "have then taken him out to the sand dunes and continued until after sunrise. 'He's a conceited liar,' Auden declared. 'How could he

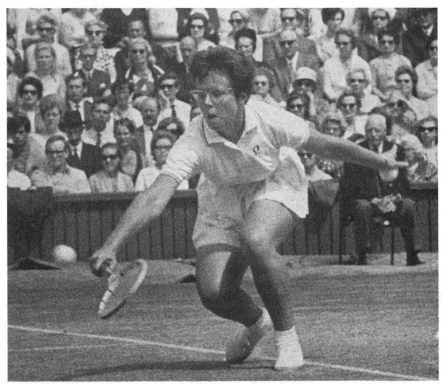

**Billie Jean King:** In tennis, love equals zero.

tury, the present writer was on a Boeing 747 en route to Houston, Texas, not exactly the most liberal world capital. When the news was announced to the passengers, a spontaneous cheer went up that lifted the plane at least another 1,000 feet. Several years later, when the story of King's problems with her former secretary-lover hit the tabloids, there wasn't a cheer to be sure, but neither did the world come to an end, as it might very well have done a dozen years before. Whatever the circumstances involved, Billie Jean King has remained a public figure, her bisexuality notwitstanding. She has not gone into hiding, she has not gone into exile. Most of her fans have not deserted her. Is the world growing up just a bit?

# 23.

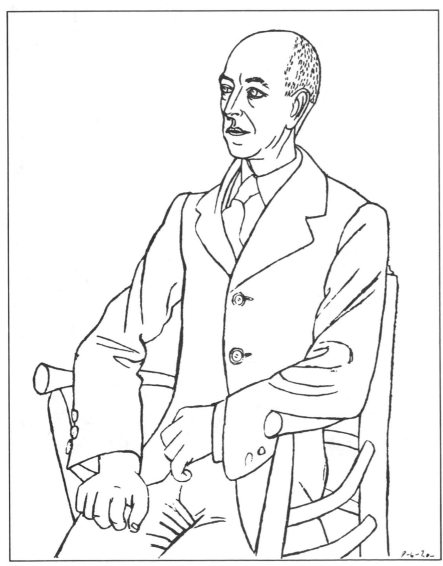

**Manuel de Falla:** How shy is shy?

**MANUEL DE FALLA, b. Cadiz, Spain, 1876.** The Spanish composer, whom Pablo Picasso considered the shyest man he had ever met, "even smaller than myself, and as modest and withdrawn as an oyster shell," was rumored to have been involved in a homosexual *ménage à trois* with composer Maurice Ravel and pianist Ricardo Viñes. De Falla became close friends with Diaghilev and Massine, with whom he collaborated on *The Three-Cornered Hat.* It was, incidentally, immediately after the first performance of this ballet that Massine announced his engagement to Lydia Sokolova, who had just performed the leading role, and was then dismissed from the Ballets Russes by the enraged Diaghilev.

# 24.

**BARUCH SPINOZA, b. Amsterdam, The Netherlands, 1632.** The great philosopher Spinoza, raised and educated in the Orthodox Jewish fashion, also studied Latin and was thoroughly familiar with European humanism. What exactly is it that caused him to be excommunicated from the synagogue when he was only twenty-four? Many writers have speculated that the horror Spinoza inspired in the Jewish community may have come not only from his espousal of advanced economic theories but also perhaps from his espousal of Greek love among impressionable students in the liberal circle where he taught. A Dutch physician, J. Roderpoort, wrote at The Hague in 1897: "Spinoza excites the youth to respect women not at all and to give themselves to debauchery." Was Spinoza merely teaching the Greek and Roman classics, with their inevitable passages on pederasty? What were Roderpoort's motives for discrediting the Jewish philospher? Was Spinoza in fact a pederast? It's all open to speculation.

# 25.

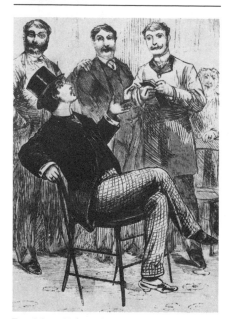

**Dr. Mary Edwards Walker:** Puttin' on the Ritz.

**DR. MARY EDWARDS WALKER, b. Oswego, New York, 1832.** Although she was called by her male enemies "the most distinguished sexual invert in the United States," Dr. Edwards, although certainly a transvestite, was not necessarily a lesbian. She was an ardent feminist, obsessed by the feminist dress-reform movement begun by Amelia Bloomer, and a mover and shaker in stirring up trouble whenever refused the right to do anything a man was permitted to do. A qualified physician, she had to force her service on an unwilling federal government during the Civil War; she eventually won a Congressional Medal of Honor for her was work; and she became the first woman in the United States permitted to dress in male attire—a right granted by Congress, no less. That she lived together with a younger feminist, Belva Lockwood, after she divorced her husband is provocative, but hardly proof that either of the two women were lesbians. Eventually, the militant Dr. Walker moved out of step with her sister feminists because her taste in dress offended them. It was one thing to wear the trousers of men—that was at least practical—but it was quite another to go whole hog as did Mary Walker. She affected shirt, bow tie, jacket, top hat, and cane. A very full discussion of this fascinating woman appears in Jonathan Katz's *Gay American History.*

# 26.

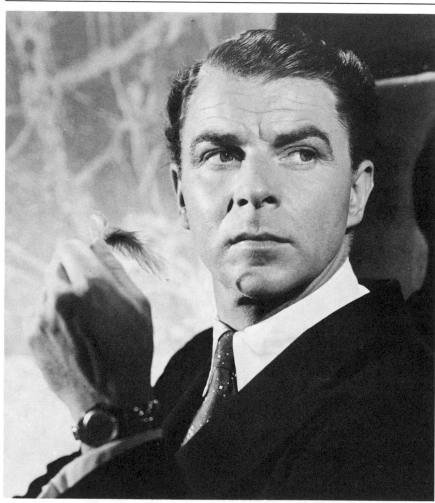

**Emlyn Williams:** A wonderful writer, a fine actor, an honest man.

**EMLYN WILLIAMS, b. Rhewl Fawr, Wales, 1905.** Although he was already known as a playwright and stage actor, Emlyn Williams became famous in 1935 for playing the baby-faced psychopathic murderer Dan in his own *Night Must Fall.* He became an international celebrity three years later when his autobiographical play *The Corn Is Green* was first performed. It has been said many times that

Williams's plays are eminently theatrical and readable, even though they are somewhat shallow, sentimental, and dependent on melodramatic effects. But these shortcomings are obviated by Williams's charm, intelligence, and moral integrity—qualities he has demonstrated also as a director and as an actor, on both stage and screen. These virtues are also apparent in Williams's two-volume autobiography, *George* (his original first name) and *Emlyn* (the middle-name he adopted for the stage). In *Emlyn*, Williams recounts the story of his love affair with an actor on the skids. It is beautifully told and, considering that Williams was a married man with several children when he wrote it, it is boldly courageous in its honesty. He also describes gay life in New York in the 1920s, including a rather hilarious scene at the Everard Baths regarding someone's false teeth coming loose in an act of fellatio. When's the last time you read a book by a living married celebrity that recounted a night at the tubs? Read Williams's autobiography. He's an honest man whose recollections can be trusted as authentic.

# 27.

**EDMUND JOHN, b. London, 1883.** Poet John came of age in the decade after the trials of Oscar Wilde and illustrates the fact that far from disappearing off the face of the globe, homosexuality simply retreated a bit further underground. A letter to one of John's young friends provides us with a very good idea of the "tone" of gay life among the pederasts of Edwardian England: "I have received your adorable illustrated letter this morning and loved it so much that I

immediately made an altar before it, lit by amber candles in copper candle-sticks, burnt incense before it, and kissed its extreme beautiful-ness."

# 28.

**RITA MAE BROWN, b. Hanover, Pennsylvania, 1944.** The woman is funny, she's deadly serious, and you'd better damn well listen to her. She's just like Molly Bolt, the heroine of her semi-autobiographical *Rubyfruit Jungle* who locks her adoptive mother in the root cellar. She's a born fighter and doesn't take any nonsense from anyone. She'd be awfully hard to take if it weren't for the fact that she's right in what she says almost all the time. And she says exactly what most people don't want to hear. Like, for example, "I don't think there is a 'gay lifestyle.' I think that's superficial crap, all that talk about gay culture. A couple of restaurants on Castro Street and a couple of magazines do not constitute culture. Michelangelo is culture. Virginia Woolf is culture. So let's don't confuse our terms. Wearing earrings is not culture, that's a fad and it passes. I think we've blown superficial characteristics out of proportion and tried to make ourselves more important than we really are . . . ." Right on, Rita Mae! Give 'em hell! No man would have the balls.

# 29.

**ROD LA ROCQUE (né Roderick la Rocque de la Tour), b. 1898.** We've already seen that Richard

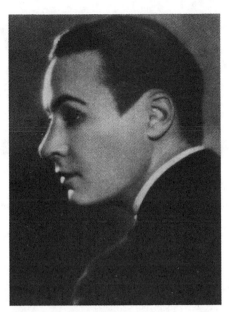

**Rod La Rocque:** Six-foot-three heart-throb of the silver screen.

Halliburton spent at least one night together with this 6'3" leading man *(see January 9),* which gives a gently ironic meaning to two of La Rocque's films, *Let Us Be Gay* (1929) and *One Romantic Night* (1930), not to mention *The Gay Bandit* and *The Coming of Amos.* And yes, Roderick la Rocque de la Tour was his real name.

# 30.

**SIR PHILIP SIDNEY, b. Penshurst, Kent, England, 1554.** The English poet and courtier was one of the leading lights of Queen Elizabeth's court and a model of Renaissance chivalry. His *Astrophel and Stella* is one of the great sonnet sequences in English and was inspired by his love for Penelope Devereaux, even though he later married Frances Walsingham. (Lest one confuse Renaissance "love" and "marriage" with the modern versions, it should be pointed out that Penelope Devereaux was twelve years old

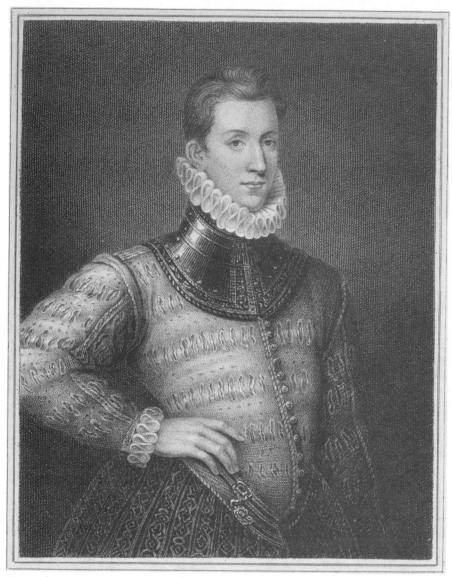

**Sir Philip Sidney:** Romantic verses to his male friends.

that he had had affairs with other men in his youth. " 'Not true!' Churchill replied. 'But I once went to bed with a man to see what it was like.' " The man turned out to be musical-comedy star Ivor Novello. " 'And what was it like?' " Maugham asked. " 'Musical' " Churchill replied.

## Other Personalities Born in November

1. **Benvenuto Cellini,** Italian sculptor, 1500
   **Antonio Canova,** Italian sculptor, 1757
   **Terence Winch,** American poet and musician, 1945

2. **Marie Antoinette,** Queen of France, 1755
   **Prince Georgi Eugenievich Lvov,** Russian nobleman who was Nijinski's first lover, 1861
   **Luchino Visconti,** Italian film-maker, 1906

3. **Vincenzo Bellini,** Italian composer, 1801

4. **Auguste Rodin,** French sculptor, 1840
   **Napier G. H. S. Alington,** 3rd Baron Alington, Tallulah Bankhead's English bisexual lover, 1896

8. **René Viviani,** French statesman, 1863
   **James Schuyler,** American poet, 1923

10. **Charles the Bold,** Duke of Burgundy, 1433
    **Wallace Rice,** American poet, 1859
    **Jennette Lee,** American writer, 1860
    **James Broughton,** American poet and filmmaker, 1879

when Sidney fell in love with her, and that Frances Walsingham was fourteen when she was married to the twenty-nine-year-old courtier. Marriages were arranged then and not made in heaven.) Sidney was in his teens when the Huguenot writer and diplomat Hubert Languet fell in love with him. Languet was thirty-six years his senior, lived with him for a time, and, when they parted, wrote passionate letters to him weekly. In his youth Sidney was strongly attached to two young men, Fulke Greville and Edward Dyer, and wrote love verses to them both, a point not lost on gay John Addington Symonds when he wrote Sir Philip's biography. Sidney died in battle at the age of thirty-two.

**WINSTON CHURCHILL, b. Blenheim, England, 1874.** In his wonderfully entertaining and informative biography of W. Somerset Maugham, Ted Morgan tells how Maugham once asked Churchill whether it was true, as the statesman's mother had claimed,

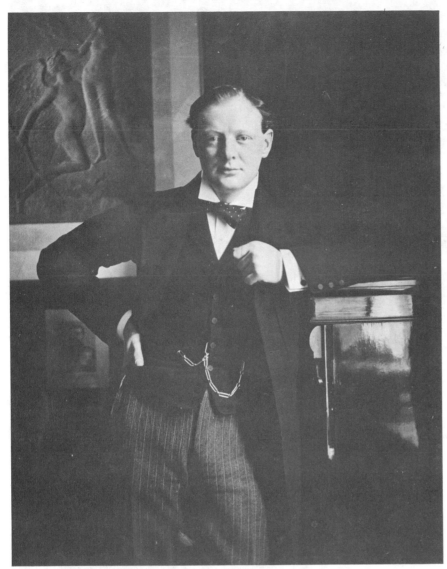

**Winston Churchill:** His mother claimed that he had affairs with men.

historian and colonial administrator, 1881
**Nathan Leopold,** (with Richard Loeb( American thrill murderer, later anthropologist, 1901

20. **Ludwig Andreas Khevenhuller,** Austrian general, 1683
**Edward Westermarck,** Finnish anthropologist, 1862
**James Pope-Hennessy,** English editor and author, 1906

21. **Harold Nicolson,** English diplomat and writer, 1886

25. **Ronald Johnson,** American poet, 1935

26. **Alma Routsong (a.k.a. Isabel Miller),** American writer, 1924
**Richard Hall,** American novelist, playwright, and critic, 1926
**Kenneth Marlowe,** American celebrity hairdresser and writer, 1926
**Arnie Kantrowitz,** American writer, 1940

27. **Fanny Kemble,** English actress, 1809

28. **Jean Baptiste Lully,** Italian-born French composer, 1632
**William Blake,** English poet and artist, 1757
**Ernst Roehm,** murdered head of Nazi S.S., 1887

13. **Ranjit Singh,** Sikh maharajah, 1780
**Kirby Congdon,** American poet, 1924

14. **William III,** King of England, 1650
**Robert S. Hichens,** English novelist, 1864
**Arthur Bell,** American writer, 1940

16. **Aleksandr Danilovich Mensh-** ikov, Russian general and statesman, 1672

17. **Il Bronzino (né Agnolo di Cosimo di Mariano),** Italian painter, 1503

19. **Pier Luigi Farnese,** Duke of Parma, 1503
**Mary Hallock Foote,** American novelist and illustrator, 1847
**Sir Ronald Storrs,** English

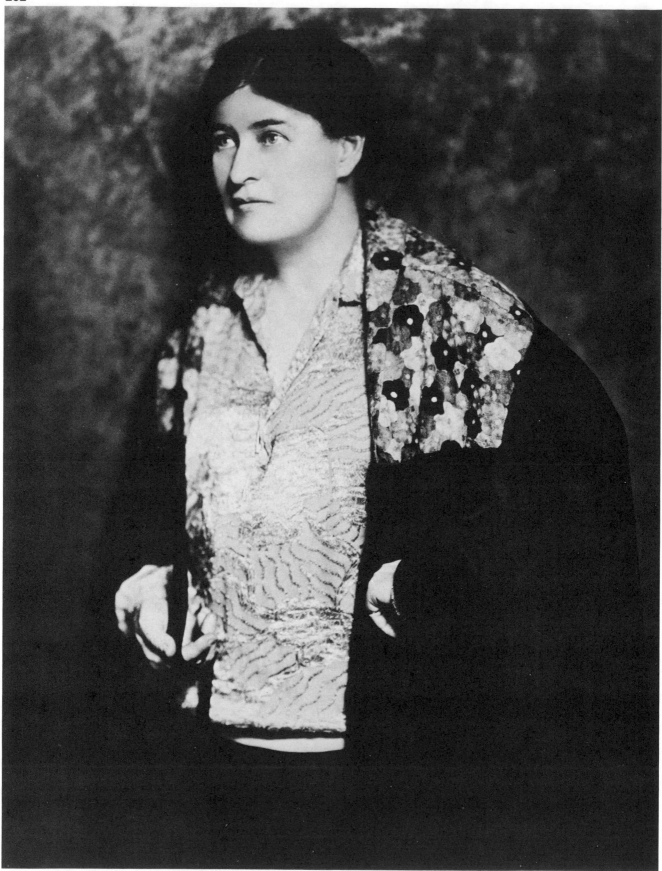

**Willa Cather:** She took every possible step to hide her "dangerous idiosyncrasy" from the world.

# DECEMBER

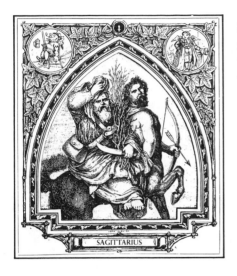

**Sagittarius** (November 22nd to December 20th) is a mutable fiery sign ruled by Jupiter. The sign has the Jupitarian qualities of strong intellect tending to express itself in more profound, philosophical ways than in the case of Gemini. Sagittarians are noted for their love of sport and outdoor life. They are restless, generous, adventurous, exuberant, and fond of travel. The fault of the sign is a tendency to become very loud and vulgarly jovial. The Sagittarian brings his reason to bear upon every phenomenon that comes under his observation. His curiosity is insatiable and his mental energy never flags. At his worst, however, he is so cerebral that his emotions are not particularly well-developed. There is, in fact, a curiously child-like transparency about Sagittarians—probably because of the absence of complex emotions such as jealousy or vindictiveness—which makes them very easy to understand.

## 1.

**REX STOUT, b. Noblesville, Indiana, 1886.** It's a mistake, of course, to assume that there's any direct relationship between the subject matter of a novelist and the novelist himself, especially since imagination is the fundamental resource of the writer. Before he turned to the detective novel in 1934, Rex Stout wrote an ambiguously gay Western in which the married hero is attracted to his assistant. The notion, though psychologically plausible, is certainly unique to the Western adventure yarn of the period and suggests an equally unusual relationship between two men that was to prove central to Stout's work over the next four decades. What exactly is the nature of the friendship, if it can be called that, between Nero

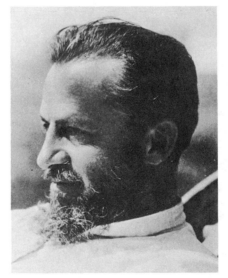

Rex Stout: Was Archie Goodwin a chubby chaser?

Wolfe, Stout's famous detective hero, and his live-in assistant Archie Goodwin? Wolfe, of course, is the most eccentric of all detectives, an elephantine genius who is both a woman-hater and almost completely dependent on his assistant who is junior sleuth, secretary, errand boy, bodyguard, bookkeeper, and chauffeur. A third member of this *mélange* housed in a brownstone on New York's West 35th Street is Fritz Brenner, the chef who prepares the gourmet meals that Wolfe prefers to women and which keep his weight at a seventh of a ton. William S. Baring-Gould's full-length biography of this fictional character, *Nero Wolfe of West Thirty-fifth Street,* doesn't touch on the fat one's sex life. But if Batman and Robin are "suspect," then what's so sacred about Nero and Archie?

## 2.

**CATULLUS (Gaius Valerius Catullus), b. Verona, Italy, c. 84 B.C.** Catullus, whose love poetry was never surpassed in ancient times, influenced a great many poets both ancient and modern. Tibullus, Propertius, Horace, and Ovid imitated his techniques, and, during the English Renaissance, English poets such as Ben Jonson and Robert Herrick attempted to capture the quality of Catullus (unsuccessfully) in English. Most of Catullus's poems are short; in a few concise lines he is able to create an experience of love, friendship, or sometimes bitterness and anger either at his mistress (whom he calls "Lesbia") or at some person he despised. Although most of his poems are about heterosexual love, a good number of them are devoted to the love of boys. These are particularly lusty, some of them very funny, and all of them explicitly sexual. (Since many editions of Catullus prudishly omit these poems, and since almost all translations are severely bowdlerized, only one edition in translation is recommended, that by Peter Whigham.) In one poem, the poet comes upon a young boy "stuffing his girl." With a wink to Venus, he "stuffs" the boy as "poetic justice." Since Catullus was a contemporary of Caesar, his pederastic poetry is characterized by the basic prejudice of the period: "taking" a boy is a manly act, but allowing another male to do unto you what you did unto him is sheer depravity.

# 3.

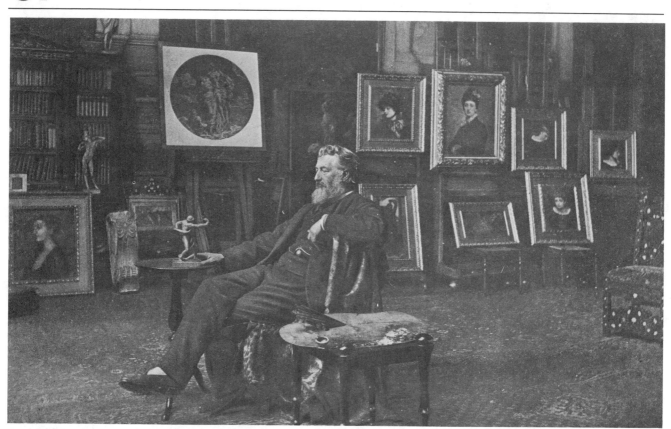

**Baron Frederick Leighton:** Propriety in art, propriety in conduct. He played by the rules.

**BARON FREDERICK LEIGHTON, b. Scarborough, Yorkshire, England, 1830.**
Leighton's painting, long in disfavor but coming back in style as more and more people learn to appreciate the Victorian Renaissance Revival, was enormously popular in his lifetime. Since Leighton's sympathies were with the Italian Renaissance tradition, his paintings—with their often mythological subjects, monumental compositions, and figures clad in classical drapery—are among the last examples of the grand traditional manner in European art. Leighton's paintings appealed to a large and influential segment of the Victorian public which craved an art of "high seriousness." Because he played by the established rules of the game, Leighton, whose homosexuality was widely known, pursued his

career and his pleasure with discretion. He died at sixty-five, the day after being made a baron, the first English painter to be so honored.

# 4.

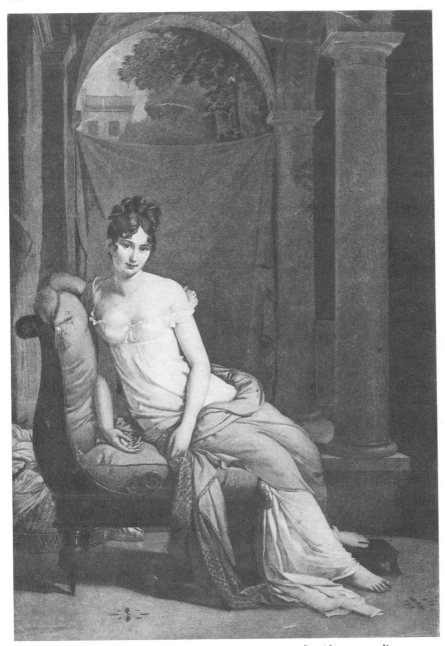

Juliette Récamier: "She fixed her great eyes upon me and paid me compliments about my figure . . . From this time on I thought only of Mme. de Staël."

**JULIETTE RÉCAMIER** (née Jeanne Francoise Julie Adélaide Récamier), b. Lyon, France, 1777. *(See April 22.)*

**RAINER MARIA RILKE, b. Prague, Bohemia, 1875.** Germany's greatest modern poet is included here only because Harold Nicolson, who knew him, and whose perception generally demands consideration and respect, believed Rilke to be gay. W. H. Auden once dismissed Rilke as "the greatest Lesbian poet since Sappho." Since Auden was not on particularly good terms with Harold Nicolson, it's more than likely that he came to his own conclusion about there being something "different" about the German poet. For many years Rilke lived in Paris, where he was secretary to the sculptor Auguste Rodin, himself supposedly gay. Since Rodin was an intimate of Diaghilev and Nijinsky, it seems highly unlikely that Rilke did not move in the same gay circle. Cocteau, for example, knew the German poet and even invented the story that Rilke had been in love with him. Once again, a good modern biography is needed. There seems to be too much "in the air" to ignore.

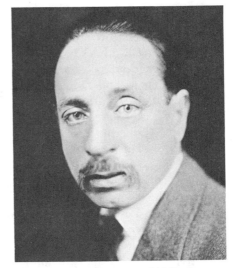

**Rainer Maria Rilke:** Harold Nicolson thought him gay.

# 5.

**CHRISTINA ROSSETTI, b. London, 1830.** Christina Rossetti,

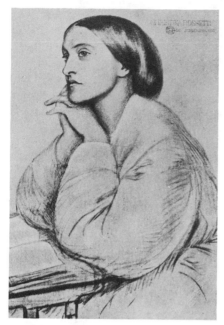

**Christina Rossetti:** Her poem speaks of "figs that fill the mouth."

religious and "delicate" (a favorite Victorian word), was the sister of poet Dante Gabriel Rossetti. The shy Christina in her simple Quakerlike dress stands in relief against the rich and intricately patterned Pre-Raphaelite tapestry which was her brother's background. Her *Monna Innominata* is one of the great sonnet sequences in English. Much of Christina Rossetti's poetry has been seen by critics from Willa Cather to Jeannette Foster as "variant," and one poem in particular, "Goblin Market," is a classic of (unconscious?) lesbian writing. The poem is convincingly interpreted in Foster's *Sex Variant Women in Literature,* and an excerpt here is sufficient for the flavor of the work. Two sisters are tempted by hideously ugly and deformed *male* goblins to eat some luscious fruit that they know to be "forbidden." One sister yields to temptation and eats the fruit, all of which is carefully selected to suggest the vagina (cherries, figs). The sister who eats goes wild, "She sucked their fruit globes fair or red . . .

sucked and sucked and sucked . . . until her tongue was sore . . . ." It's quite a poem.

# 6.

**SIR OSBERT SITWELL, b. London, 1892.** The Sitwells—Edith, Sacheverell, and Osbert—represented everything that was oh so modern to English dandies of the 1920s. Their essays, particularly those by Osbert, are rich in discussions of archaeology, architecture, painting, music, and the reverie evoked by names and places. Their culture, charm, and urbanity are recorded in Osbert's multivolume reminiscences of their patrician family and estate. Photographs of the Sitwells—particularly of Edith in her bizarre hats, all chosen for effect—are likely to put off the uninitiated from reading them. Drama critic James Agate's affectionate remark should be taken under advisement: "The Sitwells are artists pretending to be asses." Noel Coward's 1923 satire on the Sitwells—in which the sister of the "Swiss Family Whittlebot" intones, "Life is essentially a curve and Art is an oblong within that curve. My brothers and I have been brought up on Rhythm as other children are brought up on Glaxo"—resulted in a feud that lasted throughout the lifetimes of the four. Osbert Sitwell's love affair with David Horner ("his great love") is documented in John Pearson's joint biography, *The Sitwells.*

# 7.

**WILLA CATHER, b. Winchester, Virginia, 1873.** Few writers have taken such pains to destroy as

much evidence of their private lives as did Willa Cather. She believed, genuinely perhaps, that an author's biography was unimportant, that only events or people in a life that relate to incidents or characters in an author's works were relevant and worth saving. In her will she ordered that her letters were not to be quoted. She burned all the correspondence between her and the woman who is believed to have been her lover between 1901 and 1915, Isabelle McClung. She saw to it that her official biography was to be written by the friend who succeeded Isabelle McClung, Edith Lewis, thus assuring that only what was relevant (i.e., "correct") was told. All of this would actually be admirable—after all, one does not need to know Shakespeare's biography (and we don't) to appreciate his works—if it were not for the fact that such fastidious people who burn their papers generally have something to hide that in their time is considered wrong. In a sense, Willa Cather needn't have gone to so much trouble, for what little remains of the effects of her life clearly reveal her to have been a lesbian anyway. The only way to hide is never to have been born at all.

# 8.

**NORMAN DOUGLAS, b. Scotland, 1868.** Douglas was one of the liveliest, wittiest, and most original writers of his generation. His novel *South Wind* (1917) exerted a strong influence on almost every modern writer who came out of the 1920s. Douglas had discovered the joys of Capri in 1888 when he journeyed there in pursuit of a rare species of blue lizard. What he discovered there was a rare species of

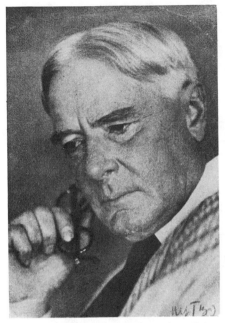

**Norman Douglas:** Even the august *Dictionary of National Biography* calls him "an ardent lover of both sexes."

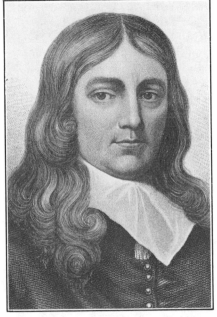

**John Milton:** His classmates called him "the lady of Christ's."

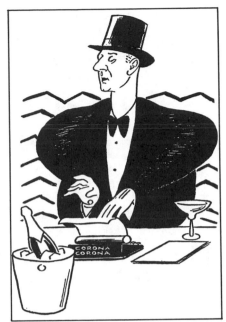

**Lucius Beebe:** Whiskey and sofa. That's right, *f.*

something else altogether. He fell in love with the island and decided to make it his "soul's operating base." *South Wind,* in part, recounts the story of how he made up his mind to leave his wife and settle in Capri to enjoy the gay life, openly and without shame. The setting of the novel is an island, like Capri, called Nepenthe, inhabited by an extraordinary group of eccentrics who, seen through the eyes of an English bishop, represent the contrast between the cultures of Northern and Southern Europe. In this satiric novel Northern (English) hypocrisy gets it between the eyes. Douglas died broke on Capri, but not before he had compiled an anthology of graffiti collected in several languages from the walls of public toilets throughout Europe.

# 9.

**JOHN MILTON, b. London, 1608.** John Milton? The great

English poet and Puritan? Nobody can say for sure that Milton was gay, but the author of *Paradise Lost* was known to his Cambridge classmates as "the lady of Christ's" and was portrayed as a repressed homosexual in Robert Graves's novel *Wife to Mr. Milton,* a classic case of it taking one to know one. As to Milton himself, we may never know, but any writer who can portray Satan as endlessly fascinating and God as a bit of a stick, can't be all bad.

**LUCIUS BEEBE, b. Wakefield, Massachusetts, 1902.** Journalist, railroad buff, dandy, and *bon vivant,* Lucius Beebe used to write a society column called "This New York," which was quite popular in the 1930s. Brendan Gill has written that the column contained so many references to Beebe's "intimate friend" Jerome Zerbe that Walter Winchell suggested it should be called not "This New York" but "Jerome Never Looked Lovelier." Beebe is said to have been fond of

inviting luscious young things to his private railroad car for what one wag described as "whisky and sofa."

# 10.

**EMILY DICKINSON, b. Amherst, Massachusetts, 1830.** Emily Dickinson is another of those pale, frail, delicate Victorian ladies whose psyches are encased in concrete, generally by their families and later by academicians. To tamper with the official versions of their lives is tantamount to spitting on the flag, with the same dire consequences. Just look at what happened to Rebecca Patterson when she dared to suggest in a biography some years back that Dickinson was a lesbian. She was fried. "What do you mean?" was the cry in the land. "How can Emily Dickinson be a lesbian? She's an American." Although there are some who think

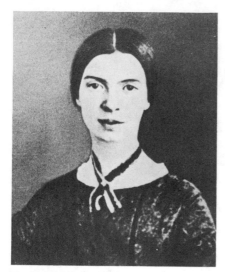

**Emily Dickinson:** Was she in love with Kate Scott Anthon, her girlhood friend?

that the great poet was in fact a lesbian, the official story remains the same as that innocently told about our lesbian grammar school teachers: their boyfriends died in World War I, so they remained old maids.

# 11.

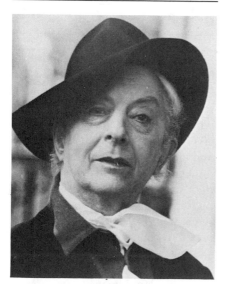

**Quentin Crisp:** A courageous life.

**QUENTIN CRISP, b. Southampton, England, 1908.** The redoubtable Quentin Crisp is proof

positive that life begins at seventy. During the Blitz, when other Britishers were convinced that civilization had come to a grinding halt, young Crisp, replete with hennaed hair and mascaraed eyes, was thanking God for the presence of G.I.'s who found him as attractive as (and infinitely cheaper than) the other London tarts. He swore then and there that he'd someday come to America, the more-than-promised land. Now, lionized as the author of the inimitably witty *Naked Civil Servant,* in high demand along the nation's sophisticated lecture circuit, and patiently awaiting a possible musical version of his unique and courageous life, he is a constant visitor to America at long last. And not a peep from the Moral Majority, which has probably mistaken him for Glora Swanson anyway.

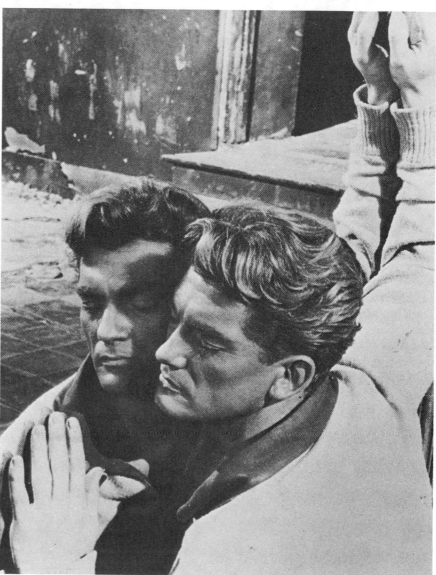

**Jean Marais:** In *Orphée,* a film by his lover, Jean Cocteau.

**JEAN MARAIS, b. Cherbourg, France, 1913.** Jean Marais was never much of an actor, and it is doubtful that he would have achieved international fame had he not become Jean Cocteau's lover, but he was, by universal acclamation, one of the most handsome men ever to appear in films. In the 1940s, when he made most of his movies for Cocteau, actors were still slicking down their hair with Kreml and Vitalis. But he changed all that. His *cheveaux fous* and athletic good looks created a new style of postwar leading man. When in 1946 he spent his time in Cocteau's *Beauty and the Beast* trapped within an ape-like costume, waiting for Beauty's kiss to turn him once again into Jean Marais, gay moviegoers around the world secretly wished that they were Josette Day who actually got to kiss the handsome actor's fur. What is perhaps most astonishing about the friendship between Cocteau and Marais is that the actor's face in profile bore an astonishing resemblance to the boys Cocteau had been sketching for thirty years before meeting him.

# 12.

**GUSTAVE FLAUBERT, b. Rouen, France, 1821.** For those who would leap to conclusions, the great French novelist made three mistakes: like Clifton Webb, he lived with his mama; he never married; and he once identified himself with the title character of his masterpiece, *Madame Bovary*—"Madame Bovary, c'est mois." What he meant by calling himself Emma Bovary, of course, was that, like his famous character, he hated bourgeois convention. As to the other two points, he seems to have had at least two intimate friendship with males, with Alfred Le Poittevin and Maxim de Camp. What's more, he seems to have gone through at least one romance typical of latent homosexuals—the impossible

dream. His friendship with the poet Louise Colet was founded on the idea that it would be impossible to win her. A. L. Rowse is convinced that Flaubert was homosexual; so are others. But there is little hard evidence.

# 13.

**MARTIAL (Marcus Valerius Martialis), b. Bilbilis in Spain, c. 38 B.C.** Martial was an urbane and witty man who is certainly the best-known writer of epigrams. He displays a great skill in adapting the form to a variety of uses. His epigrams have the precision and economy of inscriptions on monuments and tombstones, the earliest examples of the form. In a single couplet of stinging wit, Martial can expose a pretentious or foolish person. A good number of the poet's epigrams suggest not only that he was sexually promiscuous, but that he spent a fair share of his time with the boys, including Galaesus, Hyllus, Lygdus, Telesphorus, Dindymus, and Cestus. Martial, who was not married, got around. In one of his most famous epigrams, he is berated by a woman (his fictitious "wife") for sleeping with boys when, after all, he has her. Martial answers: "You use your parts, and let the boys use theirs."

# 14.

**DAN DAILEY, b. New York City, 1917.** Dan Dailey was one of 20th Century-Fox's most reliable and versatile actors. Whether he was appearing in a glossy musical as a song and dance man squiring Betty

Grable through her routines or acting in a straight dramatic role, he brightened many an otherwise undistinguished film. In fact it's hard to think of many Fox pictures made between the late '40s and late '50s that he did not appear in. Many people who were based in Hollywood or New York during those years remember his visits to the local gay bars, the polite whispers without pointing, and the path that parted like the Red Sea when he walked by. One wonders whether anyone ever so much as talked to him.

# 15.

**NERO (né Lucius Domitius Ahenobarbus), b. Rome, 37 A.D.** Nero was such a monster and so universally despised, that the stories told about him by contemporary historians are gross almost beyond belief. If the stories are in fact true, then he was second only to the great beast of the apocalypse. One tale has a carriage bearing Nero and his mother Agrippina pulling up to its destination. When the carriage door is opened, Nero gets out with his toga disheveled; mother gets out, wiping semen from her lips. It's that kind of story that gave Rome—pre-Fellini Rome at that—a bad name. Or there's the story of how the kindly emperor disposed of one wife by kicking her in the belly during the final months of her pregnancy. Contrary to popular belief, however, Nero did not fiddle while Rome burned. That was much too tame an avocation for the likes of him. He much preferred inventing his own sport—like dressing himself in animal skins and tearing at the sexual organs of prisoners tied to stakes. He was a sweet fella. When the tide turned

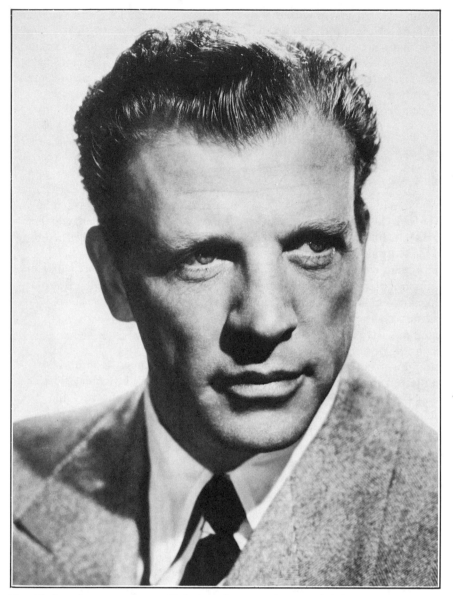

**Dan Dailey:** An actor who could do just about anything, and did.

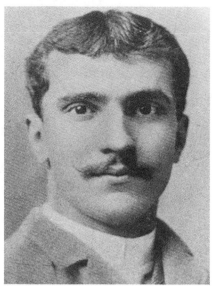

**George Santayana:** In love with a man who couldn't even remember his name.

unresponsive heterosexual who, at times, couldn't even remember his name. And it is this lifelong love—for Bertrand Russell's brother Frank—that is reflected in *The Last Puritan.* What a good-looking man Santayana was! What a sad story!

**SIR NOEL COWARD, b. Teddington, near London, 1899.** Really, now. Why waste space in telling tales about Noel Coward, when every anecdote, every affair of the heart, every Coldstream Guard kissed, is mentioned in Cole Lesley's biography of his multitalented employer, *Remembered Laughter?* Only one thing is missing from this otherwise entertaining and informative (500 pages of small type) book. Since Sir Noel seems to have laid hands on anyone he wanted, didn't he ever so much as touch his valet, Cole Lesley? Mr. Lesley is mysteriously silent on this point.

against him, he committed suicide just as he was about to be dispatched by his enemies. Supposedly, his curtain line—and a wonderful one at that—was: "What an artist is lost in me."

# 16.

**GEORGE SANTAYANA, b. Madrid, Spain, 1863.** It is frequently said that *The Last Puritan* is the best novel ever written by a philosopher. It is also one of the saddest novels in literature for it relates the story of a painfully unrequited love that was Santayana's own. The Harvard philsopher spent almost his entire life in love with an

# 17.

**DEBORAH SAMPSON, b. Plympton, Massachusetts, 1760.** Deborah

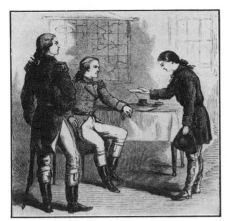

**Deborah Sampson:** On a mission to George Washington.

Sampson, masquerading as "Robert Surtlieff," was the most famous female soldier of the American Revolution. But, although her motives in fighting were patriotic, she had always shown great delight in wearing men's clothing and in drinking with the boys. For both those "offenses," in fact, she had been excommunicated from the First Baptist Church of Middleborough, Massachusetts. While in the army, Deborah Sampson developed a bit of a reputation as a ladies' man, and the stories of her exploits with women are too numerous to be anything but apocryphal. After serving seventeen months in the Continental Army (and being wounded in the Battle of Tarrytown), Deborah Sampson was honorably discharged by General Henry Knox at West Point.

**PAUL CADMUS, b. New York City, 1904.** Was there ever a painter who could render the male ass more erotic than Paul Cadmus? The artist's unique blending of realism and sexual playfulness shocked viewers in the 1930s, and *The Fleet's In,* Cadmus's suggestion of naval sexuality, caused a major scandal when the U. S. Navy ordered the painting seized. All he had done to cause such a ruckus was to paint well developed men in

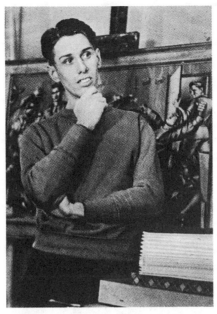

**Paul Cadmus:** He paints the *genus homo* in all its unrestrained physical exuberance.

tight-fitting Navy uniforms and to suggest that they might be interested in a couple of young women. That sailors were in pursuit of sex put the Navy in a snit. But the scandal—written up in every newspaper and magazine—made Cadmus's career. The Navy should have seen the many other works in which the sailors obviously want each other.

# 18.

**"SAKI" (H. H. Munro), b. Devonshire, England, 1890.** "Saki's" short stories at their best are extraordinarily compact and cameolike, wicked and witty, with a cruelty and a powerful vein of supernatural fantasy. They deal, in general, with the same group of upper-class Britishers, whose frivolous lives are sometimes complicated by animals—the talking cat who reveals their treacheries in love, the pet ferret who is evil incarnate.

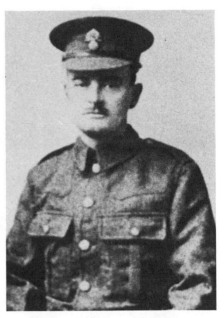

**"Saki" (H. H. Munro):** A devotee of London's Jermyn Street baths.

Now that it has been revealed that Hector Hugh Munro was gay, the stories are being re-read as allegories of the torment of remaining bottled up in a hypocritical English society. The stories are even more entertaining with this new knowledge. The *nom de plume* "Saki" was borrowed from the cupbearer in *The Rubaiyat* of Omar Khayyam.

# 19.

**BARBETTE (né Vander Clyde), b. Round Rock, Texas, 1904.** If you've seen the idiotic *Victor/Victoria* and wondered what all the fuss was about when Julie Andrews, looking very much like Julie Andrews, would sing and dance in female attire and then—as the audience went berserk—remove her wig and reveal herself to be a man, still looking very much like Julie Andrews, it was Barbette whom she was supposed to be impersonating.

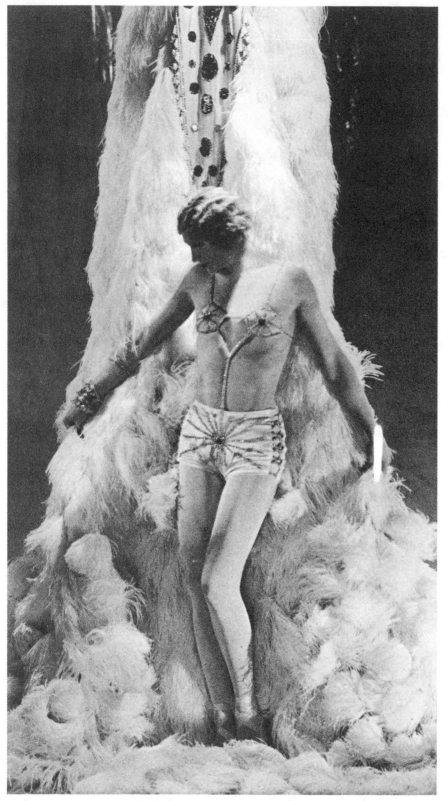

**Barbette:** *Tout Paris* was wild about the American in drag.

when, at the end, after his trapeze gig, he removed his wig and showed himself to be a man. Had he looked like Julie Andrews, it is doubtful that Jean Cocteau would have engaged Barbette for his most famous role—as a lady in a theatre box in the surrealist film, *Blood of a Poet.*

# 20.

**ELSIE DE WOLFE, b. New York City, 1860.** Elsie de Wolfe called herself the first interior decorator (she wasn't), an actress (she wasn't), and madly in love with her husband, Sir Charles Mendl (she wasn't). She was, in order of her claims, an interior decorator (certainly among the first ten thousand, but hardly the first), a clotheshorse whose abilities as a thespian never quite equalled the Parisian gowns people paid good money to see her model on the New York stage, and the lesbian lover of socialite Elizabeth Marbury (Sir Charles, who liked boys, didn't mind Elsie's past at all). With the help of Bessie Marbury, whose position among the New York 400 was unimpeachable, Elsie became decorator to the exceptionally rich. Her detractors, who thought little of her talents and less of her social climbing, simply called her "the chintz lady." No remark of Elsie's so succinctly reveals her view of herself and her world as the one she uttered when she first saw the Acropolis in Athens. "It's beige," she cried. "My color!"

# 21.

**ALBERT DEKKER, b. Brooklyn, New York, 1905.** Originally billed

For Barbette was the American female impersonator who was the toast of Paris in the late '20s, and the highlight of his act occurred

Albert Van Dekker, this actor enjoyed a long career in such motion pictures as *Marie Antoinette, Beau Geste, The Man in the Iron Mask, The Killers,* and *Suspense.* One role that immediately identifies him to movie buffs, however, is the one in which he donned those thick spectacles and reduced everyone in sight to toy size in *Dr. Cyclops.* In life, as in this film, his future was evil-starred. His was one of the more unforgettable Hollywood suicides. They found him dressed in full drag, handcuffed, and with his farewell message scrawled in lipstick.

# 22.

**THOMAS WENTWORTH HIGGINSON, b. Cambridge, Massachusetts, 1823.** This is the minister-novelist who was in love with William Henry Hurlbert. *(See July 3.)*

# 23.

**CZAR ALEXANDER I, b. St. Petersburg, Russia, 1777.** Alexander's Russia is the background for Tolstoy's *War and Peace,* so complicated is this period of European history. Basically, Alexander may be seen as the emperor of Russia who formed the coalition that defeated Napoleon and founded the Holy Alliance. The church bells that you hear at the end of Tchaikovsky's *1812 Overture* are ringing out the news of Alexander's defeat of France, which made him one of the most powerful leaders in Europe. Is it any wonder why Napoleon called Alexander "the slyest and handsomest of all the Greeks," a begrudgingly admir-

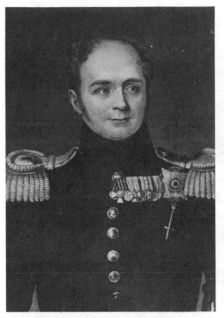

**Czar Alexander I:** The slyest and the handsomest of all the Greeks.

ing assessment of the czar's homosexuality, a contention amply supported in the documents of the period. Alexander was always shrouded in mystery. When he died, rumors persisted that he had actually fled Russia to Siberia where he became a hermit. In 1926 his tomb was opened by the Soviet government. It was empty, and the mystery remains unsolved.

# 24.

**HOWARD HUGHES, b. Houston, Texas, 1905.** He is said to have had a couple of bucks. He liked films, aviation, beautiful women, making more bucks, and, near the end, drugs. But if you're ready to accept the notion of Errol Flynn involved with Nazi spies during World War II, then you're ready to accept the story of the multimillionnaire turning over for the handsome, virile movie star—for cold cash. *(See June 20.)*

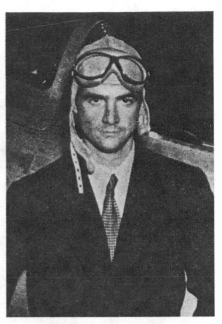

**Howard Hughes:** He flew with Flynn.

# 25.

**EPAMINONDAS, b. Thebes, 418 B.C.** Epaminondas was one of the great military geniuses of the ancient world. But since this is Christmas Day, he is included here not because of his victories in battle, but because he was revered for his moral character. He was revered, too, since he had risen from an impoverished family because of his goodness, strength, and character. He was, like other Greek warriors, homosexual—but with a difference. He never married and did not produce an heir. His delight in boys was complete in itself for him. His two favorite boys, Asopichus and Leuctra, both fell in battle, as did Epaminondas. Both, by his order, are buried with him in his tomb.

**CHRISTMAS DAY.** If you think I'm going to say what you think I'm going to say, then you're crazy Merry Christmas.

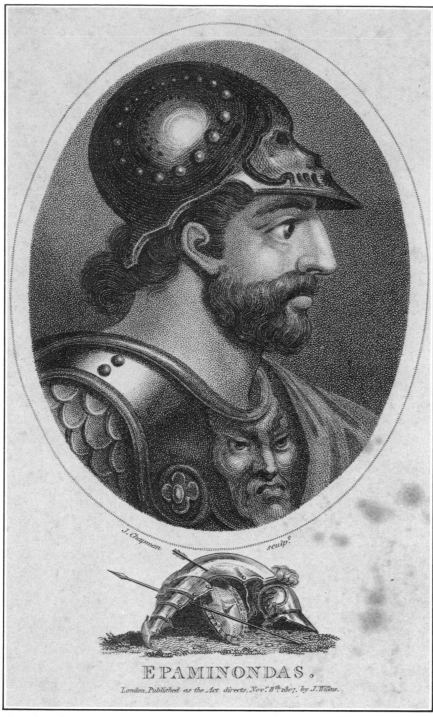

EPAMINONDAS.

*London, Published as the Act directs, Nov.ʳ 8ᵗʰ 1807, by J. Wilkes.*

J. Chapman    sculp.ᵗ

**Epaminondas:** A noble warrior, a faithful lover.

# 26.

**THOMAS GRAY, b. London, 1716.** "My life now is but a perpetual conversation with your shadow—The known sound of your voice still rings in my ears. I cannot bear this place, where I have spent many tedious years within less than a month, after you left me. . . ." So wrote Thomas Gray to a young man when he was fifty-four. Professor of Modern History at Cambridge University and one of the best-known poets of his time, he was also more than likely still a virgin. The author of "An Elegy Written in a Country Churchyard," Gray had lived most of his life with his mother, but was known to have cultivated the Platonic friendship of handsome young men. One of Professor Gray's young men introduced him to the Swiss charmer Charles de Bonstetten—and Gray was hooked. He was profoundly, deeply in love. When Bonstetten left Cambridge a year later, the poet was devastated. But the friends exchanged letters, and the young man suggested that they take a walking tour together in Bonstetten's native Switzerland. Gray was overjoyed. The trip was scheduled for the summer of 1771 and Gray wrote tireless letters of devotion while counting the ticking minutes. Finally, the time was near. He would be leaving to see his handsome young man again. The poor poet dropped dead before he had one foot out the door.

# 27.

**MARLENE DIETRICH (née Maria Magdalene von Losch), b. Berlin, 1904.** Only a bounder would suggest that you look up the silly passages on Marlene Dietrich in the incomparably silly *Here Lies the Heart* by Mercedes de Acosta. Look up the silly passages on Marlene Dietrich in the incomparably silly *Here Lies the Heart* by

## 29.

POLYCRATES, b. Samos, c. 570 B.C., By pirate raids and indiscriminate warfare, the tyrant of Samos dominated the East Aegean. He waged various wars and was, until the end of his life, victorious. His tyranny drove the philosopher Pythagoras from Samos, where Polycrates was generally hated. Eventually he was lured to Magnesia by one of his enemies and crucified. But even meanies can lose their hearts to the right boy, and Polycrates, tyrant that he was, was still a normal Greek. His special friend was the youth Bathyllus, so beautiful that Polycrates dared to erect a statue in his honor in the temple of Hera, goddess of women. Polycrates may have thought it appropriate that beautiful Bathyllus have his place among women, but his was an act of arrogance nonetheless. Almost immediately thereafter, he was crucified. Don't mess with Hera.

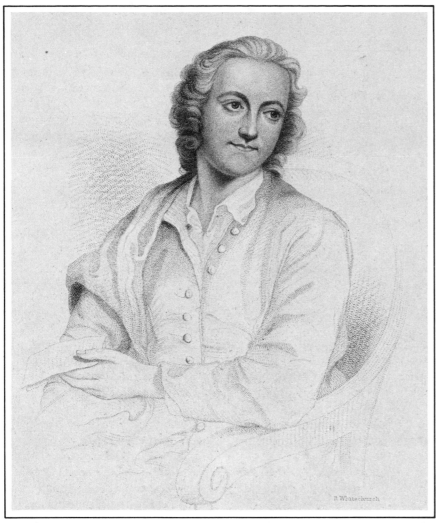

Thomas Gray: All his defenses were swept away; he was in love.

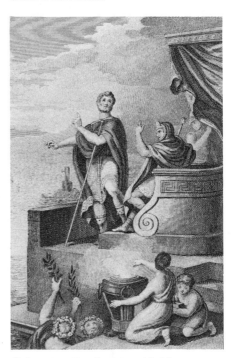

Polycrates: Don't mess with Hera.

Mercedes de Acosta. They are guaranteed to be far sillier than the silly sections on Greta Garbo. Honest.

## 28.

F. W. MURNAU (né Friedrich Wilhelm Plumpe), b. Bielefeld, Germany, 1889. The famous German director is best known for two things. Although he made such exquisite silent films as *Nosferatu* and *The Last Laugh,* his *Sunrise,* produced in Hollywood, is one of the most beautiful films ever made. His death is certainly the most bizarre in a town noted for its extraordinary ways of dying. In 1931 Murnau and his chauffeur were killed in an automobile accident. From the way the bodies had been found, it was obvious that the film director was killed, and the accident probably caused, while Murnau was blowing the driver.

# 30.

**TINY TIM** (né Herbert Khaury), b. New York City, 1923? Tiny Tim, he of the falsetto voice, stringy Charles Adams hair, ukelele, and "Tip-Toe Through the Tulips." Remember him? At the height of his momentary fame, a ghastly biography appeared in which the world learned, among other things, something of Tiny Tim's sex life.

Yes, everyone knew that Tim had married his Miss Vicky right on television (the knowing would have recognized the gay priest). But Tiny Tim, who spells out all words dealing with S-E-X, revealed the sensational news that he had once had a H-O-M-O-S-E-X-U-A-L experience in which he spilled his "S-E-E-D faster than anyone—In two seconds."

# 31.

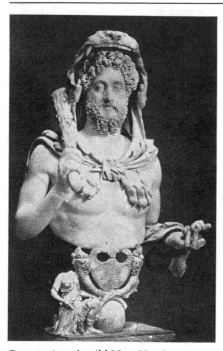

**COMMODUS** (Lucius Aelius Aurelius Commodus), d. 192. Tonight is New Year's Eve, and, after a weary journey, we are finally at the end of the gay year. To be on the safe side, why not stay home tonight and watch old Guy Lombardo re-runs on TV (the blue-haired ladies with spangled glasses are fun to watch) and spend a quiet evening in prudent memory of the emperor Commodus, who called his exceptionally well-endowed cup-bearer "my donkey," and was strangled by an over-enthusiastic wrestler named Narcissus on this day in 192 A.D. Man, Commodus really knew how to throw a wild New Year's Eve party.

**Commodus:** A wild New Year's party.

## Other Personalities Born In December

2. **Lucy Ann Lobdell,** Female transvestite "married" to another woman, 1829
   **H. Harkness Flagler,** American financier and socialite, 1870

4. **Felix V,** last of antipopes, 1383

**Thomas Carlyle,** English writer, 1795
**Samuel Butler,** English writer, 1835
**A. L. Rowse,** English historian, 1903
**John Giorno,** American poet and artist, 1936

5. **Robert Harley, 1st Earl of Oxford,** English statesman, 1661

6. **Charles Edward Sayle,** English bibliographer, editor, and poet, 1864

7. **Akiko Yosano,** Japanese poet, 1878

8. **Horace,** Roman poet, 55 B.C.
   **Christina,** Queen of Sweden, 1626
   **Charles Shively,** American poet, 1937

9. **Johann Joachim Winckelmann,** German archaeologist, 1717
   **Louie Crew,** American scholar-activist, 1936

10. **Pierre Louÿs,** French poet, 1870
    **William Plomer,** British writer, 1903

11. **Pope Leo X,** 1475
    **Francesco Algarotti,** Italian philosopher and art connoisseur, 1712
    **John Preston,** American writer-activist, 1945

15. **Vida Dutton Scudder,** American educator, 1861

17. **Ludwig van Beethoven,** German composer, 1770
    **Rev. John Francis Bloxam,** English writer, 1873
    **Bertha Harris,** American writer-activist, 1937

19. **Horace Traubel,** Whitman's Boswell, 1858
    **Jean Genet,** French novelist and playwright, 1910

20. **John Fletcher,** English playwright, 1579
    **Charles Kains Johnson,** English lawyer and editor, 1857

**22. Marc Allégret,** French film producer, 1900

**28. Manuel Puig,** Argentinian novelist, 1932
**Bryne R. S. Fone,** American scholar and writer, 1936

**29. William Carney,** American writer, 1946

## I Know They Are, You Know They Are, and They Know They Are, but Initials Will Just Have to Do

C. G., American actor
D. K., American entertainer
R. S., American actor
S. D., Spanish painter
S. S., American song writer
M. S., American children's writer
J. A., American poet
B. S., American actress
L. B., American composer
R. H., American actor
C. C., American theatrical producer
A. de S., American dancer
T. T., American actor
E. L. G., American actress
C. R., American actor
H., American singer
O. S., English stage designer
J. N., American actor
D. D. T., American composer
W. B., American actor
L. R., American singer
R. H., English dancer
A. Mc C., English actor
J. C., American writer
L. K., American dance impresario
A. R., American poet
J. N., American actor, singer
F. G., American actor
M. G., American TV personality
G. C. M., American composer
C. C., American actor and writer
J. H., American song writer
A. L., American playwright
D. R., American writer

G. C., American film director
R. T., American actor
G. H., American actor
V. J., American actor
V. H., Russian-American pianist
L. F., American dancer-choreographer
P. L., British-born American actor
L. T., American comedienne
B. S., American singer
J. K., American novelist
G. K., American actor
R. Mc D., English-born American actor
G. G., American composer
R. R., American reviewer, actor
J. R., American choreographer
R. R., American artist
E. H., American costume designer
A. D., French actor
B. L., American actor
P. S., American singer, actor
M. N., American actor, director
A. C., American composer
K. B., American comedienne
R. D., American actor
V. T., American composer
H. B., German actor
W. C., American TV actor
H. H., American actor
M. S., German actor
C. P., Canadian actor
H. L., American dancer
M. T. T., American musician
S. K., American baseball player
**and hundreds, and hundreds, and hundreds of others.**

## Credits

This book could not have been written without a dependence upon scores of biographies, most of them written during the past decade and a half. Only recently have biographers felt free to explore the homosexual backgrounds of their subjects, and one can only be grateful that our own age, if it has little else to recommend it, is at least groping cautiously towards truth. That it has taken almost a century to acknowledge the gayness of so obvious a subject as Walt Whitman would indicate how many lives of the great and not-so-great remain to be rewritten. Most of the illustrations in *The Gay Book of Days* are from the author's collection and from the voluminous files of The New York Public Library Picture Collection. The photographs of Aaron Fricke, Doric Wilson, Robert Patrick, Divine, and Quentin Crisp are by Michael Thompson, Roy Blakely, Ken Howard, New Line Cinema, and Jean Harvey respectively. I gladly acknowledge the assistance of Vicki Brooks, Michael Fiore, and Donald Rolfe, although all errors are ultimately my own.

# Bibliography

Austen, Roger. *Playing the Game: The Homosexual Novel in America*. New York, 1977.

Beurdeley, Cecile. *L'Amour Bleu*. New York, 1978.

Boswell, John. *Christianity, Social Tolerance, and Homosexuality*. Chicago, 1980.

Bullogh, Vern L. *Homosexuality: A History*. New York, 1979.

De Acosta, Mercedes. *Here Lies the Heart*. New York, 1960.

De Becker, Raymond. *The Other Face of Love*. New York, 1969.

Dover, K. J. *Greek Homosexuality*. New York, 1978.

Fone, Byrne R. S. *Hidden Heritage; History and the Gay Imagination*. New York, 1978.

Foster, Jeannette. *Sex Variant Women in Literature*. Reprint. Baltimore, 1975.

Galloway, David and Christian Sabisch, eds. *Calamus*. New York, 1982.

Garde, Noel. *From Jonathan to Gide: The Homosexual in History*. New York, 1964.

Green, Martin. *Children of the Sun*. New York, 1946.

Grier, Barbara. *Lesbiana*. Reno, Nevada, 1976.

———— and Coletta Reid, eds. *Lesbian Lives*. Baltimore, 1976.

Hunter, John Francis. *The Gay Insider*. New York, 1972.

Myers, Jeffrey. *Homosexuality and Literature*. Montreal, 1971.

Katz, Jonathan. *Gay American History*. New York, 1976.

Leyland, Winston, ed. *Angels of the Lyre*. San Francisco, 1975.

————. *Gay Sunshine Interviews*. San Francisco, 1978.

Licht, Hans. *Sexual Life in Ancient Greece*. London, 1932.

Martin, Robert K. *The Homosexual Tradition in American Poetry*. Austin, Texas, 1979.

Plummer, Douglas. *Queer People*. London, 1963.

Rogers, W. G. *Ladies Bountiful*. New York, 1968.

Rowse, A. L. *Homosexuals in History*. New York, 1977.

Ruitenbeek, Hendrik. *Homosexuality and Creative Genius*. New York, 1965.

Rule, Jane. *Lesbian Images*. New York, 1975.

Russo, Vito. *The Celluloid Closet*. New York, 1981.

Sanders, Dennis, ed. *Gay Source, A Catalog for Men*. New York, 1977.

Stambolian, George and Elaine Marks. *Homosexualities and French Literature: Cultural Contexts, Cultural Texts*. Ithaca, New York, 1975.

Tripp, C. A. *The Homosexual Matrix*. New York, 1975.

Young, Ian, ed. *The Male Muse*. Trumansburg, New York, 1973.

# Index

Ackerley, J. R., 189
Acosta, Mercedes de, 39, 50, 105, 164, 214-15
Acton, Harold, 118, 128, 133, 140-41
Adams, Nick, 121-22
Agate, James, 206
Agathon, 137-38
Agostinelli, Alfred, 121
Albee, Edward, 55, 102
Alberoni, Giulio, 61
Aldington, Richard, 156
Alexander I, Czar, 213
Alexander the Great, 71, 82, 86, 87
Algarotti, Francesco, 216
Alger, Horatio, 23, 103
Alington, Napier G. H. S., 200
Allégret, Marc, 195, 217
Altman, Dennis, 153
Alyson, Sasha, 95
Anacreon, 161
Andersen, Hans Christian, 63-64
Andros, Phil, 127-28
Anger, Kenneth, 81
Anne, Queen, 47
Anthony, Susan B., 40-41
Antinous, 28-29, 124-25
Apollinaire, Guillaume, 153, 184
Aretino, Pietro, 50, 72
Aristippus, 68
Aristophanes, 138
Armfelt, Gustaf Mauritz, 61
Arne, Thomas Augustine, 61
Arnim, Elisabeth Brentano von, 64-65
Arthur, Gavin, 57
Arvin, Newton, 153
Arzner, Dorothy, 90
Auden, W. H., 43, 46-47, 99, 130, 180, 196, 205
Augustine, St., 191-92
Augustus, Caesar, 166
Austen, Roger, 21

Babur, 47
Bacon, Sir Francis, 27
Bacon, Roger, 27
Baden-Powell, R. S. S., 47
Baez, Joan, 33
Bagoas, 86
Baker, Dorothy, 77
Baker, Josephine, 75
Baker, Dr. S. Josephine, 55, 193
Baldwin, James, 136
Bankhead, Tallulah, 32-33, 137, 186, 194-95, 200
Barber, Samuel, 61
Barbette, 211-12
Barnes, Djuna, 18, 113
Barney, Natalie Clifford, 79, 142, 184, 185
Barnfield, Richard, 103
Baron, Michel, 24

Barrie, Sir James M., 83
Barry, James Miranda, 124
Bashlow, Robert, 113
Bathyllus, 161, 215
Batten, Veronica, 142-43
Baudelaire, Charles, 67
Baxt, George, 113
Beach, Charles, 58
Beardsley, Aubrey, 90, 147-48
Beaton, Cecil, 23-24
Beauchamp, Robert Lygon, Earl, 42
Beazley, J. D., 169, 190
Beckford, William, 171-72
Beebe, Lucius, 207
Beecher, Henry Ward, 113
Beekman, Gustave, 191
Beethoven, Ludwig van, 216
Behan, Brendan, 47
Bell, Arthur, 201
Bellini, Vincenzo, 200
Benson, A. C., 77
Bentley, Eric, 169
Berg, Pierre, 136
Bernac, Pierre, 19-20, 33, 109
Berners, Lord, 169
Beza, Theodore, 113
Birkin, Andrew, 83
Birisima, George, 47
Blackwell, Antoinette, 95
Blake, William, 201
Bligh, Captain William, 158
Blitzstein, Marc, 49-50
Bloxam, Rev. John Francis, 216
Blunt, Sir Anthony, 169
Bogarde, Dirk, 60
Boccioni, Umberto, 63, 185
Bonheur, Rosa, 57-58
Bonneval, Claude, Comte de, 133
Bonpland, A. J. A., 161
Bonstetten, Charles Victor de, 18, 156, 214
Bosco, Giovanni, 153
Boswell, John, 74, 123, 158, 168
Boulanger, Lili, 153
Bouvier, John Vernou III, 88-89
Bowen, Elizabeth, 101-102
Bowie, David, 20
Bowles, Jane, 47
Bowles, Paul, 98
Bowra, C. M., 67
Boyd, Rev. Malcolm, 113
Bradley, Katherine Harris, 22, 183
Bradley, Marion Zimmer, 112
Brainard, Joe, 43, 61
Brando, Marlon, 60, 64, 179
Britten, Benjamin, 20, 109, 110, 196
Bronzino, Il, 201
Brooke, Rupert, 49, 136-37, 189-90
Brooks, Romaine, 79, 184, 185
Broughton, James, 200
Brown, Horatio Forbes, 41, 59

Brown, Dr. Howard, 77
Brown, J. G., 103
Brown, Rita Mae, 199
Browne, William Kenworthy, 61
Browning, Oscar, 33, 138, 175
Brummell, Beau, 101
Brunner, H. C., 153
Bryher, 18, 155-56
Buchanan, James, 65-66, 73
Buckingham, Bob, 15, 16, 189
Burgess, Guy, 91
Burns, John Horne, 185
Burroughs, William S., 37, 57
Burton, Richard, 191
Busoni, Ferruccio, 63
Busser, Henri, 172
Butler, Eleanor, 84
Butler, Samuel, 216
Byron, George Gordon, Lord, 27-28, 150

Cadmus, Paul, 67, 211
Caesar, Julius, 82, 123, 166, 204
Cagliostro, Alesandro, 112
Caine, Hall, 86, 173
Calamity Jane. *See* Matha Canary
Caligula, 152-53, 193
Cambacérès, Jean Jacques Régis de, 179-80
Canary, Martha, 94
Canova, Antonio, 200
Capote, Truman, 16, 23, 98, 168-69, 172, 195
Caracalla, 77
Caravaggio, 168
Carlyle, Thomas, 216
Carman, Bliss, 77
Carmines, Rev. Al, 133
Carney, William, 217
Carpenter, Edward, 57, 151-52
Carroll, Lewis, 31, 85, 103
Caryll, Mary, 84
Casa, Giovanni della, 113
Cassady, Neal, 57
Casement, Sir Roger, 155
Castlereagh, Viscount, 106-107
Cather, Willa, 60, 202, 206
Catullus, 157, 203-204
Cavafy, C. V., 70-71
Cavalieri, Tommasso, 50
Cellini, Benvenuto, 200
Chanel, Gabrielle "Coco," 146, 147
Charea, 152-53
Charles IX, 113
Charles XII, 113
Charles XIII, 156
Charles XV, 94
Charles the Bold, 200
Charles-Roux, Claire, 50
Charmus, 184
Cheevers, Harold, 53
Chevalier, Maurice, 160-61

Choisy, Abbé de, 153
Chopin, Frèdèric, 47
Christian VII, 31-32
Christina, Queen, 216
Chubb, Ralph, 38
Churchill, Sara Jennings, 185
Churchill, Winston, 24, 137, 144, 200, 201
Chute, John, 166
Clark, Don, 133
Clarke, Lige, 47
Claudius, 153
Cleopatra, 104
Clift, Montgomery, 179
Cocteau, Jean, 51, 53, 87, 118-19, 140, 146, 185, 195-96, 205, 208-209, 212
Colette, Gabrielle Sidonie, 14
Collins, Jess, 20
Commodus, 153, 216
Congdon, Kirby, 201
Compton-Burnett, Ivy, 99
Condé, Louis II de Bourbon, Prince de, 158
Connolly, Cyril, 159
Conradin, 58-59
Conklin, Margaret, 139-40
Conover, Harry, 153
Converse, Florence, 77
Cook, Eliza, 127
Cooper, Edith Emma, 22
Cooper, George 117
Corelli, Marie, 173
Cornell, Katharine, 40, 138
Correggio, 152
Corvo, Baron Frederick. See Frederick Rolfe
Cory, William, 33
Courtenay, William, 171
Coward, Noel, 146, 194, 206, 210
Cowell, Henry, 52
Crane, Hart, 18, 57, 126, 191
Crane, Stephen, 187
Crevel, René, 141, 165
Crew, Louie, 216
Crisp, Quentin, 208
Crow, Emma, 127
Crowley, Aleister, 148, 176-77
Crowley, Mart, 153
Cullen, Countee, 35, 89
Culver, Calvin. See Casey Donovar.
Cummings, E. E., 132
Curtis, Jackie, 47
Curzon, Daniel, 61
Cushman, Charlotte, 126-27
Custine, Marquis de, 61
Czerny, Carl, 47

Dailey, Dan, 209, 210
Daudet, Lucien, 140
David, Jacques-Louis, 77
David, King, 38
Dean, James, 34, 38, 122, 182
Dean, Roy, 153
Debussy, Claude, 153
Degas, Edgar, 125
Dekker, Albert, 212-13
Delacroix, Eugène, 19, 77
Delius, Frederic, 33
Demosthenes, 143
Demuth, Charles, 18
Dennis, Patrick, 87
Despenser, Hugh le, 74
De Wolfe, Billy, 41

De Wolfe, Elsie, 212
Diaghilev, Sergei, 53, 55, 56, 64, 87, 140, 148, 197, 205
Diamond, David, 42, 133
Dickinson, Anna, 41, 185
Dickinson, Emily, 207-208
Dickinson, Goldsworthy Lowes, 138-39
Dietrich, Marlene, 50, 105, 214-15
Diocletian, 27
Dior, Christian, 33
Divine, 17, 116, 180-81
Dolben, Digby Mackworth, 47
Domitian, 183, 190
Donovan, Casey, 188
Doolittle, Hilda, 156, 158
Doryphorus, 178
Dos Passos, John, 132
Douglas, Lord Alfred, 127, 181
Douglas, Norman, 81, 206-207
Dowell, Coleman, 95
Doyle, Peter, 18, 94
Duberman, Martin, 153
Dubois, Guillaume Cardinal, 169
Du Bois, Mary C., 61
Duffy, Maureen, 60
Dunant, Jean Henri, 167
Duncan, Robert, 20
Duquesnoy, Jérôme, 119
Dussek, Jan Ladislav, 47
Dworkin, Andrea, 169
Dyer, Edward 200

Eakins, Thomas, 130
Earhart, Amelia, 128, 129
Edward II, 74, 75
Eisenstein, Sergei, 33
Eliot, T. S., 167, 183
Ellerman, Annie Winifred. See Bryher
Ellis, Havelock, 36, 57
Elmslie, Kenward, 77
Eltinge, Julian, 86
Emerson, Ralph Waldo, 90, 91, 183
Eon, Chevalier d', 174
Epaminondas, 213, 214
Erasmus, Desiderius, 183
Ernest Augustus, 113
Erté, 191
Esher, Reginald Brett, Viscount, 113
Eugene of Savoy, 185
Eulenburg-Hertefeld, Philipp zu, 39

Faber, Frederick William, 113
Falla, Manuel de, 118-19
Farinelli, 33
Farnese, Pier Luigi, 201
Fassbinder, Rainer Werner, 94
Ferdinand of Bulgaria, 47
Fergusson, Gladys, 70
Ferson, Count Adelsward, 80-81
Fersen, Hans Axel, Count von, 156
Field, Edward, 113
Field, Michael, 22, 183
Firbank, Ronald, 25, 101, 106, 172
Fisher, Peter, 95
FitzGerald, Edward, 61
Flagler, H. Harkness, 216
Flanagan, William, 153
Flanner, Janet, 61
Flaubert, Gustave, 209
Flecker, James Elroy, 189-90

Fletcher, John, 216
Fletcher, Joseph, 61
Flynn, Errol, 108, 109, 213
Fone, Byrne R. S., 217
Foote, Mary Hallock, 201
Ford, Charles Henri, 141, 165
Forster, E. M., 15-16, 49, 53, 71, 110, 138, 151-52, 159, 189
Foster, Jeannette, 206
Foster, Stephen, 117
Frederick of Baden, 58-59
Frederick the Great, 29, 195
Fremstad, Olive, 61
Freud, Sigmund, 81, 190
Fricke, Aaron, 30-31
Froude, Richard Hurrell, 45-46
Fuller, Henry Blake, 33
Fuller, Margaret, 90
Fulton, James Grove, 61

Gallieni, Joseph, 77
Garber, Eric, 89
Garbo, Greta, 23, 37, 42, 50, 105, 106, 164, 215
Garde, Noel, 166
Gauguin, Paul, 13, 139, 192
Gaveston, Piers, 74
Gay, Martin, 91
Geldzahler, Henry, 133
Genet, Jean, 66, 216
George III, 99, 100
George, Stefan, 133
Gericault, Jean-Louis, 169
Germain, Lord George, 31
Gide, André, 67, 121, 127, 189, 195-96
Gielgud, Sir John, 68, 69
Ginsberg, Allen, 57, 98-99
Giorno, John, 216
Giraud, Nicolò, 28
Gloeden, Wilhelm von, 140, 162-63, 173
Goethe, Johann Wolfgang von, 150-51
Gogol, Nikolai, 61
Goldman, Emma, 113
Goodman, Paul, 169
Gordon, Charles George "Chinese," 31
Gosse, Sir Edmund, 169
Goulding, Edmund, 108
Grainger, Percy, 104-105, 133, 191
Grainger, Porter, 70
Grant, Cary, 102, 145
Grant, Duncan, 27, 49
Graves, Robert, 128, 207
Gray, Thomas, 156, 166, 214, 215
Green, Julian, 169
Greenwood, Grace, 127, 169
Greif, Martin, 37
Greville, Fulke, 200
Grieg, Edvard, 104-105, 191
Grierson, Francis, 169
Griffes, Charles Tomlinson, 169
Griffin, Walter, 153
Grillparzer, Franz, 33
Guercino, 47
Guilbert, Paul, 30
Günderode, Karoline von, 47, 64-65
Gunn, Thom, 153
Gustavus III, 33, 156
Gustavus IV, 156
Gustavus V, 105-106

Hadrian, 28-29, 124-25
Hahn, Reynaldo, 140
Haines, William, 16-17
Hall, Radclyffe, 60, 142-43
Hall, Richard, 69, 201
Halliburton, Richard, 20-21, 37, 199
Halliwell, Kenneth, 17
Hamilton, Alexander, 21-22
Hamilton, Edith, 153
Hamilton, Emma Lyon, 84-85
Hamilton, Wallace, 153
Hammarskjöld, Dag, 131-32
Hampton, Christopher, 33
Handel, George Frederick, 44-45
Hansen, Joseph, 133
Harris, Bertha, 216
Hart, Lorenz, 79-80
Harte, Bret, 149
Hartley, Marsden, 18
Hausrath, Adolf, 33
Haxton, Gerald, 30, 88
Hay, Henry, 77
Hays, Matilda, 127
Heard, Gerald, 185
Heber, Richard, 18
Heinrich of Prussia, 25
Heliogabalus, 51, 164
Henri III, 164
Henze, Hans Werner, 135
Hephaestion, 86
Herlihy, James Leo, 40
Hervey, John, 178
Hichens, Robert, 201
Hickok, Lorena, 84, 176
Hickok, Wild Bill, 91
Higginson, Thomas Wentworth, 117, 213
Hiller, Kurt, 153
Hippias, 184
Hirschfeld, Magnus, 28, 57
Hirtius, 166
Hockney, David, 133
Hoffman, Malvina, 50, 105
Hoffman, William M., 77
Hölderlin, Friedrich, 61
Holliday, Judy, 109
Holmes, Sherlock, 18-19
Hoover, J. Edgar, 16
Hopkins, Gerard Manley, 102-103
Horace, 216
Hornig, Richard, 150
Horton, Edward Everett, 48, 55
Hosmer, Harriet, 127, 170, 175
Housman, A. E., 59
Housman, Laurence, 125
Howard, Brian, 140-41
Howard, Richard, 177
Hudson, John Paul, 21, 28, 61, 75, 76, 181
Hughes, Howard, 109, 213
Hughes, Langston, 35
Humboldt, Alexander von, 155, 161
Humphreys, Laud, 185
Hunter, Tab, 116
Hurlbert, William Henry, 117, 213
Huysmans, J. K., 47

Iffland, Wilhelm August, 71-72
Inge, William, 94
Irving, Edward, 153
Isherwood, Christopher, 28, 46-47, 150

Jackman, Harold, 89
Jacob, Max, 133
Jacobs, Naomi, 132
Jagger, Mick, 130
James I, 107-108
James, Alice, 153
James, Henry, 53, 69, 110
James, William, 69
Jay, Karla, 47
Jesus, 151
Jewett, Sarah Orne, 169
Jewsbury, Geraldine, 127
Joan of Arc, 92
Jodelle, Ètienne, 132
John, Edmund, 199
John, Elton, 59
Johnson, Charles Kains, 216
Johnson, Lionel, 54
Johnson, Ronald, 201
Johnston, Jill, 95
Jonathan, Son of Saul, 37-38
Jones, Robert Hope, 47
Joplin, Janis, 26
Jorgensen, Christine, 92, 93
Jouhandeau, Marcel, 133
Jourdain, Margaret, 100
Julius III, Pope, 169

Kallman, Chester, 20
Kameny, Dr. Franklin, 95
Kantrowitz, Arnie, 201
Karl Eitel, 77
Katte, Hans von, 29
Katz, Jonathan, 22, 47, 90, 151, 198
Kaunitz, Wenzel Anton von, 35-36
Kelly, George, 24-25
Kelly, William, 121
Kemble, Fanny, 127, 201
Kennedy, William Sloan, 18
Kerouac, Jack, 58, 61
Keynes, John Maynard, 27, 49, 113, 137
Khevenhuller, Ludwig Andreas, 201
King, Billie Jean, 39, 196-97
King, Charles "Badger," 33
King, Francis, 110
King, Rufus De Vane, 65-66, 73
Kinsey, Alfred, 57, 127
Kirk, Poppy, 50
Kirkup, James, 77
Kirkwood, James, 21, 148
Kitchener, Horatio Herbert, Lord, 110
Klaich, Dolores, 153
Kleist, Heinrich von, 180
Kopay, Dave, 55, 111
Kronberger, Maximilian, 77
Krupp, Friedrich Alfred, 41, 81
Kutuzov, Mikhail I., 169

Lally, Michael, 95
Lamballe, Princess de, 169
Lamoricière, Louis Christophe, 47
Lanchester, Elsa, 115-16
Landowska, Wanda, 118
Languet, Hubert, 200
La Rocque, Rod, 21, 199
La Rue, Danny, 133
Lasalle, Ferdinand, 77
Laughton, Charles, 114, 115-16, 158
Laurencin, Marie, 50, 184-85

Laurens, John, 22
Lawrence, D. H., 38, 46, 159-60
Lawrence, T. E., 144-45
Leadbeater, Bishop C. W., 47
Lear, Edward, 85
Leduc, Violette, 66-67
Lee, Jennette, 200
Lee, Vernon, 177-78
Lehmann, John, 97-98
Leighton, Baron Frederick, 204-205
Leo X, Pope, 216
Leonardo da Vinci, 70
Leopold, Nathan, 201
Letinois, Lucien, 181
Lewis, David, 165
Lewis, Edith, 206
Lewis, Matthew Gregory, 120-21
Lewis, Sasha Gregory, 94
Leyendecker, J. C., 58
Liebig, Justus von, 94
Lifar, Sergei, 56, 62, 64, 141
Lindbergh, Charles A., 128
Lindsay, Vachel, 25, 105, 190-91
Lobdell, Lucy Ann, 216
Lockwood, Belva, 198
Loeb, Richard, 201
Loovis, David, 77
Lorca, Federico Garcia, 113
Lorrain, Jean, 111-12
Loti, Pierre, 24
Louis XIII, 169
Louÿs, Pierre, 216
Lowell, Amy, 38-39
Ludwig II, 149-50
Lully, Jean Baptiste, 201
Luxembourg, François, Duke of, 33
Lvov, Georgi Eugenievich, Prince, 200
Lyautey, Louis Hubert Gonzalve, 193, 194
Lynde, Paul, 103-104
Lynes, George Platt, 68

Mabley, Jackie "Moms," 75
McAlmon, Robert, 18, 156
McCarthy, Joseph R., 192
McClintick, Guthrie, 40, 138, 139
McClung, Isabelle, 206
McCullers, Carson, 41-42, 98
McCullers, Reeves, 42
Machiavelli, Niccolò, 94
Mackenzie, Compton, 81
McKuen, Rod, 77, 78
Maclean, Donald, 91
McNally, Terence, 188-89
McNeill, Rev. John M., 169
MacPherson, Kenneth, 156
Mahler, Gustav, 119-20
Mansfield, Katherine, 16, 159-60, 178
Marais, Jean, 208-209
Marathus, 157-58
Marbury, Elizabeth, 212
Maria Carolina, 84, 143
Mariah, Paul, 112
Marie Antoinette, 84, 85, 169, 200
Marlowe, Christopher, 46, 151, 184
Marlowe, Kenneth, 201
Marsh, Edward, 137
Marshall, John, 102
Martial, 209
Martin, Violet Florence, 113

Martineau, Harriet, 113
Mason, Daniel Gregory, 157, 195
Massine, Leonide, 56, 140-41, 197
Masters, Edgar Lee, 151
Mathis, Johnny, 169
Mattheson, Johann, 169
Maugham, Robin, 88, 89
Maugham, W. Somerset, 29-30, 49, 69, 88, 89, 185, 192, 200
Maxwell, Elsa, 22, 90-91
Mazarin, Jules Cardinal, 133
Melchior, Lauritz, 53, 56-57
Melville, Herman, 135
Mendl, Sir Charles, 212
Menken, Adah Isaacs, 104
Menshikov, Aleksandr, 201
Merrick, Gordon, 153
Merrill, George, 151
Merrill, James, 61
Merrill, Stuart, 153
Messel, Oliver, 33
Mew, Charlotte, 192-93
Micas, Nathalie, 58
Michel, Louise, 95
Michelangelo Buonaroti, 50, 151
Michelet, Jules, 153
Millay, Edna St. Vincent, 44, 190
Miller, Merle, 95
Miller, Warren, 153
Millett, Kate, 161-62
Milton, John, 207
Mineo, Sal, 21
Mishima, Yukio, 23, 52
Mitropoulos, Dimitri, 61
Molière, Jean Baptiste Poquelin, 24
Monroe, Marilyn, 97
Montezuma II, 112
Montpensier, Duchesse de, 95
Montaigne, Michel de, 47
Montesquiou-Fezensac, Robert de, 50-51
Montherlant, Henri de, 72
Morand, Suzanne, 185
More, Henry, 185
Morgan, Robin, 33
Moritz, Karl Philipp, 169
Mosher, Thomas Bird, 18
Mother Clap, 110
Muhammed II, 61
Müller, Johannes von, 17-18
Munro, H. H., 211
Murad IV, 130-31
Muret, Marc-Antoine, 68
Murnau, F. W., 215
Murry, John Middleton, 160, 178
Musser, Benjamin, 47
Mussorgsky, Modest, 61
Myers, F. W. H., 47

Napoleon Bonaparte, 143-44, 179-80, 213
Nazimova, Alla, 26, 89-90
Nero, 178, 209-210
Nerva, 190
Neuhof, Theodor, 153
Newman, John Henry Cardinal, 43, 45-46
Nichols, Beverley, 50
Nicholson, John Gambril, 185
Nicolson, Harold, 40, 52, 100, 205
Nicomedes, 123
Nightingale, Florence, 94

Nijinsky, Vaslav, 52-53, 55, 56, 140, 205
Noel, Roden, 150
Nolan, James, 169
Norse, Harold, 20, 133
North, William, 163
Novarro, Ramon, 21, 37
Novello, Ivor, 24, 69
Nureyev, Rudolf, 55

Oates, Titus, 169
O'Hara, Frank, 111
Oliver, Mary, 169
Onassis, Jacqueline Kennedy, 88, 89
Orejudas, Domingo, 133
Orleans, Charlotte, duchesse d', 82-83
Orleans, Gaston, duc d', 77
Orleans, Philippe, duc d', 169
Orlovsky, Peter, 133
Orpheus, 126
Orton, Joe, 17, 102
Owen, Elizabeth, 60
Owen, Wilfred, 137
Owles, Jim, 185
Oxford, Robert Harley, Earl of, 216

Palmieri, Mario, 33
Pangborn, Franklin, 28, 103, 104
Paquet, Felix, 161
Pasolini, Pier Paolo, 50
Pater, Walter, 137, 163
Patrick, Robert, 167-68
Patterson, Rebecca, 207
Paul I, Czar, 185
Paul II, Pope, 44
Paul VI, Pope, 146
Peabody, Elizabeth, 94
Pearce, Dr. Louise, 61
Pears, Peter, 20, 109-110, 196
Peirce, James Mills, 94
Perry, Thomas Sergeant, 33
Perry, Rev. Troy, 133
Persky, Stan, 33
Peter I, 113
Peters, Robert, 185
Petri, Egon, 63
Peyrefitte, Roger, 67, 145-46, 193
Philip II of France, 158
Philip II of Macedon, 71
Picano, Felice, 47
Pindar, 39
Pisistratus, 184
Pitt, William, 95
Pitter, Ruth, 190
Platen, August von, 182-83
Plato, 104
Plomer, William, 216
Plummer, Douglas, 110
Politian, 124
Pollitt, Herbert, 148
Polycrates, 215
Ponsonby, Sarah, 84
Pope, Alexander, 95, 178
Pope-Hennessy, James, 201
Porpora, Nicola, 153
Porter, Cole, 89, 91, 96, 102, 145
Pougy, Liane de, 79, 142, 148, 184
Poulenc, Francis, 19-20, 109, 118
Powell, John, 157, 195
Power, Tyrone, 81, 108

Powys, John Cowper, 175
Preston, John, 216
Prokosch, Frederic, 95
Proust, Marcel, 50, 67, 121, 141
Puig, Manuel, 217
Purdy, James, 133

Radiguet, Raymond, 113, 146
Raft, George, 96
Rais, Gilles de, 21, 92
Raleigh, Sir Walter, 184
Rama VI, 33
Rambova, Natacha, 25-26, 90
Rattigan, Terence, 102
Ravel, Maurice, 61, 197
Ray, Johnnie, 33
Reade, Charles, 193
Récamier, Juliette, 72-73, 205
Rainey, Ma, 70, 75, 76
Raphael, 65
Rechy, John, 52
Reed, John, 46, 181
Reich, Charles, 95
Reid, Forrest, 110
Rhodes, Cecil, 117-18
Rhys, Ernest, 125
Rice, Wallace, 200
Richard I, 158
Richard II, 18
Ricketts, Charles, 22, 172
Riley, James Whitcomb, 174, 175
Rilke, Rainer Maria, 205
Rimbaud, Arthur, 181
Rinder, Walter, 112
Rivers, Larry, 111, 153
Robbins, Harold, 89
Robertson, Ethel F. L. R., 33
Robespierre, Maximilien de, 94
Roche, Mazo de la, 33
Rochester, John Wilmot, Earl of, 67
Rodd, James Rennell, 190
Rodin, Auguste, 200, 205
Roehm, Ernst, 201
Rolfe, Frederick, 126
Romano, Giulio, 65, 72
Roosevelt, Eleanor, 84, 175-76
Rorem, Ned, 19, 181-82
Rose, Sir Francis, 146
Ross, Robert, 172
Rossetti, Christina, 205-206
Rossman, Parker G., 95
Rostand, Maurice, 148
Rothenberg, David, 153
Routsong, Alma, 201
Rowse, A. L., 67, 128, 209, 216
Rudolf II, 133
Rule, Jane, 60
Rumford, Benjamin Thompson, Count, 31, 61
Rumi, 169
Russ, Joanna, 47
Russell, Ada Dwyer, 38
Russell, Craig, 33

Sacher-Masoch, Leopold von, 33
Sachs, Maurice, 66
Sackville-West, Vita, 30, 40, 51, 52, 60, 100
Sade, Marquis de, 112
St. Laurent, Yves, 135-36

Saint-Mégrin, 164
Saint-Saëns, Camille, 19, 140, 172
Saint-Tropez, Pierre de Suffren de, 133
Saki. *See* H. H. Munro
Salaino, Andrea, 70
Saltarelli, Jacope, 70
Saltus, Edgar, 185
Sampson, Deborah, 210-11
Sand, George, 104, 115
Santayana, George, 32, 210
Sapelnikov, Vassily, 187-88
Sappho, 46
Sarton, May, 80
Satie, Erik, 87
Sayle, Charles Edward, 216
Schippers, Thomas, 61
Schlesinger, John, 40
Schneider, Maria, 60
Schubert, Franz, 33
Schuyler, James, 200
Scoppetone, Sondra, 112
Scudder, Vida Dutton, 216
Searle, Alan, 49
Sebastian, St., 26-27
Selby, Hubert, Jr., 133
Shakespeare, William, 75, 151
Shannon, Charles, 22, 77, 172
Shawn, Ted, 181
Shelley, Percy Bysshe, 153
Shively, Charles, 216
Sidney, Sir Philip, 199-200
Silverstein, Charles, 77
Simcox, Edith, 153
Singh, Ranjit, 201
Sitwell, Sir Osbert, 206
Sixtus IV, Pope, 133
Smith, Bessie, 70
Smyth, Dame Ethel, 73-74, 177-78
Spinoza, Baruch, 197-98
Sporus, 178
Solomon, Simeon, 65, 175
Somerville, Edith Anna Oenone, 94
Sophocles, 190
Spada, James, 33
Spender, Stephen, 46-47
Staël, Madame de, 72-73, 205
Stambolian, George, 77
Stanhope, Lady Hester, 61
Stebbins, Emma, 127, 169
Stein, Getrude, 17, 36-37, 60, 77, 127, 146,
    165
Stenbock, Stanislaus Eric, Count, 53-54
Steuben, Baron Friedrich von, 25, 163
Stevenson, Robert Louis, 139, 192
Steward, Samuel M., 2, 71, 127-28, 146, 181
Stiller, Mauritz, 106
Stoddard, Charles Warren, 24, 139, 174, 192
Stone, Lucy, 153
Storrs, Sir Ronald, 201
Stout, Rex, 203
Strachey, Lytton, 27, 49, 137
Strindberg, August, 33
Stuart-Young, John Moray, 61
Sturgis, Howard Overing, 32
Sullivan, Sir Arthur, 85-86

Sullivan, Harry Stack, 42
Sully, Rosalie Kemble, 127
Swinburne, Algernon Charles, 65, 104, 175
Swithinbank, Martin, 77
Symonds, John Addington, 125, 150, 173,
    200
Symons, A. J. A., 126
Szymanowski, Karol, 173-74

Talbot, Mary Anne, 47
Tasso, Torquato, 61
Tavel, Ronald, 95
Taylor, Bayard, 33
Taylor, Robert, 81
Taylor, Valerie, 169
Tchaikovsky, Modest, 94
Tchaikovsky, Peter Ilyich, 82, 188
Tchelitchew, Pavel, 141, 165
Teal, Donn, 185
Teasdale, Sara, 139-40
Tennyson, Alfred Lord, 153
Tevfik, Ahmed, 39
Thanet, 55-56
Theocritus, 83-84
Theognis, 131
Thesiger, Ernest, 33
Thomas, Carey, 17
Thompson, Dorothy, 120
Thoreau, Henry David, 122-23, 183
Thorpe, Jeremy, 77
Tiberius, 193
Tibullus, Albius, 157-58
Tilden, William, 39
Tiny Tim, 216
Tippu Sahib, 164-65
Titus, 156-57
Toklas, Alice B., 36-37, 50, 76-77, 127, 146,
    165
Tolson, Clyde, 16
Tolstoy, Count Leo, 134, 151
Tone, Gertrude Franchot, 120
Townsend, Patty, 60
Tozer, Catherine, 193-94
Trajan, 162
Traubel, Horace, 18, 216
Trefusis, Violet, 52, 100, 101
Tripp, C. A., 185, 191, 192
Troubridge, Una, 143
Tuke, Henry Scott, 103
Turing, Alan, 91, 110
Tyler, Parker, 61

Ulrichs, Karl Heinrich, 153
Umberto II, 169

Valentine, St., 39-40
Valentinian III, 133
Valentino, Rudolph, 25-26, 37, 38, 81-82
Van Vechten, Carl, 106
Veidt, Conrad, 28
Vendôme, Duc de, 132
Verdenal, Jean, 187
Verlaine, Paul, 60-61, 181
Vidal, Gore, 98, 168, 172-73, 195

Villars, Duc de, 82-83
Viñes, Ricardo, 19, 47, 197
Virgil, 185
Visconti, Luchino, 120, 200
Viviani, René, 200
Voelcker, Hunce, 113
Voltaire, 195
Vyver, Bertha, 173

Wagner, Richard, 149
Walker, Ben, 163
Walker, Dr. Mary Edwards, 198
Walpole, Horace, 120, 166-67
Walpole, Hugh, 53, 57
Walsh, David Ignatius, 191
Warhol, Andy, 153
Warren, Edward Perry, 102
Washington, George, 21-22, 25
Waters, John, 181
Watson, Dr. John H., 19
Waugh, Evelyn, 106, 183-84
Webb, Clifton, 186, 194-95
Webb, David, 133
Welles, Sumner, 185
Wescott, Glenway, 67-68
Westermarck, Edward, 201
Whale, James, 165-66
Wheeler, Monroe, 68
White, Edmund, 33
White, Patrick, 91-92
White, T. H., 92
Whitman, Walt, 18, 57, 92, 94, 151, 191,
    192
Wieners, John, 33
Wilde, Dolly, 90, 184
Wilde, Oscar, 16, 29, 53-54, 59, 86, 90,
    101, 110, 125, 137, 148, 163, 172, 173,
    178, 184, 187, 190, 196
Wilder, Thornton, 71, 127
William II Rufus, 168
William III, 201
Williams, Emlyn, 198-99
Williams, Tennessee, 55, 59-60, 98, 116-17
Wilson, Doric, 45
Wilson, Lanford, 167-68
Winch, Terence, 200
Winckelmann, Johann Joachim, 151, 216
Windham, Donald, 116-17
Winsloe, Christa, 120
Winter, George de, 18
Wittgenstein, Ludwig, 77
Woodberry, George F., 94
Woolley, Monty, 145
Woolf, Virginia, 30, 74, 189
Woollcott, Alexander, 26
Wrangler, Jack, 122
Wylie, I. A. R., 54-55, 193

Yosano, Akiko, 216
Youmans, Vincent, 169
Young, Ian, 33, 98
Young, Perry Deane, 61
Young, Stark, 185
Yourcenar, Marguerite, 29, 71, 113